Imaging Dopamine

Since its discovery 50 years ago, brain dopamine has been implicated in the control of movement and cognition, and has emerged as a key factor in diverse brain diseases such as Parkinson's disease, schizophrenia, and drug addiction. This book is an illustrated biography of the dopamine molecule, beginning with an account of its synthesis in brain, and then describing its storage, release and signalling mechanisms, and its ultimate metabolic breakdown. Using color illustrations of positron emission tomography (PET) scans, each chapter presents a specific stage in the biochemical pathway for dopamine. Writing for researchers and graduate students, Paul Cumming presents an overview of all that has been learned about dopamine through molecular imaging, a technology which allows the measurement of formerly invisible processes in the living brain. He reviews current technical controversies in the interpretation of dopamine imaging and presents key results illuminating the roles of brain dopamine in illness and health.

PAUL CUMMING is Professor in the Department of Nuclear Medicine at Ludwig-Maximilian University in Munich, Germany. He currently serves on the editorial boards of the journals *Synapse*, *Journal of Cerebral Blood Flow and Metabolism*, and *NeuroImage*.

Imaging
Dopamine

PAUL CUMMING

Ludwig-Maximilian University, Munich, Germany

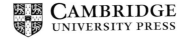

CAMBRIDGE
UNIVERSITY PRESS

CAMBRIDGE UNIVERSITY PRESS
Cambridge, New York, Melbourne, Madrid, Cape Town, Singapore, São Paulo, Delhi

Cambridge University Press
The Edinburgh Building, Cambridge CB2 8RU, UK

Published in the United States of America by Cambridge University Press, New York

www.cambridge.org
Information on this title: www.cambridge.org/9780521790024

© P. Cumming 2009

First published 2009

Printed in the United Kingdom at the University Press, Cambridge

A catalog record for this publication is available from the British Library

Library of Congress Cataloging in Publication data
Cumming, Paul.
   Imaging dopamine / by Paul Cumming.
      p.   ;   cm.
   Includes bibliographical references.
   ISBN 978-0-521-79002-4 (hardback)
1. Dopamine.   2. Tomography, Emission.   3. Single-photon emission computed
tomography.   4. Molecular radiobiology.   I. Title.
[DNLM: 1. Dopamine.   2. Tomography, Emission-Computed. WK 725 C971i   2009]
QP563.D66C86   2009
612.8′042–dc22

                                                                2008024829

ISBN 978-0-521-79002-4 hardback

"But as if a magic lantern threw the nerves in patterns on a screen."

T. S. Eliot

To the remembrance of
Professor George Leslie Cumming (1930–1994)

Contents

The color plates are between pages 28 and 29, and pages 223 and 224.

Foreword

This book is timely and will prove useful for many researchers interested not only in the specific topic, "Imaging Dopamine," but also in more general aspects of dopamine. In neurotransmitter research, dopamine has served a spearhead function ever since its discovery in the brain half a century ago. Dopamine has also played a key role in molecular imaging research; the imaging of dopamine receptors started very early in the history of positron emission tomography.

Although this book has its focus on imaging, the full utilization of imaging techniques depends on the background knowledge gained from other methodologies, a theme that has been duly considered by the author. Thus, the various aspects of dopamine, dealing, for example, with its synthesis, storage, release, and metabolism, as well as with the enzymes and transporter proteins involved in these processes, are treated in sufficient detail to provide a well-integrated and reasonably complete picture of the very complex dopamine transmission machinery.

It should go without saying that the growth of knowledge regarding the various aspects of neurotransmission has not taken place without intervals of considerable disagreement and controversy. In the course of the past half century's intense research, many issues have been resolved, whereas others are still being debated. I am pleased to find that the author has devoted some space to historical aspects, starting out with a scheme of the dopamine nerve terminal published by me in 1966. Indeed, our first experiments made in 1957 and the following years initially led to a considerable controversy, based largely on the belief prevailing at the time that the nerve cells in the brain communicated mainly by electric signaling. Thus, our proposal that the catecholamines dopamine and noradrenaline served important neurotransmitter functions in the brain was at the time hard to accept by most leaders in the field. This was evident at an international meeting in London in 1960. But only five years later, at a subsequent international meeting in Stockholm, the concept of chemical transmission in the brain had already gained considerable acceptance. This was largely due to the development of histochemical techniques, by means of which Swedish research groups had been able to visualize the neuronal localization of monoamines in the central nervous system, thus providing further evidence of their neurotransmitter function. However, very soon other controversies followed. For example, there arose a debate on whether synaptic vesicles were essential in the physiological release process or were just serving as "garbage cans."

Since those early days, the field of dopamine research has moved a long way, largely thanks to the advent of an array of powerful techniques. The early pharmacological work proposing the existence of several subtypes of dopamine receptors, "autoreceptors," and transporter proteins could be confirmed by molecular biology techniques, and their roles further elucidated by, for example, knockout techniques. The ongoing development of molecular imaging will clearly play a key role. It will continue to bridge the gap between animal and human research, and more sophisticated techniques will make it possible to record the processes underlying even the highest integrative functions of the brain. The present book will serve as an important guide for many researchers in this endeavor.

Arvid Carlsson

Acknowledgments

The author thanks those who knowingly or unknowingly made this work possible, including: Ariel Ase, Peter Bartenstein, Isabelle Boileau, Per Borghammer, Evgeny Budygin, Arvid Carlsson, Paul B. S. Clarke, Anne, Steven, and Eva Cumming; Paul Deep, Doris Doudet, Charles Gerfen, Gerhard Gründer, Joel Harrison, Per Hartvig, Eva Honoré, Irene Kon, Yoshitaka Kumakura, Hiroto Kuwabara, Christine Laliberté, Nanna Lind, Wayne R. Martin, Patrick and Edith McGeer, Ole Munk, Søren Dinesen Østergaard, Steen Jacobsen, Svend Borup Jensen, Kasper Pedersen, Luciano Minuzzi, Anette Moustgaard, Pedro Rosa-Neto, Oliver Rousset, Donald Smith, Gwenn Smith, Manoucher Vafaee, Ingo Vernalekan, Steven R. Vincent, Franz X. Vollenweider, Terri Whetstone, Matthäus Willeit, and Dean F. Wong.

Introduction

This book is a biography of dopamine, as illuminated by classical neurochemical methods and especially by molecular imaging with positron emission tomography (PET), or single photon emission tomography (SPET), a closely related technology.

Since the early 1980s, molecular imaging has become indispensable for the study of normal physiology, disease processes, and novel therapeutics. Using external detection with PET or SPET, the uptake and metabolism or binding of radioligands is monitored and quantified in living brain. This book summarizes the state of knowledge of the half-dozen molecular targets in the dopamine system, which have been investigated by imaging techniques. A key advantage of molecular imaging is that aspects of the life of dopamine can be studied in living brain, both in preclinical studies and in humans afflicted with neurodegenerative or psychiatric disorders in which dopamine is implicated. A key disadvantage is presented by the type of knowledge obtained by molecular imaging, which can be only indirectly informative of the step of the pathway for dopamine neurotransmission under investigation. Thus, the interpretation of molecular imaging results must always be grounded in basic aspects of the biochemistry of dopamine and the pharmacology of its binding sites.

Although several groups of dopamine neurons are found in the brain, the entire emphasis here is to be placed on the mesencephalic dopamine systems, which innervate the extended striatum and specific limbic structures of the forebrain. In the course of a long human life, perhaps 10 g of dopamine is formed in the striatum, to be gradually released in infinitesimal amounts from individual dopamine nerve terminals. Once released from synaptic vesicles to the extracellular milieu, dopamine binds to its receptors and so conveys the dopamine signal to receptive neurons. While the concentration of dopamine in synaptic vesicles is very high, the prevailing concentration of dopamine in the extracellular space, also known as the interstitial compartment, is very low, comparable to the sweetness obtained by dissolving a sugar cube in a large swimming pool. Nonetheless, dopamine at these trace concentrations plays a substantial role in brain signaling and has been implicated in diverse neurological and psychiatric disorders.

The advent of the modern era of dopamine research was announced when Arvid Carlsson showed that the *Rauwolfia* alkaloid reserpine depleted the concentration of dopamine in the brain and other tissues of rabbits. In the condition of dopamine depletion, the rabbits were incapacitated by rigid paralysis, but restoration of brain dopamine and also normal movement was obtained after treatment of the sick rabbits with the dopamine precursor, the amino acid 3,4-dihydroxy-L-phenylalanine (levodopa; DOPA) (Carlsson, Lindqvist, & Magnusson 1957). This fundamental observation ultimately led to the awarding of the Nobel Prize in Medicine (2000), shared by Arvid Carlsson, Paul Greengard, and Eric Kandell. The progress of knowledge about dopamine neurotransmission has always been led by technical innovations. For example, Carlsson's discovery of brain dopamine in the 1950s was facilitated by the colorimetric detection of dopamine in tissue extracts. During the 1960s, subsequent studies of the enzymology and biochemistry of the dopamine pathway made use of new radiolabeled enzyme substrates, which allowed more sensitive detection of the rates of enzymatic product formation. New methods for the biochemical isolation of specific enzymes in the dopamine pathway also benefited from the availability of radioenzymatic assays. In the 1970s, classical chromatographic methods for the separation and detection of dopamine and its metabolites in biological extracts gave way to high-performance liquid chromatography (HPLC). When HPLC is coupled with electrochemical detection, quantities of dopamine as low as 10 pg can be detected. This innovation of sensitivity led in the 1980s to the development of cerebral microdialysis, in which dopamine and its metabolites are sampled from the interstitial fluid of the brain and their minute concentrations measured by HPLC at sampling intervals as low as 1 min. Still greater sensitivity can now be obtained by analytic methods employing mass spectroscopy or by using in vivo electrochemical detection.

Once the requirement of dopamine for normal movement had been established, the search for the dopaminergic neurons began. Dopamine and other monoamine neurotransmitters such as noradrenaline and serotonin characteristically form fluorescent adducts in the presence of formaldehyde vapor. Fluorescence histology of thin sections of brain proved to be extraordinarily useful for the mapping of monoamine neurons in the brain (Carlsson, Falck, & Hillarp 1962). Using this technique, a dozen clusters of fluorescent neurons were identified in the brainstem, midbrain, and hypothalamus. However, the fluorescence technique could not identify the precise neurochemical nature of these monoaminergic neurons.

Inflammation and loss of pigmented neurons in the mesencephalon had been described in patients dying of post-encephalitic parkinsonism (von Economo 1931), an influenza-like pandemic that arose toward the end of World War I. On the basis of fluorescence histology, the degenerating neurons of the mesencephalon were soon identified as catecholamine neurons. It is now understood that the formation of the black pigment neuromelanin in dopamine neurons of the substantia nigra is a by-product of dopamine synthesis in those cells. Soon after the connection between von Economo's encephalopathy and degeneration of dopamine neurons was established, dopamine depletion was reported in post mortem brain specimens from patients dying with Parkinson's disease (Ehringer & Hornykiewicz 1960). This observation led in short order to the first attempts at symptomatic treatment of Parkinson's disease with DOPA (Barbeau, Sourkes, & Murphy 1962). Thus, the early 1960s saw the awakening of the modern field of neurochemical pathology and of the rational treatment of a neurodegenerative disorder.

In the 1980s, a more general mapping of neurochemical anatomy was made possible based on immunohistochemistry. In this technique, antibodies are used for the localization in thin brain sections of specific antigens, such as enzymes in the pathway for dopamine synthesis. In parallel with the development of immunohistochemistry, autoradiographic methods made possible the mapping of neuroreceptors in vitro. Finally, in situ hybridization, molecular cloning techniques, and gene knockout technology all have contributed profoundly to studies of dopamine in recent decades.

In this biography of dopamine, the events and processes in the pathway for dopamine neurotransmission are described sequentially, beginning with the formation of tyrosine in the liver and ending with the mediation of post-synaptic signaling by dopamine receptors. At each step in the pathway, the relevant biochemistry is reviewed in detail and discussed in the context of quantitative PET studies. A basic knowledge of biochemistry and molecular biology is assumed on the part of the reader, and concepts relevant to the compartmental analysis of PET studies are introduced as each class of radiotracer is considered.

For good or for ill, PET reveals biochemical processes in the crucible of the living brain, as distinct from the biochemist's test tube. However, PET, and to an even greater extent SPET, suffers from inherent limitations, in addition to financial considerations. Molecular imaging techniques have low spatial resolution, meaning that tracer uptake in small brain structures cannot be detected without loss of information. In addition, temporal resolution is low, meaning that rapid dynamic processes are difficult to study, since one may require several hours in order to arrive at an equilibrium condition. Finally, process resolution is low, meaning that it can be difficult to identify the precise biological meaning of PET results. In addition to the usual problems (common to all pharmacology) presented by unspecific drugs, molecular imaging necessarily introduces the complexities of kinetic modeling. In this context, the objective of kinetic modeling is to employ a dynamic measurement of brain radioactivity concentrations for the calculation of a physiological parameter, such as blood flow, glucose consumption, or neuroreceptor binding. While kinetic modeling may seem an obstacle to newcomers in the field of dopamine imaging, most kinetic models can in fact be understood with some calculus. Unfortunately, there is presently no didactic reference textbook on kinetic modeling. While this book does not rectify the lack of a general introduction to radiotracer kinetics, compartmental models are presented diagrammatically, so as to be understood intuitively. Detailed exposition of the actual mathematics underlying specific modeling procedures can be found elsewhere.

In spite of the lack of mathematical presentation, the book is thematically all about modeling. The entire pathway for dopamine transmission in living brain can be compared to a model kit. The constituent parts have mostly been identified and their connectivity has been established. Results of PET studies, in conjunction with biochemical studies in vitro, have assigned magnitudes to the several components of the dopamine system. While the instructions for assembly are presently missing, it can be hoped that the coming decades will see the realization of a comprehensive model of dopamine transmission with inestimable heuristic value for the understanding of human disease. In addition, dopamine imaging is now enabling the development of a neurochemical typology, in which human personality and predispositions are understood in terms of neurochemical substrates.

1

The life history of dopamine

1.1.   A brief overview of the dopamine pathway

The life history of a dopamine molecule begins in the liver, with the synthesis of the precursor tyrosine, and ends in the kidney, with the elimination of the conjugated dopamine metabolites to the urine. Only during a brief and specific interval in its life can a dopamine molecule engage in its proper function, which is the mediation of signaling via activation of dopamine receptors. The chemical structures of molecules in the dopamine biosynthesis and catabolic pathway are illustrated in Figure 1.1. This scheme does not include the catecholamines noradrenaline and adrenaline, for which dopamine is a precursor, since these substances might properly serve as the topic of another book.

As presented in Figure 1.1, all the reactants and enzymes in the dopamine pathway seem to be present in the same space. However, in the living organism, molecules and chemical reactions normally occur within strictly segregated spaces, known as metabolic compartments. Transfer of a molecule in the dopamine pathway from one compartment to another may be strictly impeded by diffusion barriers, or may occur via carrier-mediated facilitated diffusion or by ATP-driven active transport. Thus, the schematic pathway for dopamine synthesis in the living organism should be projected onto a model containing cellular compartments. The model proposed by Carlsson (1966) illustrates the blood, extracellular space, intracellular space, and vesicles as distinct compartments (Figure 1.2). Enzymes and transporters conduct the transfer of mass from one compartment to another, here represented as arrows. The purpose of this book is to quantify the diverse processes implied in this diagram.

Tyrosine is formed in the liver from the essential amino acid phenylalanine by a specific hydroxylase (EC 1.14.16.1), or may be derived from dietary sources.

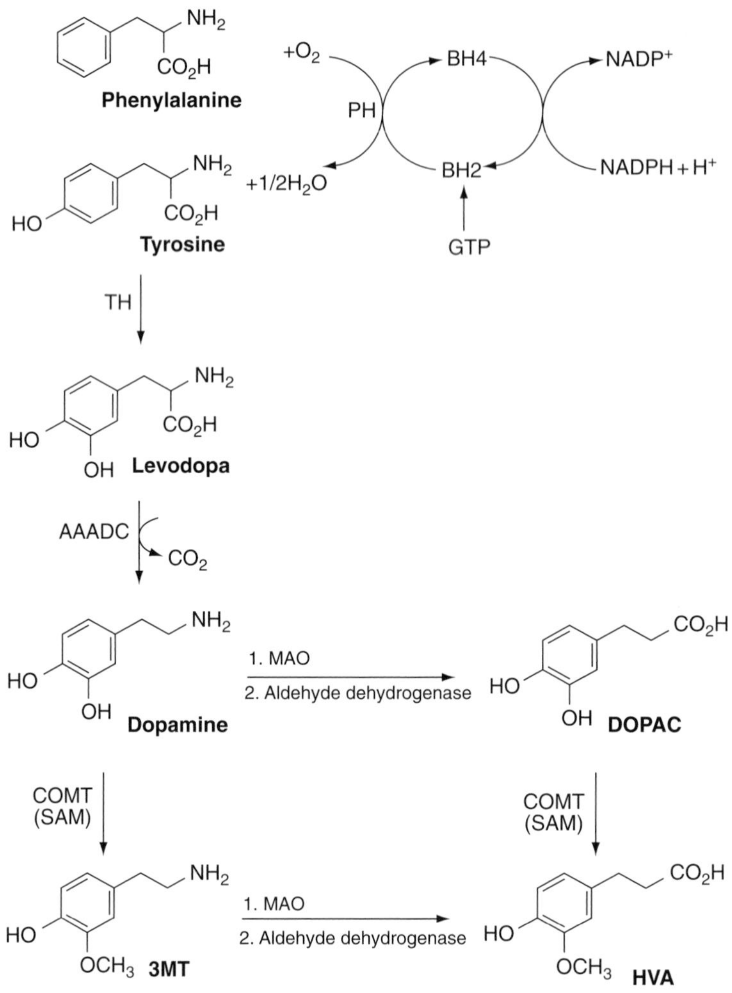

Figure 1.1 The pathway for the synthesis and catabolism of dopamine. PH, phenylalanine hydroxylase; BH2/BH4, dihydro- and tetrahydrobiopterin; TH, tyrosine hydroxylase; AAADC, aromatic amino acid decarboxylase; MAO, monoamine oxidase; COMT, catechol-O-methyltransferase; SAM, S-adenosylmethionine; 3MT, 3-methoxyryramine; DOPAC, dihydroxyphenylacetic acid; HVA, homovanillic acid.

Upon entry into the blood plasma compartment, tyrosine is delivered to the corporal tissues. Entry of tyrosine into the brain is impeded by the blood–brain barrier, which restricts access of many solutes to the brain. However, a facilitated diffusion carrier for tyrosine and other large neutral amino acids (LNAAs) is present in the capillary epithelium of the blood–brain barrier. The common carrier for LNNAs functions like a revolving door, transferring its substrates in and out of the brain. This process eventually establishes equilibrium between the blood and the

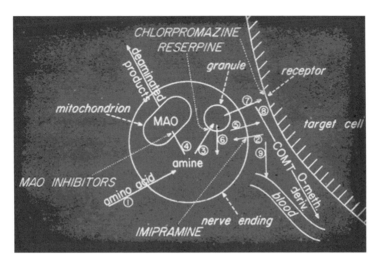

Figure 1.2 Schematic diagram of the dopamine synapse presented by Professor Arvid Carlsson in 1966. Processes in the pathway for dopamine are expressed as numbered arrows, including (1) entry of the amino acid precursor into the dopamine terminal, (2,5) bidirectional transfer of dopamine across the plasma membrane, (3) transfer of cytosolic dopamine into vesicles, and (4) oxidative deamination, and (7) binding at post-synaptic receptors. Reproduced with the kind permission of Professor Arvid Carlsson, University of Gothenburg. (For color version, see plate section.)

brain concentrations of tyrosine and its other substrates, with the key specification that concentration gradients cannot be generated by facilitated diffusion.

Once in the brain, tyrosine can be incorporated into proteins, or may serve as a precursor for the biosynthesis of DOPA within catecholamine neurons. This latter process is catalyzed by tyrosine hydroxylase (TH: EC 1.14.16.2). Under ordinary conditions, TH is nearly saturated with tyrosine in the brain; consequently, the rate of tyrosine hydroxylation is determined by the intrinsic activity of the enzyme, such that TH is classically considered the rate-limiting step for the synthesis of dopamine and other catecholamines. Regulation of TH activity is mediated by the changes in the affinity of TH for its rate-limiting co-substrate tetrahydrobiopterin (BH_4), which is modulated by phosphorylation of specific amino acid residues in the TH enzyme. In addition, dopamine and other end products, as well as synthetic amino acids, can modulate the activity of TH by simple competition at the catalytic site.

Several possible fates are available for cerebral DOPA, whether it is formed in situ from brain tyrosine, derived from circulation in the course of replacement therapy for Parkinson's disease, or while entering the brain as an exogenous substrate in the course of a positron emission tomography (PET) study. DOPA can be exported from the brain to blood via the common carrier for the LNAAs, or it can be a substrate for catechol-*O*-methyltransferase (COMT: EC 2.1.1.6) in the brain, yielding the inert metabolite O-methyldopa (OMD). The majority of DOPA formed within catecholamine neurons is normally decarboxylated by aromatic L-amino acid decarboxylase (AAADC: EC 4.1.1.28), yielding dopamine. However, the alternate metabolic fates for DOPA in the brain indicate that TH is not the sole and committed step in the synthesis of dopamine. Consequently, the modulation of AAADC activity can influence the branching ratio for DOPA metabolism, and therefore contribute to the overall regulation of dopamine synthesis.

Once formed in the cytosol or intracellular space of a dopamine neurone, dopamine is transferred by active transport into synaptic vesicles, which express the vesicular monoamine transporter type 2 (VMAT2). So long as dopamine is retained within the synaptic vesicle, it is protected from catabolism, but unbound cytosolic dopamine is rapidly metabolized by the successive actions of monoamine oxidase (MAO: EC 1.4.3.4) and COMT. This forked path of dopamine catabolism can proceed either way, although the major branch of dopamine metabolism in rat brain certainly proceeds first by oxidative deamination, yielding dihydroxyphenylacetic acid (DOPAC), which is subsequently O-methylated to yield homovanillic acid (HVA). Together, DOPAC and HVA are known as the acidic metabolites. A smaller fraction of dopamine in the brain is first O-methylated to produce 3-methoxytyramine (3MT), which is subsequently deaminated by MAO to yield HVA. The acidic metabolites are directly eliminated from the brain by a facilitated diffusion process that is inhibited by probenecid. Alternately, the acidic metabolites can be conjugated by aryl-sulfotransferase (EC 2.8.2.1) prior to diffusion from the brain into the cerebrospinal fluid (CSF) and thence to the bloodstream.

The active transport of cytosolic dopamine results in a very high concentration gradient across the vesicular membrane. The flux of dopamine into the vesicle is driven by a proton gradient established by the ATPase activity of VMAT2. A normally functioning dopamine vesicle thus resembles a mitochondrion acting in reverse; here, the consumption of ATP is used to maintain a proton gradient. The ATP-dependent dopamine storage is poisoned by the reserpine alkaloids, resulting in degranulation and massive efflux of stored dopamine into the cytosolic compartment. Because energy must be expended to maintain the dopamine concentration gradient across the vesicular membrane, degranulation is an early consequence of cerebral ischemia. Under normal physiological conditions, depolarization of the dopamine fiber encourages the fusion of a vesicle with the plasma membrane, accompanied by release of the vesicular contents into the interstitial fluid of the brain.

In the interstitial space at the site of vesicular fusion, the dopamine concentration is transiently very high, but rapidly declines as dopamine passively diffuses away from the fiber. In the striatum, interstitial dopamine is efficiently transferred back into the dopamine fiber, where it can once again run the gauntlet of MAO or be stored in vesicles for re-use. The plasma membrane dopamine transporter (DAT) facilitates the reuptake of interstitial dopamine back into the dopamine fiber. This transport process is driven by an inward sodium gradient across the polarized plasma membrane, but is not directly coupled to energy consumption. Cocaine, amphetamine, and other psychostimulants enhance the interstitial dopamine concentration in striatum by actions at the DAT. However, the relatively sparse dopamine innervation of the frontal cortex is poorly endowed with DAT, such that simple diffusion and the activity of COMT may have greater influence on interstitial dopamine concentrations. The consequent slower clearance of interstitial dopamine in the cortex results in a more prolonged action over a greater volume of tissue following an exocytosis event, a phenomenon known as volume transmission.

Once released into the interstitial space, dopamine can interact with two broad classes of G-protein-linked receptors, known as D_1-like and D_2-like receptors. In the striatum, both classes of receptors are located on medium spiny neurons, although D_2-like receptors also occur on presynaptic dopamine terminals, where they serve as "feedback" autoreceptors regulating dopamine synthesis and release. Whereas the functional aspects of dopamine D_1-like receptors are poorly understood, a great deal is known about D_2 receptors. For example, major beneficial effects of antiparkinsonian medications are mediated by activation of dopamine D_2 receptors. However, activation of dopamine D_2 receptors is a double-edged sword. Whereas it is abundantly clear that idiopathic Parkinson's disease is neurochemically a dopamine deficiency, the discovery that antipsychotic drugs antagonize D_2 receptors supports the hypothesis that schizophrenia is associated with a functional over-activity of these receptors.

Based on research during the past five decades, it has become possible to assign numbers or quantities to the arrows depicted in Figures 1.1 and 1.2. The activities of the enzymes catalyzing the steps in the pathway for dopamine synthesis and catabolism can be measured in biological samples, and the density of binding sites and transporters for dopamine can be quantified in membranes and thin sections from the brain. Corresponding assays can be obtained in living brain by measuring the uptake of radiolabeled tracers for dopamine synthesis and binding sites. In effect, PET is an extension of classical neurochemical techniques for quantifying aspects of the pathway for dopamine transmission, with the key distinction that PET results can be obtained non-invasively in the brain of living subjects, animal or human. As such, PET is a repudiation of the old canard that biochemists are "watch smashers," striving to understand a complex and subtle mechanism by first grinding it up with detergent in a pestle and mortar and then passing the resultant paste through a chromatographic column.

1.2.   A brief account of the blood–brain barrier

The brain is nourished by solutes arriving in the arterial blood and passing across the microvascular epithelium. Unlike the capillary cells of most other tissues, those in the brain form tight junctions, thus restricting the diffusion of molecules between the cerebral and the vascular compartments. Whereas proteins and most sugars are entirely restricted from diffusion across the barrier, gases such as oxygen and small lipophilic molecules can diffuse freely across the cells of the vascular epithelium. The tight junction is no barrier at all to water, which enters the brain on the arterial side and quickly returns to circulation on the venous side of the cerebral vasculature. Consequently, the water content of the brain is constantly being exchanged with "fresh" water derived from the plasma.

The blood–brain barrier is not just a physical barrier, but can actively exclude certain molecules from the brain by a process driven by the consumption of ATP. The extrusion of molecules from the brain is mediated by p-glycoprotein, which is a member of a large family of ATP-binding cassette transporters. The presence of this enzyme has been a major obstacle in the development of anti-HIV and antineoplastic compounds with activity in the central nervous system (Ebinger & Uhr 2006). The p-glycoprotein was originally understood to have a polarized distribution on the abluminal side of the capillary epithelium, but is now known to be expressed throughout the capillary cells and in perivascular astrocytes (Bendayan *et al.* 2006). Very recently, it has become possible to measure the concentration of p-glycoprotein in human brain using the PET ligand [^{11}C]verapamil (Bart *et al.* 2003). Administering cyclosporin to block the p-glycoprotein reveals that many PET radioligands are substantially extruded from the living brain (Ishiwata *et al.* 2007).

The selective permeability of the blood–brain barrier for DOPA and other large neutral amino acids relevant to the pathway for dopamine synthesis is mediated by a specific entity in the capillary epithelium known as the common transporter for the LNAAs. This protein is a member of a family of solute carriers; the sequence cloned from a rat tumor line predicts 12-transmembrane domains and an amino acid composition rich in cysteine residues (Kanai *et al.* 1998). The transporter permits the equilibration between plasma and brain of several substrates, including phenylalanine, tyrosine, DOPA, and OMD. Each of the ten or so endogenous LNAA substrates has an intrinsic permeability per unit surface area of the capillary bed, but in the living brain, the transporter is nearly saturated by the sum of its endogenous plasma substrates (Pardridge & Oldendorf 1977). Consequently, competition from other LNAAs in plasma generally reduces the influx of labeled amino acid for studies of dopamine synthesis in living brain.

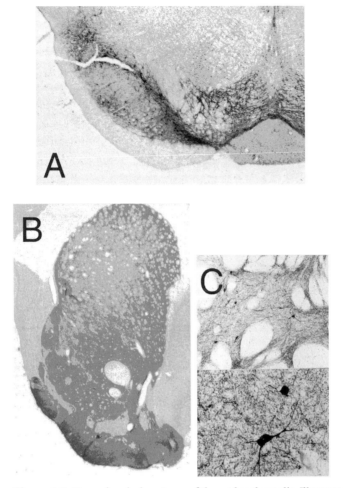

Figure 1.3 Neurochemical anatomy of the rat basal ganglia. Illustrated are
(A) TH-positive neurons in the rat substantia nigra and ventral tegmental area, (B) fibers
innervating the extended striatum, and (C) NADPH-positive neurons in the striatum at
(upper) low and (lower) high magnification. Reprinted with kind permission of Professor
Steve R. Vincent, University of British Columbia. (For color version, see plate section.)

1.3.   Neurochemical anatomy of the nigrostriatal pathway

Dopamine cells of the mesencephalic substantia nigra are large pigmented
neurons, measuring approximately 50 μm across the soma. About 10 000 dopamine neurons could dance on the head of a pin. Their pigmentation is due to the
presence of neuromelanin granules in the cytoplasm. It is generally assumed that
the population of pigmented cells is identical in number to the cells labeled in
immunohistochemical studies with antisera against TH (Figure 1.3A). In general, it

is surprisingly difficult to count neurons, even when they are intensely stained. In order to provide unbiased estimates of cell numbers, it is therefore necessary to use stereological methods. Based upon unbiased stereological methods, the dopamine neurons of the substantia nigra number approximately 10 000 in the rodent, and some 200 000 in the non-human primate (Stark & Pakkenberg 2004). In monkeys with a severe syndrome of acquired parkinsonism, only 50 000 neurons remained (Poyot et al. 2001). In the young adult human, the total number of pigmented neurons was 300,000–400,000 per side, declining in abundance by 7–10 % per decade of normal aging (Cabello et al. 2002; Ma et al. 1999). In the latter citation, it was also determined that the mean volume of surviving TH-positive neurons increased with age, suggesting either greater vitality of large neurons or hypertrophy of surviving neurons. However, it will be seen that natural attrition of dopamine neurons contributes to the pathogenesis of Parkinson's disease.

A syndrome of parkinsonism can be induced in laboratory animals receiving intracerebral injections of the dopamine analog 6-hydroxydopamine (6-OHDA). This toxin can evoke nearly complete loss of the dopamine innervation (Javoy et al. 1976). Selective toxicity of 6-OHDA for dopamine neurons is obtained by pretreatment with the noradrenaline uptake inhibitor imipramine (Roberts, Zis, & Fibiger 1975), and the dopamine cells can themselves be protected by pretreatment with DAT blockers. Pretreatment with free radical scavengers protects sympathetic fibers from 6-OHDA toxicity (Cohen et al. 1976). Together, these findings suggest a "Trojan horse" mechanism of 6-OHDA toxicity, wherein the toxin must first gain favored access to the catecholamine fibers via DAT, and then cause cellular damage by the formation of cytotoxic radicals and interrupted Ca^{2+} homeostasis.

While 6-OHDA does not cross the blood–brain barrier, accidental exposure to the meperidine analog 1-methyl-4-phenyl-1,2,5,6-tetrahydropyridine (MPTP) resulted in a syndrome of acquired parkinsonism among intravenous drug users (Langston et al. 1983), a finding which was extended to a primate model (Burns et al. 1983). There soon emerged the understanding that MPTP is a pro-toxin, which is metabolized by MAO-B in brain. The metabolite MPP+ accumulates in the dopamine neurons via DAT, in a manner similar to 6-OHDA. Within the dopamine fiber, MPP+ wreaks metabolic havoc, by releasing Ca^{2+} from mitochondria (Frei & Richter 1986) and blocking the rotenone-sensitive complex I of the mitochondrial respiration chain (Richardson et al. 2007). In effect, the poisoned dopamine neuron is asphyxiated from the inside. It is suspected that similar mechanisms underlie the natural attrition of dopamine neurons and also the accelerated degeneration leading to idiopathic Parkinson's disease.

The product of the homeobox gene *Pitx3* is a key neutrophic factor in the differentiation and survival of mesencephalic dopamine neurons during development. In adult Pitx3-deficient *aphakia* mice, there is a nearly complete absence of the ventral tier of dopamine neurons in the substantia nigra pars compacta, with associated loss of innervation to the dorsal striatum (van den Munckhof *et al.* 2003). However, the dopamine neurons of the ventral tegmental area (VTA) and their innervation of the nucleus accumbens remain nearly intact in these mice. The *aphakia* mice thus mimic idiopathic Parkinson's disease, in which the dopamine innervation of ventral striatum is also relatively spared. Co-expression of the calcium-binding protein calbindin seems to protect the mesolimbic neurons in Pitx-deficient mice from degeneration (Korotkova *et al.* 2005). Once again, calcium homeostasis is implicated in the propensity of dopamine neurons toward premature death.

There is an anatomical and biochemical fine structure in the forebrain dopamine innervations. The dopamine neurons of the ventral part of the substantia nigra innervate the dorsal striatum in patches and in a thin band lying just beneath the corpus callosum. Part of this structure can be discerned in TH immunohistochemical staining of the rat striatum, which is most dense in the thin subcallosal strip (Figure 1.3B). In contrast, the neurons of the VTA and the dorsal aspect of the substantia nigra make a more diffuse innervation of the so-called matrix of the extended striatum, in which the patches are embedded like islands (Figure 1.4).

Most neurons resident in the striatum are medium spiny projection neurons expressing the inhibitory neurotransmitter gamma-aminobutyric acid (GABA) and neuropeptides. In rodent and also monkey striatum, those medium spiny neurons expressing dopamine D_1 receptors co-express the neuropeptide substance P, while those expressing dopamine D_2 receptors co-express enkephalin (Aubert *et al.* 2000). The D_1-responsive neurons project directly to the internal segment of the globus pallidus and to the substantia nigra, whereas the D_2-responsive neurons constitute the indirect output pathway of the striatum, projecting to the external segment of the globus pallidus. Via an extra synapse in the subthalamic nucleus, the two pathways converge in the internal segment of the globus pallidus, which gives rise to projections to the thalamus, and thence to the cerebral cortex. Presumably, motor output from the cerebral cortex is shaped and modulated by the loop passing through the basal ganglia, in which dopamine exerts a substantial influence.

The patch–matrix segregation of the dopaminergic innervation respects a consistent functional and neuroanatomical segmentation of the neostriatal mosaic between limbic and sensorimotor processing (Gerfen 1992). Patch neurons are innervated by the limbic cortex and project back to the dopamine cell bodies, whereas matrix neurons receive sensorimotor inputs and project to the substantia nigra pars reticulata, subjacent to the dopamine neurons (Figure 1.4).

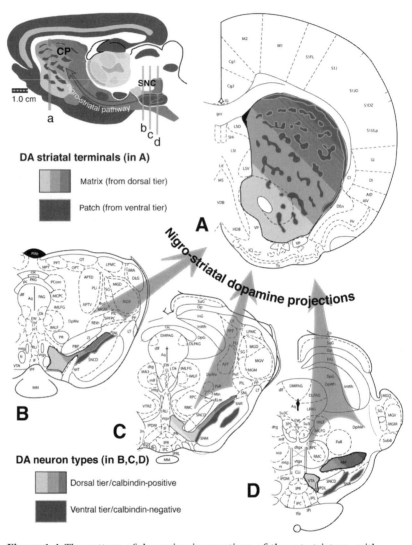

Figure 1.4 The pattern of dopamine innervations of the rat striatum, with segregation of the patch and matrix compartments. Diagram reprinted with kind permission of Dr. C. Gerfen, National Institutes of Health. (For color version, see plate section.)

The patch compartment is characterized by the presence of calbindin, high density of μ-opioid receptors, and by the relatively sparse activity of the enzyme acetylcholinesterase. The patches also contain notably higher activity of NADPH diaphorase (Sandell, Graybiel, & Chesselet 1986), which is the enzyme responsible for synthesis of the gaseous neotransmitter nitric oxide (Hope *et al.* 1991). These same NADPH-positive striatal interneurons (Figure 1.3C) tend to co-express the neuropeptides somatostatin and neuropeptide Y (Rushlow, Flumerfelt, & Naus 1995). The large acetylcholine neurons constitute an additional class of striatal interneurons, which, together with the nitric oxide neurons, modulate plasticity in the excitatory projection from the cerebral cortex to the projection neurons of the striatum (Centonze *et al.* 1999). The construction of an integrated model of the functioning of the striatal mosaic, which incorporates all of these features and connectivities, may be a task for the next 50 years in the history of dopamine.

1.4.   Physiology of dopamine neurons

Dopamine neurons, like all neurons, are normally polarized, with a resting membrane potential of approximately –70 mV. This polarization is maintained by the activity of the Na+/K+ ATPase, which is the major drain of metabolic energy in living brain tissue. In brain slices and in living brain, identified mesencephalic dopamine neurons exhibit spontaneous activity, depolarizing more or less randomly at an average rate of 3–4 Hz. It has been argued that the tonic or prevailing interstitial concentration of dopamine in terminal fields such as the striatum is mediated by tonic release, under the regulation of excitatory input from the cerebral cortex. However, dopamine neurons can characteristically switch into a mode known as "burst firing," which results in transient increases in dopamine release, and which is absolutely dependant on depolarization of the neurons (Grace 1991). In this scenario, the signaling capacity of dopamine neurons is determined by the dynamic range in the attainable interstitial dopamine concentrations, extending from the low tonic concentration to the transient phasic increases, which are terminated by reuptake or catabolism of the interstitial dopamine.

The maintenance of burst firing is not an intrinsic property of isolated dopamine neurons, but is mediated by the excitatory amino acid glutamate, and requires input from neurons in the nearby laterodorsal tegmental nucleus (Lodge & Grace 2006). Among the factors known to evoke burst firing of VTA neurons in rat brain include non-specific stimuli such as brushing a whisker (Freeman & Bunney 1987), or forced immobilization, which is a considerable stressor for awake rats (Anstrom & Woodward 2005). As noted above, members of a key class of effective antipsychotic drugs are dopamine receptor antagonists. Whereas acute treatment with these drugs stimulates the spiking and burst firing of dopamine neurons, prolonged treatment causes the neurons to become quiescent, a phenomenon known as "depolarization block" (Grace *et al.* 1997). Since the time course of this inactivation in rats seems to match with the several weeks' interval before optimal response of patients with schizophrenia, the onset of depolarization block may be a crucial mechanism in the therapeutic action of antipsychotic medication.

1.5.   The post-synaptic effects of dopamine

Dopamine receptors mediate intracellular effects via guanosine triphosphate (GTP)-binding proteins, commonly known as G-proteins. Receptor agonism stimulates the G-protein to exchange guanosine diphosphate (GDP) with GTP, which causes a dissociation of the receptor-G-protein complex. The free G-protein retains its GTP for a time, until its intrinsic GTPase activity decomposes the GTP, releasing the G-protein to reform its association with the receptor. While free from the receptor complex, the G-proteins interact with target molecules. In the case of dopamine D_1 receptors, the main signaling is mediated by G_s, which stimulates the activity of adenylate cyclase enzyme in the cytosol. Thus, agonism of D_1 receptors stimulates the formation of the intracellular second messenger cyclic AMP (cAMP), which in turn stimulates a specific phosphorylation of the intracellular phosphoprotein DARPP32 by a specific protein kinase (Bibb *et al.* 1999). The signal transduction pathway for D_2 receptors is more obscure, but appears to be largely mediated by inhibition of cAMP generation.

Signaling in dopamine-responsive neurons can be assessed by detecting the expression of the immediate early gene product, c-fos. This protein is readily detected in neurons using specific antisera. Full expression of c-fos in rat striatum is mediated by a synergistic activation of D_1- and D_2-like receptors (Keefe & Gerfen 1995), which is paradoxical, since the two receptor types are thought to be largely segregated in different populations of striatal neurons. It may be that interneurons mediate cross talk between striatal medium spiny neurons, such that integration of inputs from D_1 and D_2 receptors is obtained.

This brief account of the biochemical and neuroanatomical pathways in the signal transduction of dopamine is certain not to satisfy the fundamental question, "What does dopamine do?" During the past 50 years, brain dopamine has been firmly linked to the phenomenology of reward. Amphetamine, cocaine, nicotine, and most other addictive drugs increase dopamine release, especially in the ventral striatum; intracerebral self-administration studies in rats highlight the shell of the nucleus as the locus for rewarding properties of many drugs (Di Chiara *et al.* 2004). However, it would be erroneous to suppose that the dopamine release is synonymous with the reward itself. Observations of the firing rate of single dopamine neurons in conscious monkeys have led to a re-conceptualization of the relationship between dopamine and reward. In these monkeys, the rate of firing of dopamine neurons increases transiently when an unexpected reward (a taste of fruit juice) is presented. However, as the animal learns to perform a rewarded task consistently, the episodes of increased cell firing decline (Hollerman & Schultz 1998). Finally, the rate of cell firing increases only when an expected reward fails to materialize. In this context, dopamine mediates associative learning by broadcasting a prediction error, i.e. a deviation from the expected outcome. This allows the animal to adjust its behavior so as to optimize the chances of obtaining reward on another occasion. In general, the basal ganglia are composed of parallel circuits, each linked to discrete specialized input/output channels (Alexander & Crutcher 1990). If dopamine mediates neuronal coding of prediction errors, this may manifest in plasticity of mesolimbic circuits involved with motivation and reward whilst modulating the output of sensorimotor cortical regions controlling muscle tone and voluntary movement. The muscular rigidity of Parkinson's disease is thus a default state, occurring in the absence of correct feedback modulation of muscle tone. By extension, it might be supposed that anhedonia arises from uncoupling of prediction error signaling in the mesolimbic dopamine system: the salt loses its savour.

1.6.   A brief introduction to molecular imaging

Dopamine and an extensive cast of characters in the life of dopamine can be visualized and quantified in living brain by molecular imaging. The starting point of molecular imaging is the synthesis of a radiopharmaceutical, i.e. a drug carrying within its molecular structure a radioactive isotope. In the case of PET, this isotope must first be prepared using a cyclotron and then hastily incorporated into the radiopharmaceutical, which is then purified for intravenous injection in the living subject. On entering the blood stream, the radiopharmaceutical is carried to every tissue and organ of the body. On entering into the brain, the drug may be retained for some time, especially if it interacts with some biochemical pathway or encounters binding sites for which it has high affinity.

Wherever the drug goes, it carries a source of radioactivity. Inexorably, the radioisotope undergoes physical decay, releasing energetic particles. In the case of PET, the released particle is a positron, the positively charged counterpart of the common electron (antimatter is not science fiction, but a routine matter at PET–cyclotron facilities around the world). This positron soon encounters a nearby electron, with catastrophic consequences for both particles. With nothing to overcome their electrostatic attraction, they merge and instantly annihilate. All the energy which was bound up in the mass of the two particles ($E = mc^2$) is released in a flash of light emanating from the point of annihilation. More specifically, there are two flashes of light, with two high-energy photons traveling in opposite directions. These photons, known as gamma rays, have the electromagnetic properties of ordinary light, but inhabit an entirely different domain of energy and can easily pass through the human body or, for that matter, a sheet of lead.

The mode of radioactive decay of single-photon emission computed tomography (SPECT) isotopes is different, resulting in a single photon of somewhat less energy than those arising from positron annihilation. These formidably energetic photons pass unperturbed through the brain, but they are not completely unstoppable. Certain materials can capture these photons and transfer their energy into a cascade of more ordinary photons, which then activate a photoelectron multiplier. The tomograph consists of circular rings of these detectors, positioned so that the subject's head is near the center of the aperture of the detector ring. Perhaps millions of decay events are registered, and the spatial pattern of the radiation field is calculated. Modern PET scanners have thousands of detectors; the final calculation of the image is consequently a task for high-speed computers. The end result of this calculation is a three-dimensional image or map showing the radioactivity concentration within each image element (pixel or voxel). A series of successive images are collected in the minutes or hours after injection of the radiopharmaceutical, in order to capture the dynamic process of uptake.

The tomograph detects radioactivity, but the subject of interest is biochemistry. It is the task of kinetic modeling to transform the dynamic emission recordings into an estimate of some biochemical process in living brain. The application of PET to this task dates to the first investigations of cerebral glucose metabolism with the radiotracer [^{18}F]fluorodeoxyglucose (Phelps *et al.* 1979), which followed soon after publication of the ground-breaking autoradiographic method for quantitation of cerebral glucose consumption in living rats (Sokoloff *et al.* 1977). The underlying biochemical principle of these studies is that radioactive glucose analogs enter the pathway for natural glucose consumption in the brain. Using instrumentation and modeling methods derived from the earlier work on glucose metabolism, the first PET investigation specifically of dopamine in human brain was carried out using the dopamine receptor ligand N-[^{11}C]methylspiperone (Wagner *et al.* 1983). In subsequent years, thousands of radioligands have been tested for molecular imaging of enzymes and receptors relevant to dopamine and other neuroactive substances.

2

Enzymology of tyrosine hydroxylase

2.1.   Molecular biology and enzymology

Basic aspects of the biochemistry of TH have been investigated in considerable detail. Alternative post-transcriptional splicing of the cloned cDNA for human TH gives rise to four distinct messages (Kaneda *et al.* 1987). Of these, the TH type I resembles in sequence most closely the single transcript expressed in rat (Grima *et al.* 1987). When purified from tissue, the TH enzyme is associated with dopamine and possesses a bright blue-green color due to the complex between iron(III) and the catecholamine. Purified in the absence of catecholamines from transgenic bacteria, the enzyme is light green due to the complex between iron(III) and several histidine residues close to the active site (Ramsey, Hillas, & Fitzpatrick 1996). When purified to homogeneity, human TH type I expressed in *Escherichia coli* is a tetrameric protein of subunits with molecular mass of about 60 kDa (Nakashima *et al.* 1999), consistent with the native tetramer from rat, human, and bovine sources (Oka *et al.* 1982; Rosenberg & Lovenberg 1983).

The catalytic cycle for TH requires the reduction of iron(III), which has a half-life of 1 s in the presence of reduced biopterin (Ramsey, Hillas, & Fitzpatrick 1996), also known as tetrahydrobiopterin (BH_4). Tyrosine hydroxylation requires the reaction between equimolar amounts of molecular oxygen and BH_4, or certain synthetic reducers such as 2-amino-4-hydroxy-6,7-dimethyltetrahydropterin ($DMPH_4$) and 6-methyltetrahydropterin ($6MPH_4$). Indeed, the reaction rate is faster for $6MPH_4$ than for the endogenous compound, BH_4 (Lazar *et al.* 1982; Lazar, Mefford, & Barchas 1982). The order of the sequential formation of the quaternary complex of enzyme, BH_4, tyrosine, and oxygen has not been fully defined (Bullard & Capson 1983). The activity of TH in vivo results in the production of equimolar amounts of the product DOPA and oxidized biopterin, which can be recycled by the dihydrobiopterin nicotinamide adenine dinucleotide (NADH) reductase. Indeed, regeneration of BH_4 in PC12 cells is accelerated in the presence of NADH (Vrecko *et al.* 1997).

The initial step, the de novo synthesis of biopterin, is catalyzed by the GTP cyclohydrolase, which is consequently crucial for DOPA synthesis. Thus, certain cells in mouse brain which transiently express TH in the absence of GTP cyclohydrolase fail to produce DOPA (Nagatsu *et al.* 1997). A number of other hydroxylase enzymes also make use of BH_4. For example, tyrosine is formed in the liver by phenylalanine hydroxylase, which can be irreversibly inhibited with *p*-chlorophenylalanine (*p*CPA), at a dose not altering TH activity in brain (Gal & Whitacre 1982). However, cerebral synthesis of serotonin is highly sensitive to the inhibition of tryptophan hydroxylase by *p*CPA (Koe & Weissman 1968).

Mechanical homogenation of rat brain tissue in a medium containing a high concentration of sucrose is used to prepare a subcellular fraction known as synaptosomes. This preparation retains much of the biochemical machinery of living dopamine terminals. TH in synaptosomes from rat striatum can synthesize DOPA from phenylalanine by a two-step process involving the sequential synthesis, release, and rebinding of tyrosine (Katz, Lloyd, & Kaufman 1976). Experiments in synaptosomes from rat brain have suggested that one third of brain dopamine may be derived from phenylalanine (Kapatos & Zigmond 1977). The activity of TH can also be studied in slices of brain tissue maintained in an oxygenated medium. Superfusion of slices from rat striatum with a medium containing 25 μM of phenylalanine, but no tyrosine, can sustain dopamine synthesis, although not so well as when tyrosine is added to the medium (Milner, Irie, & Wurtman 1986). However, in a microdialysis study of the release of dopamine in living rat striatum, a low dose of phenylalanine ($200\,mg\,kg^{-1}$, i.p.) transiently increased dopamine release, while a high dose ($1000\,mg\,kg^{-1}$, i.p.) decreased dopamine release (During, Acworth, & Wurtman 1988b). Similarly, the formation of DOPA in rat retina was reduced after treatments increasing the serum concentration of phenylalanine ten-fold (Fernstrom, Baker, & Fernstrom 1989). Thus, phenylalanine supplementation can stimulate dopamine synthesis in vivo, but when given at a high dose, competitive inhibition of TH by the less-preferred substrate is the predominant effect.

2.2.   Disorders of tyrosine hydroxylase

Elimination of TH activity by the knockout technique is lethal in utero at mid-gestation (Zhou, Quaife, & Palmiter 1995), but mouse fetuses can be rescued by administration of DOPA to the pregnant dams, and can then survive post-natally. Evidently, the catecholamines are required for critical aspects of embryonic development, but the basis of this requirement is unclear. It may be, for example, that transient expression of TH modulates neuronal differentiation and migration. Traces of catecholamines were detected in the brain and sympathetic tissue of pigmented mice lacking TH. However, nervous tissue from an albino strain of these mice also lacking the tyrosinase enzyme required for neuromelanin synthesis was entirely devoid of catecholamines (Rios *et al.* 1999). This reveals the absolute requirement for an intact default pathway for rescue of DOPA synthesis in TH knockout mice.

Classical phenylketonuria is due to a deficiency in the activity of hepatic phenylalanine hydroxylase. The progressively debilitating neurological symptoms of untreated phenylketonuria are due to the neurotoxic effects of reactive metabolites of phenylalanine, and are also related to a profound deficiency of dopamine, noradrenaline and serotonin in the brain. Strict control of dietary phenylalanine intake from the earliest post-natal period is essential for normal development of children with phenylketonuria. Defects in the dihydropteridine reductase or in the pathway for the de novo synthesis of BH_4 from GTP likewise result in syndromes resembling classical phenylketonuria, but which are unresponsive to the control of dietary phenylalanine (Kaufman 1987). Autoradiography experiments in vivo suggest that most brain BH_4 is formed in brain by de novo synthesis (Hoshiga *et al.* 1993), and is not derived from circulation. This phenomenon likely accounts for the difficulty in restoring neurotransmitter synthesis by BH_4 replacement therapy. Somewhat more favorable stimulation of cerebral neurotransmitter synthesis seems possible with the synthetic co-substrate $6MPH_4$, due to its greater penetration into the central nervous system (Kapatos & Kaufman 1981). Once in the brain, biopterins enter neurons by passive diffusion (Anastasiadis, Kuhn, & Levine 1994).

In general, the regional brain concentration of BH_4 is highest in the striatum and other regions with high TH activity (Sawada *et al.* 1987), suggesting that the expressions of TH and GTP cyclohydrolase genes are normally linked by common transcription factors. Hereditary progressive dystonia, also known as DOPA-responsive dystonia or Segawa's disease, is characterized by early childhood onset of dystonia with marked diurnal variation. The symptoms are wonderfully responsive to treatment with low doses of DOPA. A deficiency of the enzyme GTP cyclohydrolase is now understood to underlie most cases of Segawa's disease (Ichinose *et al.* 1994), although recessive mutations of TH with low specific enzyme activity have been reported in several families (Ludecke *et al.* 1996; Nygaard 1995). Pharmacological blockade of the cyclohydrolase decreased the TH activity throughout rat brain (Suzuki *et al.* 1988), providing a method for modeling Segawa's disease. While deficiency in the GTP cyclohydrolase activity disease results in inadequate synthesis of dopamine, noradrenaline, serotonin, and other neuroactive substances, the clinical features are largely resolved by oral DOPA therapy alone. This observation suggests that either dopamine is uniquely indispensable for normal brain function or that the dopamine neurons are constitutionally more dependant on normal availability of BH_4. In vivo microdialysis studies reveal that BH_4 can stimulate directly the synthesis and release of dopamine, apparently by acting at a stereospecific recognition site in the brain (Koshimura *et al.* 1995).

2.3.   Regulation of activity

Most estimates of the tyrosine concentration required for half-saturation of TH in vitro (12–50 µM) are lower than the free tyrosine concentrations usually present in living brain tissue (100 µM), predicting nearly complete saturation of the enzyme with this substrate in vivo (Table 2.1). Indeed, the concentration of dopamine in microdialysates from rat striatum was unaffected by five-fold elevations in brain tyrosine concentration (Westerink & de Vries 1991). However, the association of TH with membranes apparently influences its affinity for tyrosine. Thus, phospholipase treatment of the enzyme resulted in a substantial decline in its affinity for tyrosine (Kuczenski 1983). Solubilization of the TH enzyme also increased its affinity for BH_4 co-factor, and increased the catalytic activity.

While TH is normally saturated with tyrosine, the rate of catecholamine synthesis in nervous tissue can be stimulated by tyrosine supplementation under special circumstances of pharmacological activation. For example, tyrosine supplementation can further enhance the excess production of DOPAC in the brain of rats treated with haloperidol or amfonelic acid (Fuller & Snoddy 1982), and can enhance dopamine release in methylphenidate-treated nucleus accumbens slices (Woods & Meyer 1991), or potassium-stimulated rat retina (Gibson 1992). Neurotoxic lesions to the substantia nigra notably increased the synthesis of DOPAC and HVA in the striatum following tyrosine administration, but only in those rats with the most substantial dopamine denervations. Thus, the few remaining dopamine cells were metabolically abnormal with respect to their dependence on tyrosine availability (Melamed, Hefti, & Wurtman 1980). It can be assumed that a similar state of affairs prevails in cases of advanced Parkinson's disease. Under conditions of stimulation of TH with haloperidol, the concentration of tyrosine in rat striatum decreased by almost 30% (Westerink & Wirix 1983). However, the concentration was still greater than 100 µM, which should maintain near saturation of TH. Nonetheless, the several

Table 2.1. *Some biochemical properties of TH*

Item	Quantity	Unit	Reference
Molar weight of monomer recombinant human TH isozyme	60 000	Daltons	Almas *et al.* 1992
Ferric iron per monomer recombinant rat enzyme	0.7	Atoms	Nakashima *et al.* 1999
Ferric iron per monomer recombinant rat enzyme	0.6	Atoms	Ramsey, Hillas, & Fitzpatrick 1996
pH optimum of phosphorylated bovine striatum TH	6.6	pH	Lazar *et al.* 1982
pH optimum of non-phosphorylated bovine striatum TH	6.1		
Concentration of TH in rat striatum	1	μM	Reinhard & O'Callaghan 1991
Homospecific activity (HSA) of TH from rat striatum	0.5	*	Reinhard & O'Callaghan 1991
HSA of TH from human striatum	0.7	*	Nakashima *et al.* 1999
HSA of TH from normal human caudate	1.5	*	Mogi *et al.* 1988
HSA of TH from parkinsonian caudate	7		
Affinity of rat adrenal gland TH for tyrosine	12	μM	Mueller, Thoenen, & Axelrod 1969
Affinity of rat striatum TH for tyrosine	15	μM	Stone 1980
Affinity of rat striatum TH for tyrosine	54	μM	Zivkovic, Guidotti, & Costa 1974
Affinity of membrane-bound rat striatum TH for tyrosine	7	μM	Kuczenski 1983
Affinity of phospholipase-treated rat striatum TH for tyrosine	48		
Free tyrosine concentration in rat striatum	97	μM	Groppetti *et al.* 1977
Free tyrosine concentration in rat striatum	103	μM	Heffner & Seiden 1980
Affinity of rat adrenal TH for phenylalanine	300	μM	Ikeda, Levitt, & Udenfriend 1967
Basal affinity for rat striatum TH for biopterin	1000	μM	Lazar, Mefford, & Barchas 1982
After haloperidol treatment	160		
Affinity of non-phosphorylated bovine striatum TH for biopterin	200		
Affinity of phosphorylated bovine striatum TH for biopterin	88		
Biopterin concentration in human caudate	2	μM	Sawada *et al.* 1987
Biopterin concentration in rat striatum	1	μM	Levine, Kuhn, & Lovenberg 1979
Inhibition of bovine caudate TH by dopamine, K_i with respect to biopterin	20	μM	Bullard & Capson 1983
Inhibition by bovine caudate TH by iodo-tyrosine, K_i with respect to tyrosine	62	nM	Bullard & Capson 1983
Inhibition by bovine adrenal TH by α-methyl-ρ-tyrosine (AMPT), K_i with respect to tyrosine	17	μM	Udenfriend, Zaltzman-Nirenberg, & Nagatsu 1965
Affinity for bovine caudate TH for oxygen	2	μM	Oka *et al.* 1982

Note: * HSA is the number of DOPA molecules formed per second per molecule of TH enzyme purified to homogeneity.

reports of potentiation of dopamine synthesis by tyrosine supplementation suggest that the affinity of TH for tyrosine in living brain may be lower than that seen in vitro, such that saturation is not as complete as is generally held to be the case.

Kinetic studies of TH indicate very low affinities for the co-substrate BH_4 ($K_m = 100$–$1000\,\mu M$) relative to the concentrations typically measured in the striatum (1–$2\,\mu M$; Table 2.1). It follows that the TH reaction rate should be sensitive to altered BH_4 concentrations. Indeed, the rate of DOPA synthesis and the dopamine concentration in rat striatum were substantially increased after intracerebroventricular administration of BH_4 (Miwa, Watanabe, & Hayaishi 1985), as was the outflow of dopamine in microdialysates following addition of BH_4 to the perfusion medium (Koshimura *et al.* 1990).

2.4.   Autoreceptor modulation of activity

As mentioned above, haloperidol and other blockers of dopamine D_2 receptors acutely increase the rate of formation of dopamine metabolites in rat striatum (Carlsson & Lindqvist 1963). This key observation reveals that TH activity, and consequently dopamine synthesis and metabolism, is tonically suppressed by the occupation of feedback autoreceptors by dopamine. The pharmacological blockade of these autoreceptors consequently relieves in part the tonic inactivation of TH mediated by interstitial dopamine, resulting in increased dopamine synthesis. Another model for studying autoreceptor regulation is presented by dopaminergic amacrine cells of the mammalian retina. Stimulation of amacrine cells with light activates TH by increasing the affinity of the enzyme for BH_4, as expected. However, kinetic analysis of the TH activity as a function of BH_4 concentration showed a biphasic relationship, suggesting that roughly equal proportions of TH enzyme are normally found in high- and low-affinity states (Iuvone *et al.* 1982). Thus, it is the state of equilibrium between high- and low-activity forms of TH that is ultimately modulated by the autoreceptors.

Whereas autoreceptor regulation of TH activity is characteristic of nigrostriatal dopamine fibers, this is much less evident in the projections from the VTA to the medial prefrontal cortex (Chiodo *et al.* 1984). Autoreceptor regulation is entirely absent in the dopamine neurons resident in the median eminence of the hypothalamus (Demarest & Moore 1979). The variable association between autoreceptor regulation and impulse control of dopamine synthesis is consistent with the greater capacity of tyrosine supplements to stimulate dopamine synthesis in specific brain regions. For example, the mesocortical dopamine neurons are characterized by a high rate of burst firing, and a high dopamine turnover rate (Bannon & Roth 1983). These same neurons also exhibit a notable increase in DOPA synthesis after a low dose of tyrosine ($25\,mg\,kg^{-1}$, i.p.), a treatment which failed to influence tyrosine hydroxylation in the nucleus accumbens or the striatum (Tam *et al.* 1990). The mesolimbic dopamine system may normally occupy an intermediate state with respect to autoregulation, such that tyrosine supplements at high doses ($250\,mg\,kg^{-1}$, i.p.) increased the concentration of dopamine in microdialysates to a greater extent in the nucleus accumbens than in the striatum (During, Acworth, & Wurtman 1988a). Furthermore, stimulation of dopamine synthesis with haloperidol potentiated the extra dopamine release in the ventral striatum produced by intraperitoneal tyrosine administration (During, Acworth, & Wurtman 1989). In summary, the availability of tyrosine in the brain is not always sufficient to maintain dopamine synthesis across the entire dynamic range of neuronal activity.

Autoreceptor regulation of TH activity from rat striatum becomes evident between the 4th and the 28th post-natal day (Crawford, McDougall, & Bardo 1994; Hedner & Lundborg 1985). However, haloperidol failed to elicit an increase in TH activity in the striatum from aged rats (Fine, Masserano, & Weiner 1986), suggesting that functional uncoupling of autoreceptors occurs late in life. GABA agonists (Gale *et al.* 1978) and stable antagonist analogs of substance P, when injected into the substantia nigra, prevent the BH_4-mediated activation of TH by antipsychotic drugs (Melis & Gale 1984). These latter findings suggest that the autoreceptor regulation of dopamine synthesis is opposed by GABA and facilitated by substance P. Since these are precisely the neurotransmitters found in the striatal neurons projecting back to the dopamine cells, this biochemical finding may reveal a long pathway by which dopamine release in terminal fields modulates dopamine synthesis or neuronal activity in the cell body.

2.5.   Phosphorylation of tyrosine hydroxylase

Phosphorylating conditions for TH can be obtained in vitro by incubation of brain protein in a medium containing Mg^{2+}, ATP, cAMP, and purified cAMP-dependent protein kinase. After treatment under these conditions, the affinity of TH from rat striatum for BH_4 was high (0.1 mM) throughout the pH range 5.8–6.2, but there remained some activation at subsaturating BH_4 concentrations at higher pH (Pradhan, Alphs, & Lovenberg 1981). At neutral pH, phosphorylation of TH from bovine striatum with a cardiac muscle protein kinase reduced the affinity for BH_4 and also increased the maximal velocity of the enzyme (Lazar *et al.* 1982). Thus, the ability of phosphorylation to stimulate TH in vivo is sensitive to the availability of the BH_4 co-factor, and possibly to unknown effects of pH regulation in the enzymatic compartment. Maximal activation of TH from rat striatum by haloperidol occurred when approximately one third of the enzyme was phosphorylated (Lazar, Mefford, & Barchas 1982), suggesting that the maximal extent of phosphorylation may be higher in the retina, as cited above.

Potassium-evoked depolarization of synaptosomes from rat striatum results in the incorporation of several phosphate residues into the amino acid sequence of TH (Haycock 1987). The activation of TH in the striatum following pharmacological blockade of impulse flow and dopamine release was associated with phosphorylation primarily at Ser40 (Lew *et al.* 1999). Activation of TH produced by incubation with purified protein kinase C (PKC) apparently occurs by the same mechanism as does the cAMP-dependent phosphorylation (Albert *et al.* 1984). However, the calcium/calmodulin-dependent activation of TH in the presence of ATP and Mg^{2+} at pH 7.0 is independent of cAMP-dependent protein phosphorylation (Iuvone 1984), and is associated with phosphorylation at a different serine residue of the TH polypeptide (Atkinson *et al.* 1987). This calcium/calmodulin-dependent phosphorylation may be physiologically relevant to the activation of TH occurring upon depolarization, when intracellular Ca^{2+} concentrations are transiently increased.

In addition to the above pathways, TH obtained from adrenal chromaffin cells is also phosphorylated by a cGMP-dependent protein kinase, a signaling pathway that is activated by the gaseous messenger nitric oxide (Rodriguez-Pascual *et al.* 1999). The contribution of this pathway to the regulation of neuronal TH has yet to be demonstrated. Conditions promoting carboxymethylation inhibit TH by reducing the affinity of the enzyme for BH_4 (Mann & Hill 1983). However, the physiological significance of this observation has not been investigated.

After cessation of transient cAMP phosphorylating conditions, activated TH reverts to the inactive form with low affinity for BH_4. This spontaneous process was apparently mediated by a phosphatase enzyme present in crude preparations (Vrana & Roskoski 1983). Three phosphatase activities could be detected in extracts from rat striatum (Nelson & Kaufman 1987). Of these, one could dephosphorylate [^{32}P]-labeled TH that had been phosphorylated by a cAMP-dependent protein kinase. The other phosphatases preferentially recognized TH that had been phosphorylated by a Ca^{2+}/calmodulin system. Thus, separate enzymes subserve the dephosphorylation and inactivation of TH stimulated by depolarization-dependent and cAMP-dependent activations. Given the variety of opposing factors in living tissue, the activity of TH is poised at an intermediate state of activation under normal physiological conditions.

TH is directly inhibited by its substrate tyrosine and by catechol congeners (Table 2.1). The inhibition of TH from PC 12 cells (Laschinski, Kittner, & Brautigam 1986) by dopamine ($K_i = 1$–$5\,\mu M$) and other catecholamines occurs by simple competition between dopamine and the tyrosine substrate. Furthermore, a key sequence necessary for the allosteric inhibition of TH by dopamine has been identified in the N-terminus of the enzyme (Nakashima *et al.* 1999). As noted above, phosphorylation of TH stimulates the enzyme and increases the optimal pH toward the physiological pH. In human TH, this regulation is mediated by cAMP-dependent phosphorylation at subunit Ser40, which decreases the affinity for dopamine (Almas *et al.* 1992). Thus, end-product inhibition at physiological pH is disabled in the activated and phosphorylated enzyme (Okuno & Fujisawa 1985).

The ex vivo inhibition of TH by apomorphine has usually been attributed to a feedback mechanism mediated by agonism of autoreceptors on nigrostriatal dopamine fibers (Van Zwieten-Boot & Noach 1975). However, the results of some apomorphine studies should be interpreted in light of the observed potent and direct inhibition of TH by apomorphine (Laschinski, Kittner, & Brautigam 1986). Thus, blockade by apomorphine of the increased affinity of rat brain TH for BH_4 occurring after transection of the nigrostriatal pathway (Lew *et al.* 1999) might be due in part to simple competitive inhibition of TH by apomorphine.

2.6.   Transcriptional regulation

TH is expressed in several distinct populations of neurons, in adrenal chromaffin cells, and in sympathetic ganglia of the adult rat, and can be transiently expressed in other cell-types during development. Several *cis*-response elements are present in the flanking sequences of the mammalian tyrosine TH gene, including the cAMP response element, and the AP1 motif mediating responses to nerve growth factor (Harrington *et al.* 1987). The activation of the enzyme adenylate cyclase by forskolin or by cAMP itself both result in phosphorylation of numerous targets, including various serine residues of the TH enzyme, as discussed above. With respect to transcriptional control of TH, PKA phosphorylates a specific soluble protein which (in the phosphorylated state) increases the expression of TH by binding to the cAMP response element regulating gene expression (Yamamoto *et al.* 1988).

Pheochromocytoma cells are a tumor of the adrenal chromaffin cells that have been extensively employed as a model of gene regulation. Lines of pheochromocytoma cells deficient in PKA have constitutively low expression of the TH gene, and consequently have low enzyme activity. Furthermore, the normal induction of TH expression in the presence of cAMP and other cyclic nucleotides is absent in these cells (Kim *et al.* 1993). Phorbol esters stimulate TH expression via the phosphorylating enzyme PKC, independently of the PKA-dependent pathway (Kim *et al.* 1994).

In transgenic mice with a substantial over-expression of human TH in nigrostriatal neurons (Nakahara *et al.* 1993), the rate of DOPA synthesis in living striatum remained normal, although the TH activity was greatly elevated when measured in vitro. This discrepancy seemed most consistent with end-product inhibition of the enzyme in vivo. The transcriptional regulation of TH is not identical in all monoamine neurons. For example, depletion of catecholamines with reserpine for 3 days results in greatly elevated levels of the message for TH in the noradrenergic locus ceruleus, moderate increases in the VTA neurons, but no acute effect in the substantia nigra (Pasinetti *et al.* 1990). These differences may be related to the differing requirements of these cell types to respond dynamically to changing demands for catecholamine synthesis.

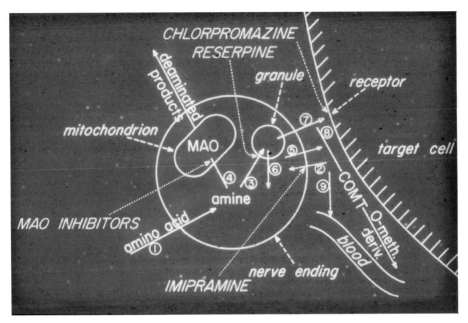

Figure 1.2 Schematic diagram of the dopamine synapse presented by Professor Arvid Carlsson in 1966. Processes in the pathway for dopamine are expressed as numbered arrows, including (1) entry of the amino acid precursor into the dopamine terminal, (2,5) bidirectional transfer of dopamine across the plasma membrane, (3) transfer of cytosolic dopamine into vesicles, and (4) oxidative deamination, and (7) binding at post-synaptic receptors. Reproduced with the kind permission of Professor Arvid Carlsson, University of Gothenburg.

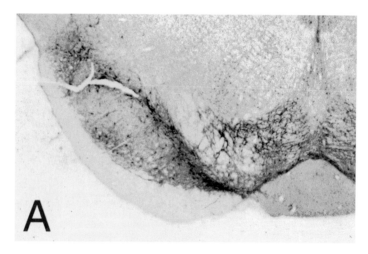

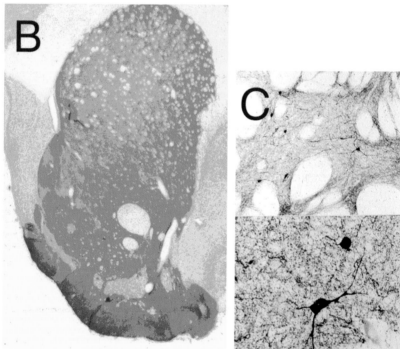

Figure 1.3 Neurochemical anatomy of the rat basal ganglia. Illustrated are
(A) TH-positive neurons in the rat substantia nigra and ventral tegmental area,
(B) fibers innervating the extended striatum, and (C) NADPH-positive neurons in the
striatum at (upper) low and (lower) high magnification. Reprinted with kind
permission of Professor Steve R. Vincent, University of British Columbia.

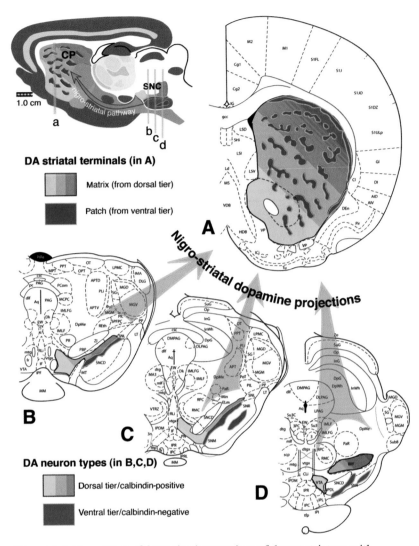

Figure 1.4 The pattern of dopamine innervations of the rat striatum, with segregation of the patch and matrix compartments. Diagram reprinted with kind permission of Dr. C. Gerfen, National Institutes of Health.

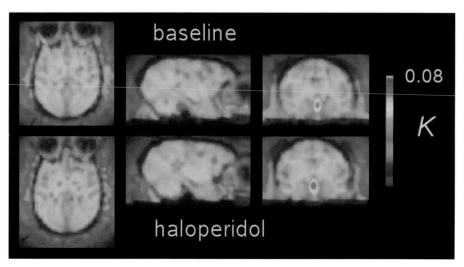

Figure 3.4 Parametric maps of the net blood brain clearance of $[^{11}C]$tyrosine (K_{in}^{Tyr}, ml g^{-1} min^{-1}) in a rhesus monkey. The animal was scanned first in a baseline condition, and again at 1 h after treatment with haloperidol (50 µg kg^{-1}). Parametric maps are co-registered to an MR-based atlas of monkey brain. Courtesy of Professor Per Hartvig, Uppsala University PET Centre.

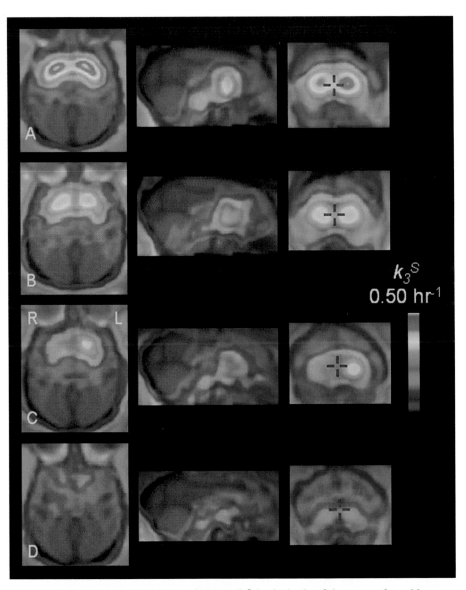

Figure 5.3 The utilization of FDOPA (k_3^s) in the brain of rhesus monkeys. Mean parametric maps are shown for (A) normal young ($n = 6$), (B) normal aged ($n = 4$) rhesus monkeys, (C) aged monkeys with unilateral intracarotid infusion of MPTP ($n = 3$), and (D) monkeys of intermediate aged with systemic MPTP administration ($n = 6$), all calculated relative to a reference tissue input by the method of Hartvig. Mean parametric maps are co-registered to the MR template, shown as gray-scale in the horizontal plane images. The cursor in the coronal plane images indicates the position (0,10,10) in the MR coordinate system. Reproduced with permission from Doudet *et al.* (2006a).

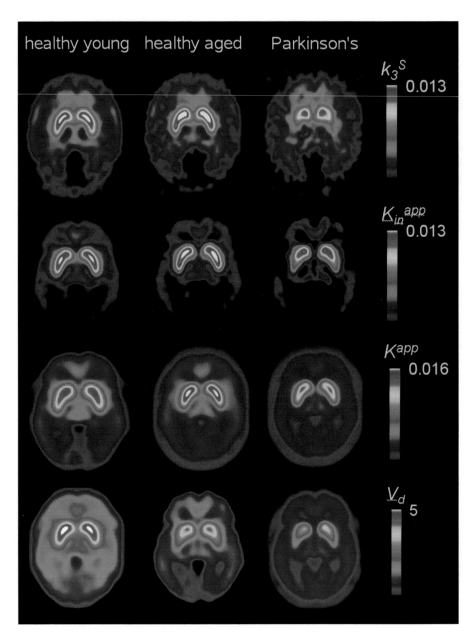

Figure 5.4 Mean parametric maps of FDOPA utilization relative to a reference tissue input (Hartvig k_3^S, min^{-1}), or arterial input (K_{in}^{app}, K^{app}; ml g^{-1} min^{-1}), and the steady-state FDOPA storage (Kumakura V_d; ml g^{-1}). Image courtesy of Dr. Yoshi Kumakura, Tokyo University.

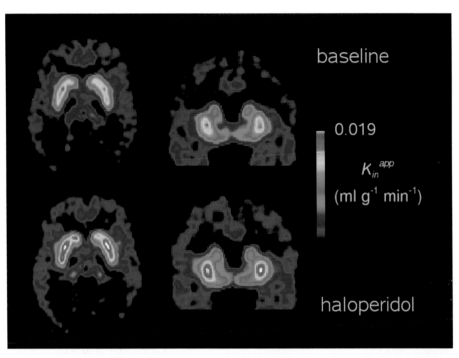

Figure 5.5 Effect of haloperidol treatment on FDOPA utilization in human brain. Mean parametric maps show the magnitude of the FDOPA net blood-brain clearance (K_{in}^{app}) in a group of (n = 9) healthy male subjects, scanned first in a baseline condition, and after acute treatment with haloperidol. Image from data presented in Vernaleken *et al.* (2006).

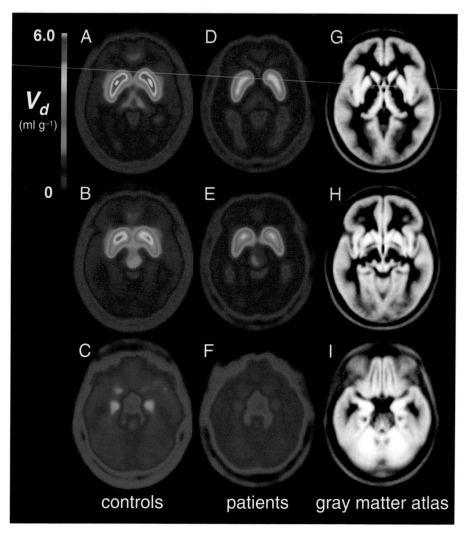

Figure 5.7 The steady-state storage of FDOPA (V_d, $\mathrm{ml\,g^{-1}}$) in the brain of unmedicated patients with schizophrenia and healthy age-matched control subjects. Reproduced with permission from Kumakura *et al.* (2007b).

3

The assay of tyrosine hydroxylase

3.1. Accumulation of DOPA after treatment with NSD 1015

3.1.1. General aspects

In the previous chapter, the kinetics of TH in vitro has been discussed in detail. It is clear that the net activity of TH under physiological conditions must be determined by the multiplicity of regulatory factors prevailing in the living brain. This chapter reviews and contrasts the several methods developed for the assay of TH in living brain. In vitro assays of TH activity are based on the formation of product in a reaction vessel under controlled conditions. However, there is no known mechanism for sequestering or concentration of DOPA in living brain. Basal concentrations of DOPA in brain are normally low because of its unimpeded diffusion back into circulation, and because of the high activity of AAADC relative to that of TH. The normally prodigious activity of cerebral AAADC in the brain of living rat is substantially blocked by treatment with the irreversible enzyme inhibitor *m*-hydroxybenzyl-hydrazine (NSD 1015), which forms a hydrazone derivative with the pyridoxal phosphate co-factor of AAADC. This blockade is essentially complete in rat brain when the drug is administered at a dose of at least $50 \, \mathrm{mg \, kg^{-1}}$ (Watanabe 1985). In the absence of AAADC activity, DOPA formed from tyrosine then accumulates in the brain tissue (Carlsson *et al.* 1972). This accumulation appears to be linear with time, from which the rate of DOPA synthesis can be calculated by linear regression. Since DOPA is formed from brain tyrosine by a first-order kinetic process, the fractional rate constant corresponding to the TH activity (k_{TH}, $\mathrm{min^{-1}}$) can be calculated by simple division of the observed DOPA synthesis rate by the brain tyrosine concentration, which generally remains fairly constant during the experiment.

Table 3.1. *Pharmacological modulation of levodopa synthesis at 30 min after NSD 1015 treatment*

Basal DOPA synthesis rate (pmol g^{-1} min^{-1})	Percentage change evoked by treatment	Treatment and reference
67	+230	Haloperidol, 2 mg kg^{-1} (Carlsson, Kehr, & Lindqvist 1976)
167	+200	Haloperidol, 0.5 mg kg^{-1} (Nissbrandt *et al.* 1988)
67	−58	Pargyline, 75 mg kg^{-1} (Carlsson, Kehr, & Lindqvist 1976)
467	−50	Apomorphine, 0.5 mg kg^{-1} (Reches *et al.* 1985)
633	−60	Apomorphine, 1 mg kg^{-1} (Bean *et al.* 1988)
367	+200	GBL, 750 mg kg^{-1} (Johnson *et al.* 1993)
300	230	GBL, 750 mg g^{-1}, mouse (Watanabe 1985)
500	−50	8-OHDPAT, 0.3 mg kg^{-1} (Johnson *et al.* 1993)
253	+60	Reserpine 0.25 mg kg^{-1}, ventral striatum (Ahlenius, Ericson, & Wijkstrom 1993)
317	−42	Medetomidine, 30 µg kg^{-1} (Koulu *et al.* 1993)
267	−24	Aged rats relative to young rats (Venero, Machado, & Cano 1991)
33	(5HTP synthesis)	(Tappaz & Pujol 1980)

Note: Results are for DOPA in rat striatum, except where otherwise specified. Identification of some treatments: medetomidine, α_2 receptor agonist; GBL (γ-butyrolactone), an inhibitor of impulse flow of dopamine cells; and 8-OHDPAT, serotonin 5HT$_{1A}$ receptor agonist.

There has been general agreement among researchers over several decades about the magnitude of DOPA synthesis in the striatum; the mean baseline DOPA synthesis rate in rat striatum based on NSD 1015 studies (Table 3.1) is close to 400 pmol g^{-1} min^{-1}. Since the brain concentration of free tyrosine is close to 40 µM, the activity of TH relative to its substrate must consequently be 0.01 min^{-1} in the striatum, a figure which is very close to the estimate obtained by following the metabolism of [^{3}H]tyrosine in living striatum, as described below. This means that precisely 1% of free tyrosine in striatum is hydroxylated with every minute, which explains why TH activity does not normally deplete its precursor, given the continued entry of tyrosine from blood. Microdissection of the rat brain has allowed the estimation of DOPA synthesis rates in specific nuclei of the mesencephalon, amygdala, and hypothalamus (Kilts *et al.* 1987). Results of these studies show that the basal rate of DOPA synthesis has an approximately 30-fold range between the lowest rate, in the cerebral cortex, and the highest rate, in the substantia nigra pars compacta, home of the dopamine neurons.

Serotonin is formed by the sequential actions of tryptophan hydroxylase and AAADC. Thus, the NSD 1015 method also allows the monitoring of the rate of synthesis of 5-hydroxytryptophan, the immediate precursor of serotonin. Using this method, it is seen that the activity of tryptophan hydroxylase in brain has a 200-fold range from lowest (cerebellum) to highest (dorsal raphe nucleus) (Tappaz & Pujol 1980). In striatum, the rate of 5-hydroxytryptophan accumulation is approximately one-tenth the rate of DOPA accumulation (Table 3.1), which indicates the relative densities of the dopamine and serotonin innervations in that structure.

3.1.2.   *Caveats of the NSD 1015 method*

The NSD 1015 method is implicitly a steady-state model, meaning that its valid use requires that AAADC blockade does not otherwise perturb the pathway for catecholamine synthesis. However, NSD 1015 is not an entirely specific inhibitor of AAADC, since concentrations greater than $1\,\mu M$ also inhibit MAO in vivo (Hunter, Rorie, & Tyce 1993), which might have consequences for the regulation of TH activity. Furthermore, low concentrations of NSD 1015 can evoke release of dopamine from slices of rat striatum by an unknown mechanism (Dluzen, Reddy, & McDermott 1992). NSD 1015 is also reported to increase the concentration of tyrosine in rat brain (Dyck 1987), and to increase the concentration of tyrosine and some other branched-chain amino acids in plasma, apparently due to inhibition of hepatic tyrosine aminotransferase (Hilton, Fonda, & Hilton 1998). It is also assumed that NSD 1015 does not significantly perturb the activity of TH, either by direct inhibition, or by removing the end-product inhibition of TH after dopamine depletion. Thus, the validity of the NSD 1015 method is subject to certain reservations related to changes in the steady-state condition.

Assays of TH activity based on the accumulation of DOPA assume that the blocked decarboxylation pathway is the only fate available for metabolism. In other words, the measured accumulation must account for all the DOPA synthesized in the interval of the experiment. However, DOPA is cleared from the brain by processes other than decarboxylation, with a net half-life close to 15 min (Westerink, de Vries, & Duran 1990), presumably via facilitated diffusion back into the circulation, as noted above. This uncorrected efflux of DOPA from the brain means that the NSD 1015 method must result in underestimation of the true rate of DOPA synthesis in vivo (Nissbrandt *et al.* 1988). It is therefore certain that the true rate of DOPA synthesis in living striatum exceeds the canonical value of $400\,\mathrm{pmol\,g^{-1}\,min^{-1}}$.

3.1.3.　Regulation of DOPA synthesis by autoreceptors

The NSD 1015 method has frequently been used as an index for testing the pharmacological regulation of TH activity in vivo, especially in studies of the modulation of dopamine synthesis by presynaptic autoreceptors. In general, any treatment altering the activation of presynaptic dopamine receptors will produce feedback alteration in the activity of TH, and of the release of dopamine. Very low doses of the dopamine autoreceptor agonist apomorphine $(30 \, \mu g \, kg^{-1})$ inhibited tyrosine hydroxylation in rat striatum (Carlsson, Kehr, & Lindqvist 1977). Although it is noted above that apomorphine can inhibit TH directly, inhibition of DOPA synthesis by apomorphine was blocked by local injection of pertussis toxin. This toxin acts by ADP-ribosylating the G_i and G_o subtypes of G-proteins, consequently inactivating them; it therefore seems likely that the apomorphine modulation is linked to dopamine $D_{2/3}$ receptors (Bean *et al.* 1988). Furthermore, blockade of dopamine catabolism with pargyline decreased TH activity, while blockade of dopamine autoreceptors with haloperidol increased the rate of tyrosine hydroxylation in rat striatum (Carlsson, Kehr, & Lindqvist 1976), as expected for receptor-mediated feedback regulation. Whereas haloperidol is an antagonist of both D_2 and D_3 receptors, studies with selective D_3 agonist 7-OHDPAT show that specifically these receptors are critical in the feedback regulation of DOPA synthesis (Ahlenius & Salmi 1994).

Because pargyline blocks both forms of MAO, it can be predicted that interfering with dopamine catabolism results in increased occupancy of the autoreceptors controlling DOPA synthesis. Indeed, chronic treatment with MAO-B selective inhibitor deprenyl decreased the rate of DOPA formation by 40% in rat striatum (Lamensdorf & Finberg 1997), suggesting that MAO-B contributes importantly to the modulation of dopamine catabolism. Also, consistent with autoreceptor regulation, the rate of accumulation of DOPA in rodent striatum was greatly potentiated by axotomy, i.e. cutting of the ascending fibers (Kehr 1974), or by the occlusion of all dopamine receptors with the alkylating agent EEDQ (Crawford, McDougall, & Bardo 1994). Treatment of rats with γ-butyrolactone, an inhibitor of impulse-dependent dopamine release, also increased DOPA formation (Walters & Roth 1974). Thus, the NSD 1015 method supports the notion, introduced above, that TH activity in living brain is normally poised somewhere in the middle of its dynamic range, between the upper limit evident after blockade of autoreceptors, and the lower limit occurring during full agonism of presynaptic autoreceptors.

The feedback inhibition of TH provoked by apomorphine was potentiated by chronic reserpine intoxication, suggesting the occurrence of sensitization of dopamine autoreceptors after a prolonged period of dopamine depletion (Reches *et al.* 1985). Furthermore, a single reserpine treatment results in the activation of DOPA formation lasting several days, but the duration of the linear DOPA accumulation after γ-butyrolactone was then reduced to about 15 min, rather than the usual 2 h (McMillen & Shore 1980), again suggesting sensitization of the autoreceptors. Similarly, the expected stimulation of the DOPA following chronic reserpine treatment was paradoxically reversed by treatment with the dopamine antagonist remoxipride (Ahlenius, Ericson, & Wijkstrom 1993). Together, these observations suggest that dopamine autoreceptors can become supersensitive after brief or prolonged dopamine depletion, a finding surely relevant to the occurrence of motor fluctuations during DOPA treatment for Parkinson's disease.

The response of DOPA synthesis rate to the pharmacological blockade of impulse flow is not identical in all brain regions endowed with a catecholamine innervation. Treatment with γ-butyrolactone trebled the rate of DOPA synthesis in the caudate nucleus, doubled the rate in olfactory tubercle and nucleus accumbens, and only slightly increased the rate in the substantia nigra pars compacta. This treatment was without effect on DOPA synthesis in the amygdala, even though apomorphine could produce some reductions in DOPA accumulation in that structure (Kilts *et al.* 1987). Likewise, DOPA synthesis in medial prefrontal cortex is unresponsive to blockade of impulse flow with γ-butyrolactone (Galloway, Wolf, & Roth 1986), but apomorphine could nonetheless reduce the rate of DOPA synthesis and the rate of catabolism of dopamine. The authors suggested that the end-product inhibition of TH in cortex predominates over the effects of autoreceptor-mediated regulation when impulse traffic is interrupted. In summary, autoregulation of DOPA synthesis is less distinct in extrastriatal structures.

3.1.4.   Other factors regulating DOPA synthesis

The NSD 1015 method has been used to test the effects of diverse pharmacological agents on the activity of the pathway for dopamine synthesis. For example, the inhibitory amino acid GABA and the GABA-B agonist baclofen did not change the basal production of DOPA in striatal slices, but partially inhibited the depolarization-evoked stimulation of DOPA synthesis (Arias-Montano, Martinez-Fong, & Aceves 1991, 1992). These findings support the claim that Ca^{2+} influx, which is antagonist by inhibitory substances, normally contributes to the mechanism of depolarization-induced activation of DOPA synthesis. Likewise, incubation of slices from rat striatum with the excitatory amino acid *N*-methyl-ᴅ-aspartic acid (NMDA) caused a dose-dependent doubling of DOPA production, although this could be only partially blocked with baclofen (Arias-Montano, Martinez-Fong, & Aceves 1992). Acute ethanol increased DOPA synthesis in the nucleus accumbens but not in the dorsal striatum (Blomqvist *et al.* 1993). Conversely, a high dose of an inhibitory substance, the GABA-A agonist diazepam (1 mg kg^{-1}), reduced the rate of DOPA synthesis in the limbic forebrain, including the olfactory tubercle and nucleus accumbens, without significantly altering the rate in the dorsal striatum (Biswas & Carlsson 1978). These findings thus indicate a particular vulnerability of mesolimbic DOPA synthesis to GABA-ergic modulation.

The selective α_2-adrenergic agonist medetomidine (Koulu *et al.* 1993) and the selective serotonin 5HT$_{1A}$ agonist 8-OHDPAT both inhibited DOPA synthesis in rat striatum to the same extent as did dopamine autoreceptor agonist apomorphine (Johnson *et al.* 1993). These pharmacological studies indicate that entirely different classes of G-protein-linked receptors can modulate DOPA synthesis, perhaps by converging on common intracellular second messenger systems. Acute cocaine treatment, which blocks the reuptake of interstitial dopamine and also serotonin, reduced DOPA synthesis in the nucleus accumbens, caudate nucleus, and medial prefrontal cortex, with con-comitant inhibition of 5-hydroxytryptophan hydroxylation in the same regions (Baumann *et al.* 1993). In contrast, treatment with buspirone, a selective partial agonist of serotonin 5HT$_{1A}$ autoreceptors, profoundly inhibited the synthesis of 5-hydroxytryptophan in rat brain, but was without effect on DOPA synthesis, as expected, given its greater pharmacological specificity (Tunnicliff *et al.* 1992). However, acute treatment with amperozide, a selective serotonin 5HT$_{2A}$ antago-nist, acutely stimulated DOPA synthesis in limbic structures, including the nucleus accumbens, olfactory tubercle, and amygdala (Pettersson *et al.* 1990), suggesting that serotonergic heteroceptors exert a tonic inhibition of TH. In contrast, chronic administration of amperozide via an osmotic minipump failed to alter DOPA synthesis in any brain region (Adell & Myers 1995).

Acute activation of DOPA synthesis in rat striatum by low doses of estradiol is attributed to a decline in end-product inhibition, presumably a consequence of phosphorylation of the TH enzyme (Pasqualini *et al.* 1995). Castration had no effect on the rate of DOPA synthesis in the striatum and nucleus accumbens of male rats. Nonetheless, the inhibition of DOPA synthesis evoked by a low dose of apomorphine was potentiated by castration, indicating that androgens can enhance the sensitivity to agonists of presynaptic autoreceptors (Klint *et al.* 1988).

3.2.   Superfusion of living striatum with [^{3}H]tyrosine

Whereas the NSD 1015 method is based on the progressive synthesis of DOPA from its natural precursor, radioisotope methods provide an alternate approach for measuring the activity of TH. Dopamine synthesis in living striatum has been tested using superfusion experiments in which [³H]tyrosine was introduced into the brain interstitial fluid via a "push-pull" cannula. In this method, the radioactive precursor mixes with the native tyrosine in the brain, and becomes available as a substrate for TH (Leviel, Gobert, & Guibert 1989). By definition, the concentration of [³H]tyrosine divided by the total mass of tyrosine in a volume of tissue equals the *specific activity*. If [³H]tyrosine is supplied to brain continuously by superfusion, the specific activity of tyrosine sampled at the site of superfusion will eventually approach an equilibrium, reflecting the complete mixing of labeled and unlabeled substances. One can then assume that local de novo synthesis of dopamine incorporates radioactivity at the same specific activity present in the tyrosine pool in brain (correcting, of course, for the halving of specific activity from the loss of a ring-tritium with each ring-hydroxylation). However, Leviel *et al.* (1989) found that the specific activity of interstitial [³H]dopamine collected during superfusion with [³H]tyrosine was initially higher than the specific activity calculated for the entire concentration of non-radioactive dopamine in the tissue. This delay to equilibrium reveals the presence in striatum of a large pool of "old" dopamine sequestered in synaptic vesicles.

After blockade of TH with the competitive inhibitor α-methyl-*para*-tryosine (AMPT), the concentration of dopamine in rat striatum declines, indicating a half-life for vesicular dopamine of 1 or 2 h. Several half-lives would be required to obtain complete equilibrium between newly formed [³H]dopamine and the vesicular pool. Nevertheless, the specific activity of extracellular [³H]dopamine rapidly becomes fairly stable during superfusion experiments, reflecting the rapid entry of newly synthesized dopamine into the extracellular space. Within minutes of the addition of AMPT to the superfusion medium, the specific activity of extracellular [³H]dopamine in cat striatum began to decline with a half-life of about 30 min, while the total dopamine concentration began to decline with a half-life of 60 min (Leviel & Guibert 1987). This observation further supports the notion that new dopamine is used first, while old dopamine is, in a manner of speaking, cellared like old wine. The specific activity of the acidic metabolite [³H]DOPAC declined in parallel with that of [³H]dopamine after synthesis blockade with AMPT, again suggesting that older, unlabeled dopamine is recruited for exocytosis prior to its metabolism by MAO (Leviel, Gobert, & Guibert 1989). The slowly declining specific activity of [³H]DOPAC with time after AMPT treatment implies that old dopamine was being mobilized for release via transit through the cytoplasm. This implies that dopamine from old vesicles is recycled by degranulation, followed by repackaging in new vesicles after a perilous second transit through the cytoplasm. However, this interpretation is based on the assumption that the labeled compounds were sampled from volumes of tissue affected to the same extent by local infusion of 0.1 mM AMPT. In fact, the concentration of DOPAC in the interstitial fluid had declined by half only at 3 h of AMPT superfusion, suggesting that DOPAC measured at the site of the push-pull cannula may arise from a distal site unaffected by the TH inhibitor. Thus, spatial inhomogeneity of metabolite pools emerges as a limitation in this use of the superfusion method.

3.3.   Intracerebroventricular infusion of [³H]tyrosine

The blood–brain barrier can be circumvented by direct injection of agents or tracers into the CSF, which fills the ventricular space and communicates directly with the interstitial fluid. Thus, radioactive catecholamines are formed in brain after intracerebroventricular infusion of [³H]tyrosine. As in the push-pull cannula technique, the specific activity of these compounds in extracts from rat striatum can be calculated by first assaying dopamine and its metabolites by HPLC with electrochemical detection, and then using scintillation spectroscopy to measure radioactivity in the HPLC fractions. Based on this approach, the ratio of the concentration of [³H]dopamine to the specific activity of [³H]tyrosine in the striatum has been used as "conversion index," indicative of the rate of neurotransmitter turnover. During operant behavior in which rats have been trained to work by pressing a lever for water reinforcement, the magnitude of this conversion index in the striatum increased in proportion to the individual rat's rate of response, indicating that the rate of dopamine synthesis was coupled to behavior (Heffner & Seiden 1980). However, the total brain dopamine concentration was unaffected during behavior, indicating that steady-state concentrations were maintained in the presence of increased consumption of dopamine.

Five minutes after intracerebroventricular infusion of [³H]tyrosine, the specific activity of [³H]DOPAC in the striatum was much higher than that of [³H]dopamine (Groppetti *et al.* 1977), suggesting that the newly synthesized [³H]dopamine was not being immediately equilibrated with a secure storage pool, as also suggested by the results of push-pull cannula experiments described above.

3.4.   Intravenous injection of [³H]tyrosine

Superfusion studies can perturb cerebral metabolism at the site of the push-pull cannula, and intracerebroventricular perfusion may also result in the occurrence of concentration gradients for [³H]tyrosine and its metabolites within the brain. Studies with intravenous bolus injection of [³H]tyrosine may be more reflective of normal physiology, in which brain tyrosine is derived from the circulation (van Valkenburg *et al.* 1984). This approach has been used to test modulation of dopamine synthesis by opiates (Smith *et al.* 1972). Here, the specific activity of [³H]dopamine formed in mouse brain after intravenous [³H]tyrosine injection was doubled by acute treatment with morphine, showing that morphine acutely stimulates dopamine turnover. Repeated injections of morphine resulted in tolerance to the stimulation of dopamine synthesis by the opiate.

The specific activity of [³H]dopamine in rat striatum reached a peak about 40 min after the intravenous bolus [³H]tyrosine injection (Lippens *et al.* 1988). However, the specific activities of the acidic dopamine metabolites [³H]DOPAC and [³H]HVA did not reach an early peak, and failed to decline after 40 min, as would have been expected if the [³H]dopamine mixed immediately with the neurotransmitter pool subject to catabolism. This finding seems somewhat in contrast to the observations based on the push-pull cannula or intracerebroventricular infusion methods, possibly due to the indeterminate [³H]tyrosine input in those studies. With intravenous [³H]tyrosine administration, the input for brain catecholamine synthesis can be measured in arterial blood samples, and the pathway becomes more amenable for compartmental modeling.

3.5.   Modeling the metabolism of [³H]tyrosine

A compartmental model of the fate of tyrosine entering into brain is presented in Figure 3.1. Tyrosine in plasma is delivered to the brain capillary bed at a rate defined by the local cerebral blood flow, or perfusion rate, F (ml g^{-1} min^{-1}), multiplied by the arterial plasma concentration. The initial clearance of [³H]tyrosine from the blood to brain occurs by a process of facilitated diffusion, which is defined as the product of the unidirectional blood–brain clearance, K_1^{Tyr} (ml g^{-1} min^{-1}), and the plasma tyrosine concentration. The magnitude of K_1^{Tyr} divided by the total blood flow, F, is defined as the extraction fraction of tyrosine at the blood–brain barrier. Based on experiments presented below, the magnitude of the extraction fraction is approximately 10%; the remainder of the tyrosine arriving in the arterial side passes directly into venous circulation without ever having entered the brain.

The LNAA transporter in the blood–brain barrier behaves as a revolving door, facilitating the bidirectional transit of its substrates between the brain and the blood. However, this process cannot establish or long permit the occurrence of a concentration gradient for tyrosine between blood and brain. Therefore, free tyrosine in the brain is constantly returning to the blood at the rate defined by the product of its concentration in the brain and the fractional

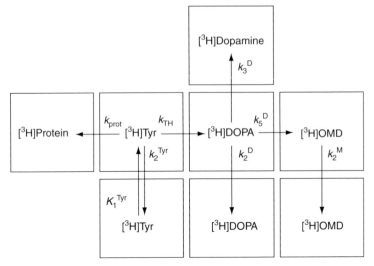

Figure 3.1 Compartmental model for the cerebral uptake and metabolism of [³H]tyrosine ([³H]Tyr). The amino acid in circulation is transferred to the brain at unidirectional clearance K_1^{Tyr} (ml g⁻¹ min⁻¹). Once in the brain, [³H]tyrosine is exported back to plasma (k_2^{Tyr}, min⁻¹), is incorporated into protein at rate constant k_{prot} (min⁻¹), or is a substrate for TH (k_{TH}, min⁻¹). The [³H]DOPA formed in the brain is exported to plasma (k_2^D, min⁻¹), is a substrate for COMT in the brain (k_5^D, min⁻¹), or (unless blocked by NSD 1015) is a substrate for AAADC (k_3^D, min⁻¹). The [³H]OMD formed in the brain is cleared to circulation (k_2^M, min⁻¹) by the common transporter for the other LNAAs.

rate constant for the elimination of tyrosine from the brain, k_2^{Tyr} (min⁻¹). Alternately, tyrosine in the brain can serve as a precursor for the synthesis of brain proteins by a series of steps including the reversible transfer to the aminoacyl transfer RNA, and the subsequent incorporation into brain proteins. This trapping in the brain is essentially irreversible if one considers an autoradiography or PET experiment lasting much less than the half-life of brain proteins. The overall fractional rate constant for the incorporation of brain tyrosine into brain protein is defined as k_{prot}^{Tyr} (min⁻¹) in the present compartmental model. If tyrosine is not returned to circulation or incorporated into protein, it may be a substrate for TH in the brain. Then it will be hydroxylated at a rate constant defined by the local activity of the TH enzyme (k_{TH}, min⁻¹), which is a fractional rate constant defined in terms of the Michaelis–Menten constants for the enzyme,

$$k_{TH} = \frac{V_{max}[Tyr]}{(K_m + [Tyr])},$$

where V_{max} is the maximal activity of the TH enzyme (at the prevailing concentrations of BH_4 and oxygen in living brain), [Tyr] is the concentration of free tyrosine in brain, and K_m is the affinity of TH for tyrosine. Since the brain concentration of free tyrosine is some five-fold greater than the K_m measured in vitro, TH is assumed to be nearly saturated by tyrosine in living brain (although this assumption was called into question in the preceding chapter). In this scenario, the only way to increase DOPA synthesis is to modulate the affinity of the enzyme for BH_4, as discussed in the preceding sections. In catecholamine fibers, DOPA would normally by decarboxylated at rate k_3^D (min^{-1}), but pretreatment of rats with NSD 1015 reduces the activity of AAADC to essentially zero. In this circumstance, the rate of transformation of tyrosine in the brain to DOPA is indeed determined by the TH activity, but the brain concentration of DOPA is also influenced by the rate of its elimination from the brain by processes other than decarboxylation. This must entail at least two mechanisms: export back to circulation (k_2^D) as noted above, and also the activity in situ of COMT, which is here defined as k_5^D (min^{-1}).

The fate of [³H]tyrosine in living rat brain can be followed by radiochemical fractionation of brain and plasma extracts taken from rats at intervals following tracer injection (Cumming *et al.* 1998). Temporal changes in the concentrations of radiolabeled compounds measured in plasma and in the brain during 45 min of [³H]tyrosine circulation were used to estimate the magnitudes of some of the processes illustrated in Figure 3.1 (Table 3.2). Surprisingly, the baseline rate constant for TH activity relative to [³H]tyrosine in rat striatum was somewhat less than estimates based on turnover of non-radioactive compounds. This

Table 3.2. *Kinetics of [³H]tyrosine uptake and metabolism in rat brain*

Tissue and condition	K_1^{Tyr} (ml g^{-1} min^{-1})	k_{cl} (min^{-1})	k_{TH} (min^{-1})	k_{prot} (min^{-1})
Striatum				
Baseline	0.058	0.144	0.0048	0.028
Haloperidol	0.053	0.108	0.0204	0.014
Cortex				
Baseline	0.062	0.146	0.0008	0.032
Haloperidol	0.063	0.114	n.d.	0.016

Note: The unidirectional blood–brain clearance (K_1^{Tyr}) and the net elimination rate constant from brain (k_{cl}) for [³H]tyrosine were calculated in rats pretreated with a centrally acting AAADC inhibitor. Temporal changes in the concentrations in brain of the enzymatic product [³H] levodopa were used to calculate the TH activity (k_{TH}) relative to [³H]tyrosine derived from the circulation. The rate constant for incorporation of [³H]tyrosine into brain protein (k_{prot}) was also calculated. Data from Cumming *et al.* 1998.

discrepancy suggests violation of the assumption that [³H]tyrosine administered intravenously becomes fully mixed with the precursor pool in the brain. Indeed, the amount of dopamine synthesis in brain slices incubated in a tyrosine-free medium can greatly exceed the decline in tissue-free tyrosine content (Buyukuysal & Mogol 2000). These observations together suggest the presence of a large storage pool of brain tyrosine with slow turnover, even though this scenario seems at odds with the nature of the blood–brain barrier, which does not permit the maintenance of a concentration gradient. It may be that recycling of tyrosine from brain protein constitutes a significant precursor pool for catecholamine synthesis. Consider the following calculation: If brain is 10% protein by weight, of which 5% is tyrosine, a mean turnover of brain protein every 10 days would provide an internal tyrosine source comparable in magnitude to the rate of DOPA synthesis in the striatum.

3.6.   Autoradiography in vivo with tyrosine: an introduction to the analysis of PET data

In principle, the TH inhibitor and substrate AMPT might enter the pathway for dopamine synthesis, while remaining excluded from protein synthesis. However, the distribution of [¹⁴C]-AMPT in living rat brain was nearly homogeneous, apparently due to its low rate of biotransformation in catecholamine fibers (Cumming *et al.* 1994). Incubation of rat brain slices with tritiated α-fluoromethyltyrosine did result in the labeling of individual neurons from the rat locus coeruleus (Bezin *et al.* 2000). Using this tracer, it was possible to detect pharmacological activation of TH in the perikarya within minutes of treatment with RU 24722, a phasic activator of catecholamine turnover.

Also, in principle, [¹¹C]tyrosine could be used for PET studies of dopamine synthesis in living brain. The results for [³H]tyrosine in rat striatum presented in Table 3.2 (Cumming *et al.* 1998) show that the incorporation of [³H]tyrosine into brain protein must exceed by ten-fold the rate of [³H]catecholamine synthesis in living rat striatum. Thus, the specific signal due to the dopamine pathway is likely to be indiscernible in PET studies with [¹¹C]tyrosine, being projected upon a background of extensive protein synthesis. However, pretreatment with haloperidol resulted in substantial enhancement of [³H]DOPA formation in rat striatum, approaching the rate for protein synthesis. Indeed, in the haloperidol condition, the incorporation of [³H]tyrosine into rat brain protein actually declined. These findings in rats predict that haloperidol challenge might result in a detectable catecholamine signal in [¹¹C]tyrosine PET studies of living striatum.

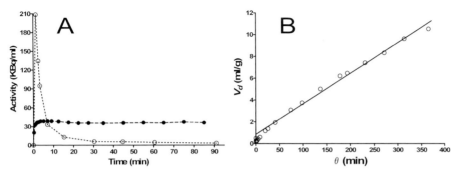

Figure 3.2 Kinetics of [^{11}C]tyrosine uptake in the striatum of monkey measured by PET. (A) The arterial input of [^{11}C]tyrosine as a function of time reaches an early peak after intravenous injection, and rapidly declines due to distribution throughout the body, and due to peripheral metabolism, whereas the brain concentration of radioactivity derived from [^{11}C]tyrosine reaches a plateau within 10 min. (B) The linear graphical analysis of [^{11}C]tyrosine reveals a brief initial phase dominated by unidirectional blood–brain clearance (K_1^{Tyr}), followed by a prolonged linear phase related to the irreversible trapping of tracer in the brain protein (K_{in}^{Tyr}); the ordinate intercept corresponds to the equilibrium V_d for LNAAs, close to 1 ml g^{-1}.

The concept of TH activation was tested in a PET study of a rhesus monkey, which underwent [^{11}C]tyrosine (200 MBq, i.v.) scans at baseline, and again after treatment with haloperidol (0.3 mg kg^{-1}). In both conditions, positron emission was recorded during 90 min after tracer injection. As is typical of dynamic PET scans, a series of static recordings were made sequentially, every minute for the first few minutes, then every 5 min, and finally every 10 min. In addition, a series of arterial plasma samples were collected, and the concentration of untransformed [^{11}C]tyrosine was measured by HPLC. Knowing the total brain radioactivity concentration and the arterial plasma inputs as a function of time (Figure 3.2A), it now becomes possible to calculate the distribution volume (V_d) of the tracer as a function of circulation time; V_d is simply the ratio of the brain radioactivity to that in blood, and consequently has units of ml g^{-1} (Figure 3.2B).

In spite of its simple definition, the concept of V_d is tricky, being reminiscent of the telephone box of Dr. Who, which is much larger on the inside than it seems from the outside. Yet, distribution volume is all that can be measured with PET, and provides the sole basis for calculations based on kinetic modeling. This stands in contrast to the [^{3}H]tyrosine studies, in which all labeled compounds were measured by HPLC. The concept of distribution volume can be understood using the hungry chicken model (Figure 3.3). In this model, two chickens consume an identical input of feed. While the fat chicken retains

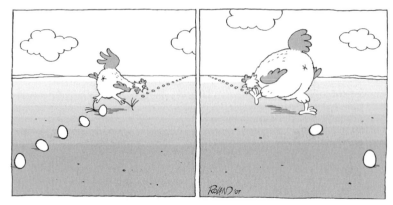

Figure 3.3 The hungry chicken model of distribution volume. Two hungry chickens consume the same input, but deposit eggs at inherently different rates. Their body masses reflect the composite of those internal processes resulting in the retention of mass derived from the same input. In analogy to a PET experiment, the lean chicken corresponds to a brain region with low specific binding of the tracer, whereas the fat chicken represents a region of high specific binding. If the trapping process were irreversible, both chickens would continue to grow forever, but if the trapping process were reversible, the chickens would eventually reach a constant weight, i.e. a state of equilibrium.

most of this mass, the lean chicken returns most of what it consumes. We cannot be certain what internal process accounts for this difference; all we know is that the volumes of the two chickens differ. The hungry chickens also illustrate the distinction between reversible and irreversible trapping: in the former case, the chicken will eventually reach a stable weight, whereas, in the latter, a chicken will continue to increase in volume so long as the input is available.

Returning to the case of $[^{11}C]$tyrosine, if the low baseline activity of TH is ignored for the present, the concentration of radioactivity in the brain is determined by only three factors: the unidirectional blood–brain clearance (K_1^{Tyr}), which has units of cerebral blood flow (ml g^{-1} min^{-1}), and the fractional rate constants for the return of brain $[^{11}C]$tyrosine back to circulation (k_2^{Tyr}, min^{-1}) and for the irreversible trapping in brain protein (k_{prot}, min^{-1}). The composite of these kinetic steps is known as the net blood–brain clearance of $[^{11}C]$tyrosine (K_{in}^{Tyr}, ml g^{-1} min^{-1}), which can be expressed as

$$K_{in}^{Tyr} = \frac{K_1^{Tyr} k_{prot}}{(k_2^{Tyr} + k_{prot})}.$$

This is a special case of the Gjedde–Patlak graphical analysis for irreversible trapping of $[^{18}F]$fluorodeoxyglucose in metabolically active tissue

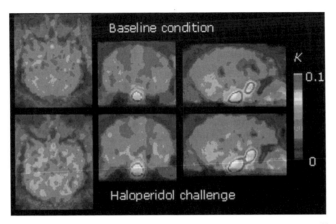

Figure 3.4 Parametric maps of the net blood brain clearance of [^{11}C]tyrosine (K_{in}^{Tyr}, ml g^{-1} min^{-1}) in a rhesus monkey. The animal was scanned first in a baseline condition, and again at 1 h after treatment with haloperidol (50 µg kg^{-1}). Parametric maps are co-registered to an MR-based atlas of monkey brain. Courtesy of Professor Per Hartvig, Uppsala University PET Centre. (For color version, see plate section.)

(Gjedde 1981; Patlak & Blasberg 1985; Patlak, Blasberg, & Fenstermacher 1983). In this graphical analysis, the total distribution volume of the tracer in brain relative to the arterial concentration ($V_{d(T)}$) is plotted as a function of normalized tracer circulation time, known as *theta*. The normalization of the arterial input is obtained by integrating the area under the input curve, and dividing by the instantaneous concentration at time (T), i.e. the end of the integration interval. This operation results in a transformation of the arterial input into units of time. In general, the magnitude of *theta* is systematically less than the real laboratory time, as can be seen by comparison of the abscissas of Figures 3.2A and 3.2B. Unlike the arterial input, in which the [^{11}C]tyrosine concentration is constantly changing, each interval of *theta* entails a constant exposure of the blood–brain barrier to the radiotracer. It is this property of the transformation of the arterial input to units of theta that allows the linear graphical analysis of net tracer uptake in brain.

Close inspection of the plot of V_d as a function of *theta* (Figure 3.3B) reveals two linear phases. The first occurs during the first few minutes of the study, when unidirectional clearance (K_1^{Tyr}) is the predominant process. The magnitude of this uptake in monkey striatum (0.05 min^{-1}) was almost identical to that calculated for [^{3}H]tyrosine in rat striatum, with the advantage that the parameter was estimated in a single monkey, rather than a large population of rats. The product of K_1^{Tyr} and the arterial concentration of endogenous tyrosine (100 µM, which is nearly constant during the entire PET experiment) is equal to the total flux of tyrosine into monkey brain. After about 10 min, the concentration of free [^{11}C]tyrosine in monkey brain approaches equilibrium with the arterial concentration, whereupon the Gjedde–Patlak slope declines toward the second linear phase, which corresponds to the magnitude of K_{in}^{Tyr}, and remains perfectly linear so long as the assumption of irreversible trapping is not violated. The product of the net clearance in monkey brain (0.03 min^{-1}) and the arterial concentration of endogenous tyrosine is equal to the rate of trapping of [^{11}C]tyrosine as brain protein.

The magnitude of K_{in}^{Tyr} can be calculated by linear regression for every image element of the PET scan, known as *voxels*. By this means, a parametric map was generated, in which the magnitude of K_{in}^{Tyr} is presented for each of approximately one million cube-shaped voxels comprising the three-dimensional PET space. The magnitude of K_{in}^{Tyr} was uniformly close to 0.03 ml g^{-1} min^{-1} throughout the monkey brain (Figure 3.4A). "Hot spots" can be seen in the pituitary gland and in the basilar vasculature of the brain. Hypothesis predicted that haloperidol treatment should have increased the magnitude of k_{TH} to such an extent that [^{11}C]dopamine synthesis might be visible in the activated striatum, projected upon the uniform background of protein synthesis. As it were, the chicken should have become fatter due to increased retention of radioactivity. However, the treatment did not discernibly increase the [^{11}C]tyrosine K_{in}^{Tyr} in the striatum or any brain region (Figure 3.4B). Thus, the PET method is unable to detect catecholamine synthesis in monkey striatum, even in a pharmacologically stimulated condition. The rate of dopamine synthesis in living brain consequently remains unknown.

4

Enzymology of aromatic amino acid decarboxylase

4.1. Kinetic properties of AAADC in vitro

DOPA and other substrates are decarboxylated by aromatic amino acid decarboxylase (AAADC), some biochemical properties of which are summarized in Table 4.1. AAADC purified from pig kidney occurs as a homodimer, with two catalytical sites, each of which binds a single pyridoxal phosphate (Vitamin B6) (Dominici *et al.* 1990). The pyridoxal phosphate co-factor is essential for catalytic activity, and the majority (80%) of AAADC in rat brain normally occurs as the holozyme (Kawasaki *et al.* 1992), endowed with an equimolar amount of pyridoxal phosphate. Pyridoxine is transferred across the blood–brain barrier by a saturable process and is phosphorylated in the brain by a specific kinase; brain pyridoxal phosphate concentrations can be increased by peripheral loading with pyridoxine (Spector & Shikuma 1978).

AAADC substrates form reversibly a Schiff base with the pyridoxal phosphate group. The consequent withdrawal of electrons from the amino acid moiety weakens the carbonyl bond, encouraging the irreversible loss of carbon dioxide, which is followed by release of the decarboxylated amine and recycling of the co-factor for the next catalytic cycle. Electrophilic substituents on the α-carbon decrease the reaction rate for AAADC substrates. In the case of the "suicide substrate" α-fluoromethyl-DOPA, an irreversible covalent bond is formed with the holozyme, resulting in a permanent loss of catalytic activity of the enzyme (Maycock, Aster, & Patchett 1980). Another suicide inhibitor, NSD 1015 (the α-hydrazine derivative of DOPA), is commonly used for the assay of DOPA synthesis, as reviewed in Chapter 5.

AAADC can decarboxylate several aromatic L-amino acids, including 5-hydroxytryptophan, tyrosine, phenylalanine, and histidine, although the

Table 4.1. *Some kinetic properties of AAADC*

Item	Quantity	Unit	Reference
Molar weight of monomer from bovine adrenal medulla	56 000	Dalton	Albert, Allen, & Joh 1987
Bovine striatum	56 000	Dalton	Siow & Dakshinamurti 1990
Human pheochromocytoma	50 000	Dalton	Ichinose *et al.* 1985
pH optimum for dopa, rat brain	6.7	pH	Siow & Dakshinamurti 1990
pH optimum for dopa, human pheochromocytoma	7.0	pH	Ichinose *et al.* 1985
Homospecific activity, human pheochromocytoma	500	Mol dopa min^{-1} mol AAADC^{-1}	Ichinose *et al.* 1985
Homospecific activity, bovine adrenal medulla	5	*	Albert, Allen, & Joh 1987
Homospecific activity, bovine striatum	88	*	Siow & Dakshinamurti 1990
K_m for DOPA, human pheochromocytoma	45	μM	Ichinose *et al.* 1985
K_m for DOPA, rat retina	57	μM	Hadjiconstantinou *et al.* 1988
K_m for DOPA, mouse striatum	33	μM	Hadjiconstantinou *et al.* 1993
K_m for DOPA, pig kidney	190	μM	Christenson, Dairman, & Udenfriend 1970
K_m for 6-[^{18}F]fluoro-DOPA, rat striatum	100	μM	Cumming *et al.* 1988
K_m for 2-[^{18}F]fluoro-DOPA	982	μM	
K_m for 5HTP, human pheochromocytoma	67	μM	Ichinose *et al.* 1985
K_m for 5HTP, pig kidney	100	μM	Christenson, Dairman, & Udenfriend 1970
K_m for 5HTP, pig kidney	50	μM	Lovenberg *et al.* 1963
K_m for 5HTP, cat brain	8	μM	Bouchard & Roberge 1979
K_m for pyridoxal phosphate, rat retina	47	nM	Hadjiconstantinou *et al.* 1988
K_m for pyridoxal phosphate, mouse striatum	180	nM	Hadjiconstantinou *et al.* 1993
V_{max} for DOPA, mouse striatum	200	pmol g^{-1} min^{-1}	Hadjiconstantinou *et al.* 1993
V at 1 mM DOPA squirrel monkey, caudate ($n=3$)	290±29	pmol g^{-1} min	Yee *et al.* 2000
Putamen	280±11	pmol g^{-1} min	
Nucleus accumbens	139±24	pmol g^{-1} min	
Substantia nigra	230±33	pmol g^{-1} min	
MPTP 2 mg kg^{-1} treated monkey, caudate ($n=3$)	100±24	pmol g^{-1} min	
Putamen	101±25	pmol g^{-1} min	
Nucleus accumbens	135±15	pmol g^{-1} min	
Substantia nigra	229±33	pmol g^{-1} min	
V_{max} for DOPA, human caudate	11	nmol g^{-1} min^{-1}	Mackay *et al.* 1978
DOPA concentration in rat striatum	300	nM	Cassel & Persson 1992
Pyridoxal phosphate concentration, rat brain	7	mM	Spector & Shikuma 1978

Note: *The activity of purified enzyme, calculated in units of DOPA molecules formed per minute by each molecule of AAADC.

preferred substrate is DOPA (Lovenberg, Weissbach, & Udenfriend 1962). Because of the enzyme's ambivalence with respect to substrate, the term AAADC is preferred to DOPA decarboxylase (DDC), which implies substrate specificity. Most studies indicate a similar affinity (K_m) of AAADC for 5-hydroxytryptophan as for DOPA (Table 4.1). However, the maximal velocity for decarboxylation from several tissues is some ten-fold higher for DOPA than for 5-hydroxytryptophan (Christenson, Dairman, & Udenfriend 1970; Ichinose et al. 1985), indicating that the decarboxylation of DOPA is thermodynamically favored. Ring [^{18}F]fluorination of DOPA in the 6-position (6-[^{18}F]fluoro-L-dopa, FDOPA) was without effect on the decarboxylation kinetics in vitro by AAADC from rat brain. However, 2-[^{18}F]fluoro-L-DOPA had very low affinity and low reaction rate, apparently due to electron-withdrawing effects of a fluorine cis to one of the phenolic groups, which enhances ionization (Cumming et al. 1988). D-amino acids are not substrates for decarboxylation, although they can inhibit the enzyme in a time-dependent manner, apparently by transamination process at the active site (Voltattorni, Minelli, & Dominici 1983).

The relative activity of AAADC with respect to DOPA or 5-hydroxytryptophan is not uniform in bovine brain, suggesting that local factors may influence the substrate preference (Siow & Dakshinamurti 1990). Furthermore, the decarboxylation of DOPA was more sensitive to depletion of pyridoxine than was 5-hydroxytryptophan decarboxylation (Ebadi & Simonneaux 1991). This discrepancy may reflect mechanistic differences rather than the presence of distinct forms of the enzyme; conceivably the rate of transamination is not identical for the two substrates.

Tyramine and phenylethylamine are formed by the decarboxylation of their respective amino acid precursors, tyrosine and phenylalanine. Their formation in the brain is apparently catalyzed by AAADC, and the distribution of these products in the brain reflects the distribution of AAADC. For example, the concentration of p-tyramine in mouse striatum (20 nM) declined to nearly zero after treatment with the AAADC inhibitor α-fluoromethyl-DOPA (Boulton & Juorio 1983). The baseline concentrations of the tyramines, also known as trace amines, in the brain are very low because of their very rapid deamination in the absence of a mechanism for vesicular storage. While the true rate of tyramine synthesis tends to be masked by MAO, at several hours following blockade of MAO with pargyline, the concentration of tyramine in rat basal ganglia had reached 500 nM (Sardar, Juorio, & Boulton 1987).

In spite of their low baseline concentrations, the trace amine can in some circumstances act as endogenous sympathomimetic substances stimulating the release of cytosolic dopamine in an amphetamine-like manner (Knoll et al.

1996). It has been suggested that these amphetamine-like effects may contribute to the side effects, or the therapeutic benefits, of treatment with MAO inhibitors. Furthermore, a remarkable stimulation of the rates of tyrosine and phenylalanine decarboxylation in mouse striatum may contribute to the psychoactive and neurotoxic properties of benzene and other organic solvents (Juorio & Yu 1985).

4.2.   Regulation and transcription of AAADC

Molecular cloning of cDNA libraries has revealed that a single gene codes for AAADC in neuronal and non-neuronal tissues (Albert, Allen, & Joh 1987). Distinct promoters may initiate transcription in different tissues, with alternate splicing of the message differing only in the 3'-untranslated sequence (Albert *et al.* 1992; Krieger *et al.* 1991). The factors regulating AAADC expression are poorly understood, but several positive regulatory elements, including an interleukin response element, have been identified in the promoter region for human AAADC (Le Van Thai *et al.* 1993).

Exposure of pheochromocytoma cells to the AAADC inhibitor NSD-1015 increased the expression of mRNA, and also increased the concentration of AAADC protein (Li, Juorio, & Boulton 1993). After catecholamine depletion with reserpine, increased expression of messages for TH and also AAADC was evident in the adrenal medulla, where the proto-oncogenes *c-fos* and *c-jun* were also induced by the catecholamine depletion. Moderate increases in the expression of genes for the catecholamine-synthesizing enzymes were also seen in the noradrenaline neurons of the locus ceruleus after reserpine treatment, but not in the mesencephalic nigrostriatal dopamine neurons (Wessel & Joh 1992). Evidently, the factors regulating AAADC expression are not identical in all tissues, or even in all brain regions expressing the enzyme.

If depletion of catecholamine is followed by increased expression of the AAADC gene (and least in some brain regions), the expected contrary phenomenon is that inhibition of dopamine catabolism should reduce AAADC expression. Contrary to this expectation, prolonged treatment of rats with MAO inhibitors *increased* the activity of AAADC in rat brain (Campbell *et al.* 1980). Furthermore, deprenyl and some other irreversible inhibitors of MAO-B also increased the expression of AAADC in pheochromocytoma cells (Li *et al.* 1992). This cell line does not even express MAO, so some additional property of these compounds must be responsible for their effects on gene expression. It is believed that the propargyl moiety of the irreversible MAO inhibitors somehow imparts control over gene expression. Whereas, clorgyline, an MAO selective inhibitor of MAO-A, initially decreased and then increased the expression of AAADC mRNA in mouse mesencephalon, the MAO-B inhibitor deprenyl caused a transient increase in the expression of the AAADC mRNA (Cho *et al.* 1996). This effect was not paralleled with increased expression of TH mRNA and could not be attributed to increased autoreceptor occupancy following inhibition of dopamine catabolism. Thus, the biochemical basis of the complex properties of propargyl compounds on catecholamine enzyme expression remains elusive.

Exposure to light stimulates the physiological activity of dopaminergic amacrine cells in the rat retina, and rapidly increases the activity of AAADC in those cells (Hadjiconstantinou *et al.* 1988). If the known mechanisms for the regulation of TH activity serve as any indication, depolarization of amacrine cells may likewise activate AAADC by a Ca^{2+}/calmodulin-dependent phosphorylation process. However, the requirement of protein synthesis for light activation of AAADC implicates gene expression. Nonetheless, the stimulation of AAADC activity by light is reduced with α-adrenergic agonists (Rossetti *et al.* 1989) or by dopamine D_1 agonist treatment (Rossetti *et al.* 1990), consistent with a cAMP-dependent component of the pathway for activation of catecholamine synthesis in activated amacrine cells.

A rapid and transient stimulation of AAADC activity from mouse striatum is evoked by treatment with forskolin, an activator of adenylate cyclase; unlike the case in the retina, this stimulation in the striatum was due to increased reaction velocity, and did not require protein neosynthesis (Young, Neff, & Hadjiconstantinou 1993). Thus, cAMP-linked protein kinases are critical for the modulation of brain AAADC activity. Similarly, a transient stimulation of AAADC from mouse striatum could be evoked by treatment with phorbol esters, which are activators of PKC. Together, these results suggest that at least two intracellular pathways can activate AAADC in the striatum, but the molecular basis of this activation is unclear. For example, it is unknown whether phosphorylation of the native protein is responsible for regulation of AAADC. The activity of ornithine DDC, a closely related enzyme, is regulated by a Ca^{2+}/calmodulin-dependent association of the active enzyme with a proteinaceous inhibitor known as *antizyme*. It could be rapid changes in association with an (as yet) unidentified protein contributing to the acute regulation of AAADC activity.

Acute treatment with antipsychotic dopamine receptor antagonists increased AAADC activity in rodent striatum, while dopamine agonists decreased the activity (Hadjiconstantinou *et al.* 1993; Zhu *et al.* 1993). The expression and activity of AAADC in mouse striatum was increased after repeated exposure to the antisense oligonucleotide coding for the dopamine D_2 receptor (Hadjiconstantinou *et al.* 1996), perhaps also consistent with autoreceptor regulation of AAADC activity, as is well established for TH. Chronic amphetamine treatment decreased the expression of AAADC message throughout rat brain, as did treatment with the antiepileptic substance vigabatrin. However, chronic cocaine treatment was without effect on AAADC mRNA expression (Buckland, Spurlock, & McGuffin 1996). While regulation of neuronal AAADC by feedback mechanisms is well established, the dynamic range of this regulation seems less than is the case for TH.

4.3.   AAADC activity in living brain

The cellular distribution of AAADC in the brain may contribute to ambivalence in the actual site of metabolism of exogenous DOPA. For example, immunohistochemically identified serotonin fibers in rat brain can form dopamine from exogenous DOPA (Arai *et al.* 1994). Furthermore, a selective lesion of the forebrain serotonin innervation reduces the trapping of radioactivity derived from [^{3}H]DOPA in some brain regions of living rat, including the amygdala, which has a notably dense serotonin innervation (Cumming *et al.* 1997b). Thus, the cellular site of DOPA metabolism in different brain regions may be determined by the relative abundances of dopamine and serotonin fibers, although it is not immediately apparent that all dopamine formed in serotonin cells should be stored within the same neurons, to be released along with serotonin as a "false neurotransmitter." In addition, the presence of AAADC in noradrenaline fibers must be considered.

DOPA in blood plasma is reversibly transferred across the blood–brain by a common carrier for tyrosine, phenylalanine, and other LNAAs (Oldendorf & Szabo 1976). In the context of compartmental modeling of tracer uptake, it is difficult to over-emphasize that this mechanism cannot establish a concentration gradient across the capillary endothelium, but instead brings about a state of equilibrium between the brain and the plasma concentrations of the free amino acids. After entry into brain, enzymatic decarboxylation of [^{14}C]DOPA (Horne, Cheng, & Wooten 1984), [^{3}H]DOPA (Liskowsky & Potter 1985), and FDOPA (Cumming *et al.* 1987a), and the subsequent trapping of the corresponding radiolabeled dopamine in vesicles results in the progressive accumulation of radioactivity in those brain regions enriched in catecholamine fibers. This phenomenon provides the basis of the detection of AAADC activity in living brain by PET. The goal of tracer kinetic models is to extract physiological estimates from PET recordings, which show only temporal changes in the total radioactivity concentration of brain tissue, irrespective of its biotransformation. Several approaches to this goal will be elaborated in the following chapter.

4.4.   In vivo metabolism of AAADC substrates

The pathway for DOPA metabolism is summarized in kinetic terms in Figure 4.1. This schema is true for $[^3H]$DOPA, and also for the PET tracers FDOPA and β-$[^{11}C]$DOPA. As was the case for labeled tyrosine, the concentrations of each labeled molecule in the pathway for DOPA metabolism can be measured in rats by HPLC analysis of blood and brain extracts as functions of tracer circulation time. Of course, kinetic results with exogenous AAADC substrates must be interpreted with the usual caveat of tracer studies, that the tracer should become mixed in the same compartment containing the endogenous compound, in this case DOPA. In effect, it is assumed that DOPA formed naturally within the brain is not trapped in a subcompartment containing both TH and AAADC, but is free to diffuse away from the site of its synthesis, unless it encounters AAADC. Naturally, the concentration time-series cannot be obtained in single

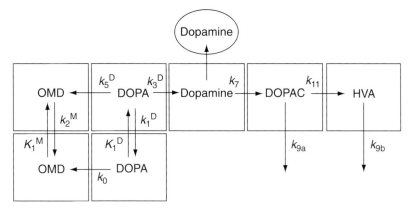

Figure 4.1 The pathway for metabolism of DOPA. After intravenous injection, the tracer is metabolized by COMT at the whole-body rate constant expressed as k_0 (min^{-1}), yielding the inert metabolite OMD. The tracer and its plasma metabolite are together transferred reversibly across the blood–brain barrier, and would establish an equilibrium defined by the ratio of the unidirectional blood–brain clearance (K_1^D, K_1^M; ml g^{-1} min^{-1}) and the respective fractional rate constants for return to circulation (k_2^D, k_2^M; min^{-1}). OMD can be formed in the brain at rate constant k_5^D (min^{-1}). In the striatum, DOPA is decarboxylated at rate constant k_3^D (min^{-1}), which is the relative activity of AAADC relative to the concentration of its substrate. The decarboxylated product dopamine is formed in the cytosol, where it can be deaminated by MAO at rate constant k_7 (min^{-1}), if not stored in synaptic vesicles, represented by the ellipse. The primary deaminated metabolite DOPAC is eliminated from the brain by conjugation and diffusion at rate constant k_{9a} (min^{-1}) or metabolized in situ by the brain COMT to form HVA, which is eliminated from the brain by the sum of conjugation and diffusion processes at net rate constant k_{9b} (min^{-1}).

experimental animals, but requires that measurements be obtained in a series of individual rats, at tracer circulation times extending over several hours, the entire range of time relevant to the cerebral metabolism of the AAADC substrate.

Having obtained a time series of [^{3}H]DOPA concentrations in arterial plasma and in brain, the magnitude of the unidirectional blood–brain clearance of DOPA (K_1^D), and also the magnitude of the sum of all the rate constants describing its elimination from brain tissue (k_{cl}^D) can be calculated. The latter kinetic term expresses the composite effects of several DOPA removal processes, including return to circulation (k_2^D), decarboxylation by AAADC in dopamine terminals (k_3^D), and O-methylation in situ (k_5^D). The relative activity of AAADC (k_3^D) is calculated from the time series of brain concentrations of [^{3}H]DOPA and the enzymatic product [^{3}H]dopamine measured during a few hours after tracer administration.

Results of a number of separate estimates of k_3^D in rat striatum are presented in Table 4.2, illustrating three key points. First, the magnitude of k_3^D is rather high, thus predicting low steady-state concentrations of DOPA in striatum. Second, the magnitude of k_3^D is somewhat higher than the sum of the other processes removing DOPA from brain (i.e. $k_2^D + k_5^D$, approximately 0.1 min^{-1}), consistent with the results based on analysis of human FDOPA scans (Gjedde et al. 1993). Indeed, the rat results suggest that approximately 75% of DOPA entering the striatum from circulation is decarboxylated in situ, and lesser proportions in the extra-striatal regions where AAADC activity is low. Finally, the existence of multiple possible fates for DOPA in living brain has important implications for the role of AAADC in the regulation of dopamine synthesis. Whereas the activity of TH sets the upper

Table 4.2. *Some estimates of the activity (*k_3^D*, min*$^{-1}$*) of AAADC*

Substrate	Striatum	Cortex	Reference
FDOPA	0.17	–	Cumming, Kuwabara, & Gjedde 1994
[^{3}H]DOPA, baseline	0.26	0.02	Cumming et al. 1995b
Acute pargyline	0.13	0.002	
[^{3}H]DOPA, baseline	0.20	0.015	Cumming et al. 1997a
Acute flupenthixol	0.44	0.013	
Acute apomorphine	0.16	0.05	
[^{3}H]DOPA, baseline	0.50	0.054	Reith, Cumming, & Gjedde 1998
Subchronic MK-801	2.0	0.54	
β-[^{11}C]DOPA, cat	0.4	–	Data from Miwa et al. 1992

Note: The magnitudes of the fractional rate constant k_3^D were calculated on the basis of radiochemical fraction of products formed from AAADC-labeled substrates in living striatum or cortex of awake rats, or in striatum of cat.

limit for dopamine synthesis in living brain, the activity of AAADC determines the "branching ratio" for the DOPA pathway in the brain. Since AAADC activity is not infinite, changes in its activity can influence the fraction of DOPA directed toward catecholamine synthesis, rather than disposal by other pathways. This imparts a potential role for AAADC in the co-regulation with TH of dopamine synthesis.

The prediction that AAADC activity in living brain can be modulated has been tested in studies of [^{3}H]DOPA metabolism measured ex vivo (Table 4.2). These studies revealed that pargyline treatment decreased the magnitude of $k_3{}^D$ in rat striatum (Cumming *et al.* 1995b), whereas pharmacological blockade of dopamine receptors increased $k_3{}^D$ (Cumming *et al.* 1997a). Both of these findings indicate modulation of AAADC in rat striatum via presynaptic autoreceptors; substantial activation of $k_3{}^D$ was seen in another study with pharmacological blockade of NMDA-type glutamate receptors (Reith, Cumming, & Gjedde 1998). The magnitude of $k_3{}^D$ is consistently ten-fold higher in the striatum than in the cerebral cortex, a proportion that is roughly consistent with the distribution of monoamine innervations. Finally, the mean of available estimates of $k_3{}^D$ in rat striatum is 30-fold higher than estimates of the magnitude of k_{TH}, indicating superabundance of the ultimate enzyme in the dopamine synthesis pathway. However, due to the presence of the alternate pathways for DOPA metabolism, this superabundance is just sufficient to ensure that the majority of brain DOPA is directed toward dopamine synthesis in the crucible of living striatum.

5

PET studies of DOPA utilization

5.1. General aspects of the quantitation of FDOPA utilization

PET recordings consist only of the total radioactivity concentration in brain volumes as a function of circulation time. How then is one to deduce the rate of decarboxylation of AAADC substrates in living brain, knowing (without the luxury of dissection and HPLC analysis of brain extracts) only the total amount of radioactivity in a volume of brain tissue and the concentration of the tracer in blood? The exogenous AAADC substrate FDOPA has been used in hundreds of PET studies. The quantitation of FDOPA uptake in brain is formally similar to the cases of fluorodeoxyglucose (FDG) and [^{11}C]tyrosine. Thus, FDOPA passes reversibly across the blood–brain barrier by a process of facilitated diffusion. In the brain, FDOPA can be trapped as non-diffusible [^{18}F]fluorodopamine at a rate defined by the local AAADC activity, k_3^D. In most PET studies, substantial amounts of the inert plasma metabolite O-methyl-FDOPA (OMFD) also enter the brain, creating a diffuse and non-specific background radioactivity on which the specific signal is superimposed. The model for FDOPA kinetics is schematically represented in Figure 5.1, which is essentially a simplification of the more detailed compartmental model, presented in the preceding chapter. The objective of this chapter is to review the various methods that have been brought to bear on the quantification of PET studies with FDOPA and other substrates for AAADC (Hoshi *et al.* 1993) and to show how these different methods illuminate different aspects of the life history of dopamine in different clinical conditions.

Since FDOPA is also a substrate for AAADC in peripheral tissues and in the blood–brain barrier, subjects for PET studies are generally pretreated with the AAADC inhibitor carbidopa, which (unlike NSD 1015) is almost excluded from passage into the brain. In this treatment condition, the major pathway for the

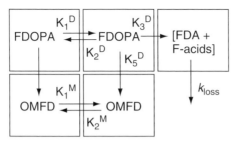

Figure 5.1 The compartmental model for FDOPA kinetics in the brain. FDOPA is reversibly transferred across the blood–brain barrier (K_1^D, k_2^D), as is the plasma metabolite OMFD (K_1^M, k_2^M). In the brain, FDOPA can be O-methylated in situ (k_5^D), or metabolized by AAADC (k_3^D). The product [^{18}F]fluorodopamine is assumed to occupy a single compartment also containing the [^{18}F]-labeled acidic metabolites, which together leave the brain by a process of simple diffusion (k_{loss}).

peripheral metabolism of FDOPA is by COMT in the liver and other tissues, yielding the inert metabolite OMFD. Concentrations of FDOPA and OMFD are measured by HPLC analysis of plasma extracts collected during the PET recording. Within 30 min of FDOPA injection, OMFD becomes the major radioactive species in the plasma of humans (Boyes *et al.* 1986), rats (Cumming *et al.* 1987a), and monkeys (Figure 5.2A). When carbidopa is omitted, several additional metabolites are present in human plasma (Cumming *et al.* 1993), and an unknown fraction of FDOPA can be metabolized by AAADC within the capillary epithelium, before ever entering the brain parenchyma.

As in the case for [^{11}C]tyrosine, the initial phase of a PET recording with FDOPA is dominated by the initial clearance of tracer across the blood–brain barrier. During the first few minutes after tracer injection, the flux of FDOPA from blood to brain greatly exceeds the rate of efflux from the brain. Consequently, the unidirectional clearance of FDOPA can be calculated by linear graphical analysis of the influx during the first few minutes after tracer injection. In a dual tracer study with serial counting of the γ and β radioactivities in blood and brain, the unidirectional blood–brain clearance of FDOPA exceeded that of [^{3}H]DOPA by about 50% (Cumming *et al.* 1995a, b). In general, the influx of large neutral amino acids to the brain is proportional to their octanol–water partition coefficient (Smith *et al.* 1987). Thus, the relatively lipophilic FDOPA is more readily transferred to the brain than is DOPA itself.

The presence of OMFD in plasma has been a problematic issue in the analysis of FDOPA scans. OMFD enters readily into the brain and eventually becomes the predominant radioactive compound in most regions of rat brain (Cumming *et al.* 1987a) and primate brain (Firnau *et al.* 1987). While the proportions of FDOPA and OMFD in the brain of experimental animals can be measured by

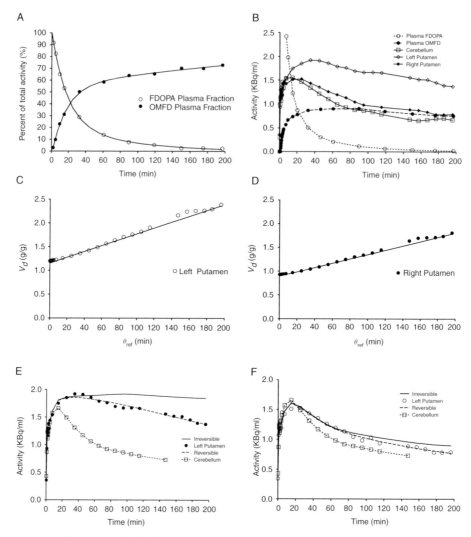

Figure 5.2 FDOPA kinetics in a monkey with unilateral MPTP-lesion to the right striatum. (A) The plasma fractions of FDOPA and OMFD as a function of circulation time, and (B) time–radioactivity curves for plasma FDOPA and OMFD along with TACs measured in the cerebellum and in the left and right putamen. Hartvig reference tissue plots show the magnitude of k_3^S on the (C) lesioned and (D) unlesioned sides. Corresponding results of compartmental analysis (E,F) show the fitting of the extended compartmental model to the entire 240-min-long recordings from putamen (broken line), and also the fitting of the irreversible k_3^D model to the initial 60 min of the recordings (solid line). The difference between the two lines corresponds to the washout of [^{18}F]fluorodopamine formed during the PET recordings. Data derived from Cumming, Munk, & Doudet (2001).

radiochemical fractionation of tissue extracts, the uncertain contribution of OMFD to the total radioactivity measured in PET experiments is a vexing matter for kinetic modeling. This recalls the state of affairs with [^{11}C]tyrosine, in which protein synthesis swamped the signal due to [^{11}C]dopamine synthesis. Since FDOPA is entirely excluded from entry into brain proteins, its major biochemical pathway in the brain is defined kinetically as k_3^D, the relative activity of AAADC with respect to FDOPA. The different methods for quantification of FDOPA metabolism in the brain are intended to identify a parameter indicative of k_3^D, isolated from interference from the background radioactivity comprised by the inert tracer OMFD. These methods must contend with another peculiar aspect of FDOPA metabolism; it shall be seen that the product [^{18}F]fluorodopamine is rapidly catabolized to acidic metabolites. These compounds diffuse from the brain, resulting in progressive violation of the assumption of irreversible FDOPA trapping. However, this property of FDOPA can also be a virtue, since the rate of elimination of [^{18}F]fluorodopamine from the brain may prove to be a more salient feature of pathophysiology of dopamine neurons than is the activity of AAADC itself.

5.2.   Methods for the quantitation of DOPA-PET studies

5.2.1.   *The reference tissue method*

Quantitative PET studies are often encumbered by the need to collect and analyze arterial blood samples, so as to obtain a metabolite-corrected arterial input function. The arterial puncture can be uncomfortable for the subject, and the handling of plasma samples adds to the cost of the PET procedure. Many researchers have consequently settled on a reference tissue method for the quantitation of FDOPA scans. The underlying assumption of this approach is that a reference region can be identified which is nearly devoid of monoamine innervations, such that it can be assumed that the local magnitude of k_3^D is nearly zero. In practice, the cerebellum and the occipital cortex have found wide use as a reference tissue in FDOPA studies. Using an anatomical template placed over the reference region, a time–radioactivity curve is extracted from the reconstructed dynamic emission recording (Figure 5.2B). This time–radioactivity curve is assumed to serve as a surrogate for the missing arterial FDOPA input, thus serving as an estimate of the precursor concentration in the brain regions of high AAADC activity. Then, the local rate of FDOPA utilization can be calculated using a graphical analysis very similar in form to the Gjedde–Patlak linearization (Bruck *et al.* 2006; Hoshi *et al.* 1993; Ishiwata *et al.* 2007), which may be termed the Hartvig analysis, after its first proponent (Hartvig *et al.* 1993). The linear regression slope of the Hartvig plot

(Figure 5.2C,D) corresponds to the activity of AAADC (k_3^s, min^{-1}) relative to the reference tissue input.

Voxel-wise parametric maps of k_3^s in normal young, aged, and MPTP-lesioned monkeys are presented in Figure 5.3. In humans with idiopathic Parkinson's disease, the magnitude of k_3^s is reduced to a much greater extent in the putamen than in the caudate nucleus, relative to the age-matched healthy control subjects (Figure 5.4). Some representative results obtained using this analysis for pig, monkey, and human are presented in Table 5.1. While the slope of the Hartvig plot is clearly sensitive to nigrostriatal degeneration, it seems not to be affected by normal aging, either in monkeys or humans. The Hartvig plot has been employed as the standard method in the multi-center clinical study of the rate of progression of Parkinson's disease (Whone *et al.* 2004). However, the Hartvig plot suffers from the defect that the reference tissue time–activity curve is defined as a surrogate for the arterial FDOPA input, but is progressively contaminated with OMFD. The contribution of OMFD to the total radioactivity in the reference region results in an over-estimation of the true FDOPA concentration in the brain, such that Hartvig slopes tend to be of lower magnitude than real net blood–brain clearances, as defined below.

5.2.2.   Arterial input Gjedde–Patlak plot

The uptake of FDOPA in the brain can also be analyzed by linear graphical analysis with respect to a metabolite-corrected arterial input. However, the entry of OMFD to the brain still presents a problem. To reduce the interference from OMFD, the time–activity curve measured in a reference region is subtracted from the total radioactivity measured in the brain (Martin *et al.* 1989). In this analysis, the linear regression slope of the plot of V_d versus the normalized arterial FDOPA input is equal to the net blood–brain clearance of FDOPA (K_{in}^{app}; ml g^{-1} min^{-1}). As in the case of [^{11}C]tyrosine, this net clearance of FDOPA is a macroparameter comprising the blood–brain distribution and the rate of irreversible trapping, here defined by the activity of AAADC. Some representative results obtained using this analysis for pig, monkey, and human are presented in Table 5.2, and mean parametric maps of K_{in}^{app} in groups of healthy young humans, healthy aged humans, and Parkinson's disease patients are presented in Figure 5.4.

5.2.3.   Compartmental analysis

If FDOPA were unmetabolized in the brain, its cerebral concentration would approach an equilibrium defined only by the ratio of unidirectional clearance (K_1^D) and the fractional rate constant for facilitated diffusion back to blood (k_2^D). The magnitude of this equilibrium distribution volume (V_e^D) is

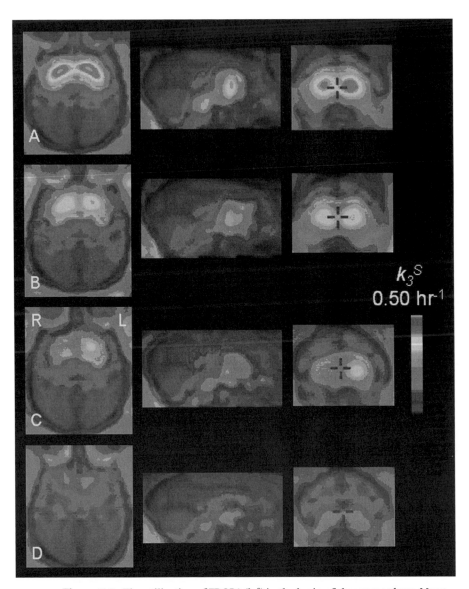

Figure 5.3. The utilization of FDOPA (k_3^s) in the brain of rhesus monkeys. Mean parametric maps are shown for (A) normal young ($n = 6$), (B) normal aged ($n = 4$) rhesus monkeys, (C) aged monkeys with unilateral intracarotid infusion of MPTP ($n = 3$), and (D) monkeys of intermediate aged with systemic MPTP administration ($n = 6$), all calculated relative to a reference tissue input by the method of Hartvig. Mean parametric maps are co-registered to the MR template, shown as gray-scale in the horizontal plane images. The cursor in the coronal plane images indicates the position (0,10,10) in the MR coordinate system. Reproduced with permission from Doudet *et al.* (2006a). (For color version, see plate section.)

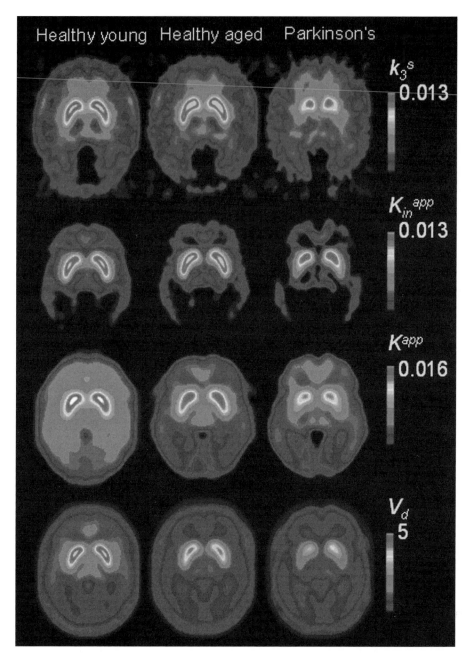

Figure 5.4 Mean parametric maps of FDOPA utilization relative to a reference tissue input (Hartvig k_3^S, min^{-1}), or arterial input (K_{in}^{app}, K^{app}; $ml\,g^{-1}\,min^{-1}$), and the steady-state FDOPA storage (Kumakura V_d; $ml\,g^{-1}$). Image courtesy of Dr. Yoshi Kumakura, Tokyo University. (For color version, see plate section.)

Table 5.1. *Cerebral kinetics of AAADC substrates calculated in brain relative to a reference tissue input*

Condition	k_3^S (min^{-1})	Reference
Monkey, [^{11}C]5HTP, whole striatum ($n = 12$)	0.007 ± 0.001	Hartvig *et al.* 1993
Monkey, β-[^{11}C]DOPA, whole striatum ($n = 12$)	0.012 ± 0.001	
Monkey, [^{11}C]5HTP, whole striatum ($n = 7$)	0.008 ± 0.002	Hartvig *et al.* 1995
Treatment with 10 mg kg^{-1} pyridoxine ($n = 5$)	0.009 ± 0.003	
Heathy rhesus monkey, FDOPA, caudate ($n = 3$)	0.0069 ± 0.0023	Poyot *et al.* 2001
Putamen	0.0077 ± 0.0018	
MPTP-lesioned monkey, caudate ($n = 3$)	0.0011 ± 0.0010	
Putamen	0.0006 ± 0.0006	
Young rhesus monkey, FDOPA, caudate ($n = 6$)	0.0056 ± 0.0018	Doudet *et al.* 2006
Putamen	0.0066 ± 0.0019	
Aged rhesus monkey, caudate ($n = 4$)	0.0047 ± 0.0011	
Putamen	0.0051 ± 0.0014	
Healthy aged human ($n = 16$), FDOPA, caudate	0.0118 ± 0.0016	Lee *et al.* 2000
Putamen	0.0109 ± 0.0013	
Parkinson's disease ($n = 35$), caudate	0.0088 ± 0.0015	
Putamen	0.0043 ± 0.0019	
Healthy human adults, FDOPA, anterior putamen		Nurmi *et al.* 2001
($n = 8$)	0.0101 ± 0.0016	
Posterior putamen	0.0099 ± 0.0010	
Caudate nucleus	0.0098 ± 0.0012	
Parkinson's disease, anterior putamen ($n = 21$)	0.0056 ± 0.0027	
Posterior putamen	0.0045 ± 0.0024	
Caudate nucleus	0.0075 ± 0.0021	

Note: Linear graphical analysis was used for the calculation of the relative activity of AAADC (k_3^S, min^{-1}). Each estimate is the mean ± SD of n estimates.

determined by the ratio of the solubilities of FDOPA in brain and blood, which is close to 0.75 ml g^{-1} in the case of [^{11}C]tyrosine, and also the inert LNAA [^{14}C]AMPT (Cumming *et al.* 1994). However, the transfer of FDOPA across the blood–brain barrier occurs in competition with other substrates for the carrier, which is nearly saturated by the sum of all its several endogenous substrates in plasma. The summed concentration of large neutral amino acids was about 500 μM in the plasma of fasted monkeys, but was elevated two-fold in a loading experiment (Stout *et al.* 1998). The individual estimates of K_1^D in the brain of monkeys declined with increasing plasma concentrations of the competitors, in a manner predicted by Michaelis–Menten kinetics for a saturable uptake process. Furthermore, the efflux of

Table 5.2. *Net blood–brain clearance (K_{in}^{app}, ml g^{-1} min^{-1}) of FDOPA in pig, monkey, and human*

Study	K_{in}^{app}	Reference
Landrace pig ($n=8$)	0.011±0.003	Danielsen *et al.* 1999
Monkey striatum, normal ($n=8$)	0.008±0.002	Melega *et al.* 1996
MPTP-lesioned ($n=4$)	0.002±0.001	
Healthy monkey putamen ($n=6$)	0.0123±0.0043	Cumming, Munk, & Doudet
With correction for lost metabolites	0.0140±0.0053	2001
MPTP-lesioned monkey putamen ($n=6$)	0.0041±0.0027	
With correction for lost metabolites	0.0070±0.0030	
Normal human, striatum ($n=16$)	0.012±0.002	Morrish, Sawle, & Brooks
		1995
Early Parkinson's, asymptomatic side ($n=11$)	0.010±0.002	
Early Parkinson's, symptomatic side	0.007±0.001	
Normal human, caudate ($n=5$)	0.016±0.005	Morrish, Sawle, & Brooks
Putamen	0.015±0.004	1996
Parkinson's disease, caudate ($n=9$)	0.011±0.004	
Putamen	0.006±0.002	
Normal human, putamen ($n=4$)	0.0095±0.0017	Rousset *et al.* 2000
And with partial volume correction	0.0159±0.0028	
Parkinson's disease, putamen ($n=4$)	0.0030±0.0015	
And with partial volume correction	0.0029±0.0020	
Normal human, putamen at baseline ($n=9$)	0.0118±0.0022	Vernaleken *et al.* 2006
And after challenge with haloperidol	0.0139±0.0034	
Normal human, caudate nucleus ($n=10$)	0.0096±0.0019	Hietala *et al.* 1999
Untreated patients with schizophrenia ($n=19$)	0.0122±0.0037	

Note: The net influx is calculated relative to a metabolite-corrected arterial FDOPA input by linear graphical analysis, following subtraction from the brain radioactivity measurements of the entire radioactivity concentration measured in a reference region.

FDOPA and other LNAAs from brain is sensitive to the sum of the concentrations of all competitors in the brain, each relative to its individual affinity for the common carrier. Consequently, the magnitude of the observed V_e^D of FDOPA in monkey brain declined from $1\,ml\,g^{-1}$ in the fasted animals to $0.4\,ml\,g^{-1}$ when the concentration of co-substrates was elevated by loading (Huang *et al.* 1998).

In treated adults with classical phenylketonuria, there was impaired utilization of FDOPA in the caudate and the putamen in the absence of motor symptoms (Landvogt *et al.* 2008). Initial clearance of the tracer to the brain was also delayed, suggesting the elevated phenylalanine levels in plasma interferes with FDOPA uptake and also decarboxylation.

With respect to distribution across the blood–brain barrier in a reference region devoid of AAADC, what is true for FDOPA is also true for OMFD. This insight led to the constrained approach for compartmental analysis of FDOPA in the presence of OMFD (Gjedde *et al.* 1991; Huang *et al.* 1991). The number of free parameters describing the blood–brain partitioning of the two amino acids is reduced from four to two by the following assumptions. First, it is assumed that the blood–brain partitioning of FDOPA at equilibrium ($V_e^D = K_1^D / k_2^D$) is identical to that of OMFD ($V_e^M = K_1^M / k_2^M$). Second, it is assumed that this partitioning is homogeneous throughout the brain. Finally, it is assumed that the magnitude of the unidirectional clearance of OMFD to that of FDOPA (q: K_1^M / K_1^D) is in a fixed ratio. Estimates of the magnitude of this permeability ratio have been obtained by experiments giving q a mean magnitude of 1.5 (Cumming & Gjedde 1998), i.e. favoring the influx of the more lipophilic OMFD. While some uncertainty may remain about the true magnitude of q, it has been shown that the compartmental analysis is quite stable to a range of physiologically plausible q values (Leger *et al.* 1998). Of course, when the enzymatic activity of COMT in peripheral tissues is pharmacologically blocked, the whole FDOPA model reduces to a scenario presented by the upper half of Figure 5.1, in which K_1^D, k_2^D, and k_3^D alone determine FDOPA kinetics in the brain. The use of COMT inhibitors in the course of clinical FDOPA studies (Ishikawa *et al.* 1996) is well tolerated, and allows considerable simplification of the kinetic model.

Unless COMT is inhibited, the compartmental analysis of FDOPA metabolism must accommodate two arterial inputs, i.e. the respective arterial time–radioactivity curves for FDOPA and OMFD. Using the constrained approach, the best fit is first obtained for the time–activity curve recorded in the cerebellum, where the magnitude of k_3^D can plausibly be fixed at zero. Results of a typical fitting for a cerebellum curve from monkey brain are presented in Figure 5.2E,F. In the final phase of the compartmental analysis, the common partition volume of the two amino acids observed in the cerebellum is used as a constraint for the fitting of K_1^D, k_2^D, and k_3^D models to the time–radioactivity curve observed in the striatum, or in some other region of high AAADC activity. In this approach, the number of parameters to be estimated in the striatum reduces to two, K_1^D and k_3^D, neglecting the contribution of radioactivity in cerebral vasculature. In practice, the model is fitted to data recorded only during the first 60 min of the experiment, so as to minimize the effects of progressive violation of the assumption that [^{18}F]fluorodopamine formed in striatum is irreversibly trapped. Fittings of this model to a time–radioactivity curve recorded in the intact striatum (Figure 5.2E) and MPTP-lesioned striatum of a monkey (Figure 5.2E) show that the model describes well the data recorded during the first hour of the PET recording, but that the extrapolated curve fitted to this data progressively overshoots the data recorded at later times. Because of the inherent instability of the model for analyzing noisy voxel-wise data, parametric mapping of the magnitude of k_3^D has not proved practical.

5.2.4.   *Steady-state estimates of FDOPA kinetics*

All of the above methods are based on the assumption that [^{18}F]fluorodopamine, once formed, is irreversibly trapped within the synaptic vesicles. However, inspection of the results of linear graphical analysis and also the compartmental modeling presented in the preceding section show that the striatal radioactivity concentrations eventually decline, indicating progressive violation of the key assumption of the incomplete model. Indeed, [^{18}F]fluorodopamine is rapidly metabolized to its diffusible acidic metabolites in the striatum of living rats (Cumming *et al.* 1987a). In order to correct for loss of mass during the PET recording, it is possible to employ an extended compartmental model, in which it is specified that [^{18}F]fluorodopamine is further metabolized to its acidic metabolites, which then are free to diffuse from the brain.

Strictly speaking, [^{18}F]fluorodopamine is not itself diffusible, but comprises a precursor pool for its diffusible metabolites. Since the FDOPA model already suffers from over-specification, stability of modeling fits is not improved by addition of yet another rate constant. Therefore, [^{18}F]fluorodopamine and its acidic metabolites are generally assumed to leave the brain as a single pool (Huang *et al.* 1991), a simplification which becomes essentially true in the hours after tracer injection, when an equilibrium develops between the two pools (Deep *et al.* 1997; Deep, Gjedde, & Cumming 1997). Then [^{18}F]fluorodopamine and its metabolites can properly be assumed to occupy a single diffusible compartment, which leave the brain at the rate established by k_{loss}.

In practice, it is difficult to obtain stable estimates of k_{loss} when FDOPA recordings of only 2-h duration are available (Danielsen *et al.* 1999). However, stable estimates of the magnitude of k_3^D corrected for loss of the [^{18}F]fluorodopamine metabolites (k_3^{D*}) can be calculated in monkeys scanned for 4 h (Cumming, Munk, & Doudet 2001), during which time the washout of metabolites becomes quite substantial. Results of representative fittings in normal (Figure 5.2E) and MPTP-lesioned (Figure 5.2F) monkey putamen show that the extended model describes very well the time–activity curve recorded during the entire 4 h. This is in contrast to the simple k_3^D model that showed progressive deviation between the extrapolated curve and the measured data. Indeed, the magnitude of k_3^D in intact monkey putamen is some 40% less than is k_3^{D*} (Table 5.3), indicating the extent of bias due to

Table 5.3. *The relative activity of aromatic amino acid decarboxylase (AAADC) with respect to FDOPA* (k_3^D, *min*$^{-1}$) *in brain of pig, monkey, and human*

Subjects	k_3^D	Reference
Healthy minipigs, whole striatum ($n = 10$)	0.047 ± 0.018	Cumming *et al.* 2001
Post-MPTP ($n = 21$)	0.021 ± 0.018	
After fetal mesencephalic grafts ($n = 23$)	0.042 ± 0.019	
Healthy monkey, whole striatum ($n = 8$)	0.065 ± 0.013	Leger *et al.* 1998
Healthy monkey, putamen ($n = 6$)	0.035 ± 0.006	Cumming, Munk, &
With correction for lost metabolite (k_3^{D*})	0.053 ± 0.005	Doudet 2001
MPTP-lesioned monkey putamen ($n = 6$)	0.029 ± 0.014	
With correction for lost metabolites (k_3^{D*})	0.028 ± 0.015	
Healthy control, caudate	0.08 ± 0.02	Kuwabara *et al.* 1995
Parkinson's disease, caudate	0.05 ± 0.02	
Healthy control, putamen	0.08 ± 0.01	
Parkinson's disease, putamen	0.04 ± 0.01	
Healthy control subjects, caudate nucleus ($n = 13$)	0.075 ± 0.005	Reith *et al.* 1994
Unmedicated patients with schizophrenia ($n = 5$)	0.10 ± 0.01	
Untreated patients with schizophrenia ($n = 9$)	0.078 ± 0.029	Grunder *et al.* 2003
And after subchronic haloperidol treatment	0.056 ± 0.009	
Healthy human, putamen ($n = 4$)	0.077 ± 0.029	Rousset *et al.* 2000
After partial volume correction	0.28 ± 0.18	
Parkinson's disease, putamen ($n = 4$)	0.044 ± 0.012	
After partial volume correction	0.056 ± 0.040	

Note: The magnitude of k_3^D was calculated using a constrained compartmental model relative to an arterial input. Except where specified, the model assumed that [^{18}F]fluorodopamine formed in brain from FDOPA is irreversibly trapped for the duration of the PET recording.

uncorrected loss of [^{18}F]fluorodopamine during the first 60 min of the PET recording.

Acquisition of 4-h long emission recordings in awake humans is extremely difficult, since such prolonged immobility is hard to tolerate, especially for patients. When such prolonged PET recordings are available, it becomes possible to re-linearize the linear graphical analysis by addition of an exponential term corresponding to k_{loss}, defined above as the rate constant for export of [^{18}F]fluorodopamine, together with its acidic metabolites, out of the brain (Cumming, Munk, & Doudet 2001; Sossi *et al.* 2004). In effect, the crooked graphical analysis is straightened by addition of the extra rate constant. Using this approach, the effects of pharmacological challenge with COMT inhibitors has been investigated in living monkeys; treatment with tolcapone, a COMT inhibitor with action in the central nervous system, reduced the magnitude of

k_{loss} by 40%, whereas a peripherally acting COMT inhibitor was without such effect (Holden *et al.* 1997). This isolated finding would suggest that COMT plays a rather greater role in the eventual catabolism of [^{18}F]fluorodopamine than has generally been appreciated. However, others report that COMT inhibitors can have intrinsic effects on FDOPA uptake and decarboxylation in living brain (Leger *et al.* 1998).

The ratio of the net tracer clearance to brain (K_{in}^{app}) to the rate constant for eventual washout (k_{loss}) corresponds to the effective distribution volume of FDOPA in the brain (*EDV*, ml g^{-1}). In other words, by considering the entire time course of a 4-h long PET recording, it becomes possible to calculate the steady-state storage capacity for the reversible trapping of FDOPA metabolites in the brain (Sossi, Doudet, & Holden 2001). Using this method in patients with Parkinson's disease showed that the magnitude of K_{in}^{app} in putamen had declined by only 27%, whereas the magnitude of EDV had declined by 65% (Sossi *et al.* 2004). Thus, the equilibrium index emerges as the most sensitive indicator of perturbed FDOPA metabolism in Parkinson's disease. However, the requirement of this method for such long PET recordings can seldom be satisfied. Therefore, an alternate method has been developed in order to estimate steady-state FDOPA kinetics using recordings of only 2-h duration (Kumakura *et al.* 2005, 2006).

The general approach for FDOPA steady-state calculations is as follows: the constrained compartmental model is fitted to the time–activity curve measured in the cerebellum, as described above. In the course of this calculation, best fits of the time–activity curves for FDOPA and OMFD in the cerebellum are estimated. The calculated brain OMFD curve is then subtracted frame-by-frame from every voxel of the original dynamic PET scan. This is in contrast to the more usual approach of subtracting the entire cerebellum radioactivity, which contains both FDOPA and OMFD, in constantly changing proportions. The more correct mathematical subtraction of OMFD isolates the brain radioactivities due to FDOPA, [^{18}F]fluorodopamine, and its acidic metabolites, without over-subtraction of FDOPA, the precursor pool for decarboxylation. Finally, the extended graphical analysis is used to calculate the magnitude of the intrinsic clearance (*K*). This clearance is inherently corrected for k_{loss}, and therefore is of somewhat greater magnitude than the conventional K_{in}^{app}, which suffers from uncorrected metabolite loss. Several estimates of the magnitude of k_{loss} (Table 5.4) predict a half-life for brain [^{18}F]fluorodopamine of approximately 2 h in the healthy striatum, similar to that seen in biochemical assays of dopamine turnover. However, it remains possible that [^{18}F]fluorodopamine preferentially traces a pool of newly synthesized dopamine with rapid turnover.

Table 5.4. *The fractional rate constant (min^{-1}) for the elimination of [^{18}F]fluorodopamine and its deaminated metabolites from brain of pig, monkey, and human*

Subjects	Fractional rate constant	Reference
Healthy pig, striatum ($n=8$)	0.0037 ± 0.0048 (k_{loss})	Danielsen *et al.* 1999
Healthy monkey, putamen ($n=6$)	0.00158 ± 0.0029 (k_{loss})	Cumming, Munk, &
	0.00358 ± 0.00071 (k_9)	Doudet 2001
MPTP-lesioned monkey, putamen ($n=6$)	0.0054 ± 0.0030 (k_{loss})	
	0.0060 ± 0.0020 (k_9)	
Healthy human, striatum ($n=10$)	0.004 ± 0.002 (k_9)	Huang *et al.* 1991
Healthy control subject, putamen ($n=3$)	0.013 ± 0.002 (k_9)	Kuwabara *et al.* 1995
Parkinson's disease, putamen ($n=3$)	0.025 ± 0.007	
Healthy control subjects, putamen ($n=6$)	0.0010 ± 0.0004 (k_{loss})	
Very early Parkinson's disease ($n=9$)	0.0018 ± 0.0011	Sossi *et al.* 2004
Advanced Parkinson's disease ($n=13$)	0.0021 ± 0.0008	
Healthy young control subjects, putamen ($n=7$)	0.0016 ± 0.0008 (k_{loss})	Kumakura *et al.* 2005
Healthy aged control subjects ($n=8$)	0.0037 ± 0.0015	
Parkinson's disease subjects ($n=5$)	0.0094 ± 0.0020	
Healthy aged control subjects, putamen ($n=6$)	0.0079 ± 0.0013 (k_{loss})	Kumakura *et al.* 2006
Early Parkinson's disease, less affected side ($n=8$)	0.0124 ± 0.0032	
And more affected side ($n=8$)	0.0167 ± 0.0032	
Healthy age-matched control subjects ($n=15$)	0.0041 ± 0.0012 (k_{loss})	Kumakura *et al.* 2007a
Untreated patients with schizophrenia ($n=8$)	0.0080 ± 0.0038	

Note: Estimates were obtained from prolonged PET recordings using an extension of the linear graphical analysis (k_{loss}) or an extended compartmental model (k_9) in which [^{18}F]fluorodopamine and subsequent metabolites are assumed to diffuse from brain.

5.3. The true activity of AAADC in living brain

Based on compartmental analysis of FDOPA uptake, the magnitude of k_3^D is generally close to $0.06 \, \text{min}^{-1}$ in the striatum of healthy humans. According to Michaelis–Menten kinetics, the magnitude of k_3^D should be close to V_{max}/K_d, which predicts a magnitude close to $1 \, \text{min}^{-1}$ on the basis of typical literature values of AAADC kinetics in vitro (Yee *et al.* 2000). The extended compartmental model presented above reveals a systematic 50% bias in the estimation of FDOPA kinetics, if [^{18}F]fluorodopamine trapping is assumed to be irreversible. However, this cannot account for the 15-fold discrepancy between PET and enzymology results; other factors in vivo must substantially attenuate the activity of AAADC with respect to exogenous substrates. On the other hand, the mean estimate of k_3^D

based on the biochemical fraction of AAADC substrates and their central metabolites formed in living striatum is 0.3 min^{-1}, i.e. closer to the predicted rate
based on enzyme kinetics. In these studies, continued decarboxylation of the
tracer during the brief post mortem phase prior to extraction of metabolites
could have resulted in some over estimation of the rate of product formation in
living brain, so ex vivo rat results cannot without reservation be identified as the
"true" AAADC activity.

Inherent limitations of the spatial resolution of PET images present an alternate explanation for the discrepancy between PET and enzymology results.
Physical intrusion of one small structure into another brain region, and the spillover of radioactivity between regions are together known as partial volume
effects. The relatively low spatial resolution of PET consequently results in brain
time–radioactivity curves that are substantially degraded by partial volume effects.
Correction for the effects of partial volume has been tested in the case of
FDOPA-PET recordings obtained with a tomograph of 6 mm resolution (Rousset
et al. 2000), which is quite large relative to the size of the human caudate and
putamen. The general approach of the partial volume correction was to assume
that the brain is composed of a small number of biochemically homogeneous
tissue types: caudate, putamen, gray matter, and white matter. Knowing the
performance of the tomograph, it is then possible to back-calculate what the
true tissue radioactivity concentrations must have been in order to produce
the observed measurements. Results of the study suggested that the rate of
FDOPA utilization is substantially underestimated due to loss of signal from the
caudate and putamen. Indeed, the corrected magnitude of k_3^D in the striatum of
normal humans was in the range of the biochemical estimates obtained by fractionation of rat striatum ex vivo. However, the correction resulted in an unaccep-
table trade-off between precision and accuracy; while the higher estimates of k_3^D
are presumably more true, it became more difficult to quantify the extent of the
loss of dopamine innervation in Parkinson's disease (Tables 5.2 and 5.3). While one
may conclude that current FDOPA studies are only semi-quantitative, it can be
hoped that this state of affairs will be improved with the advent of new tomographs with spatial resolution as low as 2 mm.

5.4.   Other substrates for PET studies of AAADC

FDOPA was the first tracer to be employed for PET studies of AAADC, but it
may not be the ideal tracer. Although AAADC does not distinguish kinetically
FDOPA from DOPA in vitro (Cumming et al. 1988), FDOPA is a superior substrate
for hepatic COMT than is DOPA itself. This preference results in the formation of

relatively larger amounts of the plasma metabolite OMFD during the interval of PET scanning (Cumming *et al.* 1995a). Because of this property, and because it is chemically identical to the endogenous compound, β-[^{11}C]DOPA might be preferable to FDOPA for PET studies. Indeed, at the end of 50-min long PET recordings, the *O*-methylated metabolite of β-[^{11}C]DOPA constituted only 25% of plasma radioactivity in the monkey, as compared to 60% in the case of FDOPA (Torstenson *et al.* 1999). Furthermore, the shorter half-life of [^{11}C] (20 min) relative to [^{18}F] (120 min) results in the absorption of less radioactivity by subjects undergoing PET scans. This latter physical property may also allow the design of pharmacological challenge studies in which the subject is scanned twice in a single session, rather than on separate days as would be required with FDOPA. Unfortunately, the relatively complex radio-enzymatic synthesis of β-[^{11}C]DOPA seems to have discouraged its widespread use.

The ambivalence of AAADC toward its several substrates presents the possibility of alternate substrates for PET studies. The utilization of the serotonin precursor [^{11}C]5HTP was slightly lower than that of β-[^{11}C]DOPA in monkey striatum (Hartvig *et al.* 1993). Addition of pyridoxine enhanced the utilization of [^{11}C]5HTP in monkey striatum (Hartvig *et al.* 1995), indicating incomplete saturation with the co-factor in vivo, at least in the case of serotonin synthesis. The pattern of uptake of [^{11}C]5HTP in brain of humans and other primates resembles the pattern of serotonin innervations (Hagberg *et al.* 2002; Lundquist *et al.* 2006). However, specificity of this tracer for AAADC specifically within serotonin terminals remains to be established on the basis of lesion studies selectively targeting the dopamine or serotonin innervations.

The FDOPA analog 6-[^{18}F]-L-*meta*-tyrosine (FMT) has been developed as an alternate tracer for AAADC, which has the advantage of not being a substrate for COMT. FMT enters the brain rapidly, eventually giving rise to a more intense labeling of the striatum than is typical of FDOPA (Brown *et al.* 1999). However, the decarboxylated product, 6-[^{18}F]-*meta*-tyramine, is not sequestered in synaptic vesicles (Endres *et al.* 1997b), but is instead rapidly metabolized by MAO, yielding the acidic metabolite [^{18}F]hydroxyphenylacetic acid (Jordan *et al.* 1998). In general, the acidic metabolites should diffuse from the brain, so it is unclear how the specific signal is retained within the living striatum. Possibly, the diffusion rate constant for this compound is very slow relative to the duration of the PET recording, but this conjecture needs to be tested by experiment.

5.5.   Pharmacological modulation of AAADC activity

Based on the results of [^{3}H]DOPA studies ex vivo, modulation of the activity of AAADC by drugs binding to autoreceptors has been tested in PET

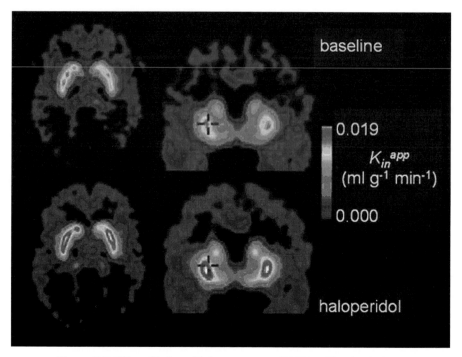

Figure 5.5 Effect of haloperidol treatment on FDOPA utilization in human brain.
Mean parametric maps show the magnitude of the FDOPA net blood-brain clearance
($K_{in}{}^{app}$) in a group of (n = 9) healthy male subjects, scanned first in a baseline condition,
and after acute treatment with haloperidol. Image from data presented in Vernaleken
et al. (2006). (For color version, see plate section.)

paradigms. Acute challenge with haloperidol significantly increased the magnitude of $K_{in}{}^{app}$ in the putamen of healthy volunteers in investigations with
FDOPA (Figure 5.5) (Vernaleken *et al.* 2006), consistent with upregulation of
dopamine synthesis. In another such study, treatment of volunteers with the
atypical neuroleptic failed to increase the striatal influx of FMT (Mamo *et al.*
2004b). However, this discrepancy may be related to the uncertain metabolic
fate of that tracer, which is not so well understood as is the case for FDOPA.
Alternately, the use of the atypical antipsychotic risperidone as the agent
of pharmacological challenge may have influenced the negative result in the
FMT study. Subchronic treatment with haloperidol *decreased* the magnitude of
$k_3{}^D$ with respect to FDOPA in the striatum of patients with schizophrenia,
consistent with downregulation of dopamine synthesis (Grunder *et al.* 2003).
This finding was interpreted to reveal the onset of depolarization block, a
putative mechanism for the delayed clinical response to classical neuroleptics
treatment. FDOPA influx was slightly reduced in putamen and amygdala of
untreated young patients with ADHD, and was 15–20% lower than normal in

patients treated with methylphenidate, consistent with pharmacological modulation of AAADC (Ludolph et al. 2008).

5.6.   Clinical FDOPA-PET studies

5.6.1.   *Age-related changes measured by FDOPA-PET*

Cell counting studies cited above generally have shown a 7–10% decline in the number of dopamine neurons of the substantia nigra with each decade of human life. In spite of this precipitous decline in dopamine neurons, the activity of AAADC from post mortem brain was only 27% lower in the caudate nucleus (but not putamen) of elderly human subjects than in the young (Kish *et al.* 1995). This observation evoked discussion about the possibility of compensatory changes in the aging substantia nigra, especially since the preponderance of PET studies with FDOPA in vivo fail to show any important decline in uptake with normal aging of humans (Cumming & Gjedde 1998). A comparison of FDOPA utilization with other PET markers for dopamine neurons revealed that the decline in k_3^s was less than that reported for VMAT2 in synaptic vesicles of patients with Parkinson's disease, suggesting that AAADC activity could increase in compensation for partial nigrostriatal degeneration (Lee *et al.* 2000). Similar findings have been observed in a multi-tracer PET study of aged and MPTP-poisoned rhesus monkeys, in which there was only a trend toward declining k_3^s with age (Figure 5.3) (Doudet *et al.* 2006). However, numerous model-based factors may underlie the difficulty in detecting age-related changes in FDOPA kinetics.

Failure of most FDOPA studies to age-related changes in dopamine metabolism may arise from the use of reference tissue methods subtraction, which results in over-subtraction of the precursor pool. This approach causes significant negative bias in the estimation of the magnitude of K_{in}^{app} (Kumakura *et al.* 2005, 2006). Using the hybrid kinetic approach of a more valid mathematical subtraction of the brain OMFD concentration, it was revealed that the conventional calculation of K_{in}^{app} conceals an underlying decline with age in the magnitude of the net blood–brain clearance. Parametric maps of the mean magnitude of the net FDOPA influx based on a more physiologically valid subtraction of the OMFD curve (K^{app}; Figure 5.4) reveal a substantial decline with normal aging, which cannot be detected in the corresponding k_3^s and K_{in}^{app} maps from the same subjects. A still more complete steady-state kinetic analysis reveals that the most significant alteration in FDOPA kinetics with normal aging is an increase in the magnitude of k_{loss}, which is not entirely compensated by the putative modulation of the rate of FDOPA decarboxylation proposed above. Parametric maps of the FDOPA steady-state V_d (Figure 5.4) clearly show a 10% decline with each decade of healthy aging, surpassed by the still-greater decline in Parkinson's disease patients, a result entirely in agreement with histological studies of cell loss in the substantia nigra. The driving force for this decline in FDOPA storage seems to be the impaired vesicular storage of the product [^{18}F]fluorodopamine. This conjecture might be confirmed in dual tracer studies with FDOPA and the vesicular ligand [^{11}C]DTBZ, a tracer to be presented in Chapter 9, below.

While it is clear that dopamine is essential for normal movement, it is unclear how much extra dopamine is used during the execution of a motor task. In other words, it is presently uncertain whether [^{18}F]fluorodopamine turnover is altered by behavioral state. Indeed, the relationship between motor or sensory activity and FDOPA utilization has scarcely been investigated. In the only study of this relationship, non-noxious electrical stimulation of the median nerve reduced the net influx of FDOPA in contralateral striatum of awake humans and anesthetized cats (Hassoun *et al.* 2005). Implicitly, this finding suggests that the rate of washout of FDOPA metabolites was increased by the stimulus, thus increasing the discrepancy between K_{in}^{app} and K. There seem to have been no direct tests for the effect of aerobic exercise or performance of fine motor tasks on FDOPA utilization and trapping.

5.6.2.   *Acquired parkinsonism and idiopathic Parkinson's disease*

The relationship between FDOPA utilization and survival of dopamine neurons is best documented with the MPTP model of acquired parkinsonism in experimental animals. Here, the quantitative PET results can be compared with subsequent post mortem histological analysis, preferably using stereological cell counting procedures. Impaired utilization of FDOPA in the striatum of MPTP-poisoned monkeys was associated with atrophy of the remaining dopamine neurons in the substantia nigra (Pate *et al.* 1993). Stereological cell counting showed that 200 000 dopamine neurons in the substantia nigra of healthy baboons had imparted an FDOPA k_3^s of 0.007 min^{-1} in the striatum. In baboons with only 67 000 dopamine neurons remaining after MPTP poisoning, the magnitude of striatal k_3^s had declined to 0.001 min^{-1} (Poyot *et al.* 2001). This relationship was less clear in animals with relatively low MPTP doses, in which declines in FDOPA utilization correlated better with striatal dopamine concentration (Yee *et al.* 2001) and with striatal AAADC activity measured in vitro (Yee *et al.* 2000) than with actual loss of dopamine neurons in the substantia nigra, measured post mortem. Indeed, the "non-linearity" of FDOPA utilization has been noted previously (Barrio, Huang, & Phelps 1997), and has been discussed above in the context of steady-state models of FDOPA kinetics. Using the alternate AAADC tracer FMT, there was general agreement between the pattern of reduced tracer influx and the topography of the remaining dopamine neurons in the brain of MPTP-treated rhesus monkey (Oiwa *et al.* 2003). In a study of xenografting in pigs with MPTP-induced parkinsonism, some functional recovery and improved FDOPA utilization were obtained in association with the survival of approximately 100 000 dopamine neurons ectopically placed in the denervated striatum (Dall *et al.* 2002). In a group of five patients dying with Parkinson's disease, cell counts in the substantia nigra correlated with results of earlier FDOPA-PET examinations (Snow *et al.* 1993); this seems to be the only instance of follow-up histological examination in human FDOPA studies.

Notwithstanding the limitations of the conventional methods for the quantitation of FDOPA utilization, the threshold of K_{in}^{app} for the emergence of parkinsonian symptoms was detected in a study of patients with early hemi-parkinsonism (Table 5.2) (Morrish, Sawle, & Brooks 1995). The rate of progression of Parkinson's disease has been investigated in a number of longitudinal PET studies. For example, the magnitude of k_3^s declined by 6% per year in the caudate and 10% per year in the putamen of a cohort of 21 subjects with Parkinson's disease, versus less than 1% per year in healthy aged subjects (Nurmi *et al.* 2001). In the REAL-PET study, the magnitude of k_3^s in the putamen declined by 6.5% per year in Parkinson's disease patients treated with the direct agonist ropinirole versus 10% per year in patients treated with the indirect agonist levodopa (Whone *et al.* 2003). This finding may reveal a neuroprotective effect of direct dopamine agonists, and could also be confounded by pharmacological modulation of AAADC, as reported in rats for another agonist, apomorphine.

The first reductions in FDOPA utilization of early Parkinson's disease are noted in the dorsal putamen; follow-up 2 years later shows a further decline in the dorsal putamen, along with additional loss in other regions of the striatum (Bruck *et al.* 2006; Ishiwata *et al.* 2007). Even in cases of advanced Parkinson's disease, the FDOPA influx is less impaired in the caudate nucleus (−45%) than in the putamen (−64%) (Broussolle *et al.* 1999). Increased FDOPA utilization in the frontal cortex has been described in two independent PET studies of early Parkinson's disease (Bruck *et al.* 2005; Rakshi *et al.* 1999). The increase in the dorsolateral prefrontal cortex was particularly notable in women with early Parkinson's disease (Kaasinen *et al.* 2001c).

In a study of 31 patients with early Parkinson's disease with a follow-up interval of 5 years, the annual declines of k_3^s were 4% in the caudate and 6% in the putamen (Hilker *et al.* 2005). A semilog transformation of the k_3^s data suggested the occurrence of an exponential decline in the integrity of the nigrostriatal pathway, and a preclinical interval of approximately 5 years. However, it has been noted that k_3^s can be consider to be a macroparameter, thus potentially having a hyperbolic relationship with the magnitude of k_3^D, the relative activity of AAADC (Borghammer, Kumakura, & Cumming 2005). Using literature values for the magnitudes of K_1^D and V_e^D, which are not themselves affected by age (Cumming & Gjedde 1998), the plot of log[k_3^s] can be replotted as the estimated k_3^D as a function of age (Figure 5.6),

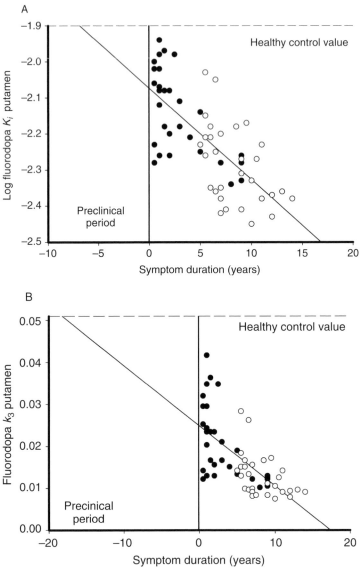

Figure 5.6 FDOPA utilization and the progression of Parkinson's disease. (A) The logarithm of magnitude of FDOPA utilization calculated relative to a reference tissue method (k_3^s) in a large cohort of Parkinson's disease subjects as a function of symptom duration (data from Hilker *et al.*, 2005) and (B) a re-analysis of the same data according to a linear model, in which the relative activity of DOPA decarboxylase (k_3^D, min^{-1}) was estimated from the magnitude of k_3^s based on population means for the blood–brain distribution of FDOPA. Solid symbols are upon entry into the study, and open symbols show results at follow-up approximately five years later. Solid lines are the linear regression slopes, extrapolated back to the corresponding estimates for healthy subjects. Figure reproduced with permission from Borghammer, Kumakura, & Cumming (2005).

predicting a preclinical interval of 15 years. This discrepancy presents the distinction between a zero-order process of disease progression, in which dopamine cells
die at a fixed rate until none remain, and a first-order process, in which the cells die
at a rate which is a function of the number of remaining cells.

The factors regulating AAADC expression in the healthy brain are poorly understood. In one genetic study of healthy subjects, the TaqI A1 allele of the dopamine
D_2 receptor, which imparts risk for alcoholism, was associated with significantly
elevated FDOPA influx in the putamen, compared with subjects having only the
A2 allele (Laakso *et al.* 2005). There have been a number of FDOPA–PET investigations of the genetics of familial parkinsonism. Echogenicity of the substantia
nigra, a non-specific marker of degeneration associated with increased iron content, was elevated in relatives of patients with sporadic Parkinson's disease, and
seemed to correlate with subclinical motor slowing, as well as with reduced
FDOPA utilization (Ruprecht-Dorfler *et al.* 2003). In a study of carriers of a mutation
of a gene at the PARK8 locus, the pattern of reduced striatal FDOPA uptake was
similar to that seen in idiopathic Parkinson's disease (Adams *et al.* 2005). Similar
patterns were also seen in carriers of the recessive *DJ-1* gene evoking early onset
parkinsonism (Dekker *et al.* 2004). Furthermore, affected members of a *parkin*
kindred, characterized by juvenile-onset parkinsonism, had reduced FDOPA utilization, as did unaffected carriers in the kindred (Khan *et al.* 2002). Indeed, a gene
dosage effect could be seen in an FDOPA study of another *parkin* kindred (Hilker
et al. 2002). Finally, members of a parkinsonian kindred with mutation of
α-synuclein (Samii *et al.* 1999) had a pattern of reduced FDOPA utilization indis-
tinguishable from that seen in idiopathic Parkinson's disease. FDOPA endopheno-
typing has been used to investigate an Amish family with high incidence of
Parkinson's disease. Using a stringent criterion of three standard deviations
below the normal mean for FDOPA uptake, several clinically suspect individuals
could be identified on the basis of PET results (Racette *et al.* 2006). Impaired FDOPA
uptake in the striatum was also predictive of the subsequent phenoconversion of
familial progressive supranuclear palsy (Tai *et al.* 2007), and was clearly evident in
patients with neuronal ceroid lipofuscinosis (Ruottinen *et al.* 1997) and Lesch-
Nyhan syndrome (Ernst *et al.* 1996), whereas a 10% reduction could be seen in
patients with restless legs syndrome (Ruottinen *et al.* 2000). In summary, results of
most genetic studies of parkinsonism show similar disturbances in presynaptic
dopamine function, irrespective of the underlying genetic abnormality resulting
in the nigrostriatal degeneration.

5.6.3.   *Other clinical FDOPA studies*

Increased activity of AAADC especially in the caudate nucleus of
unmedicated patients with schizophrenia was an early finding in the history

of quantitative FDOPA studies (Reith *et al.* 1994). This finding has since been replicated in independent studies with FDOPA (Hietala *et al.* 1999), with notably large increases present in the ventral striatum (McGowan *et al.* 2004). In studies with β-[^{11}C]DOPA, increased influx was seen throughout the striatum, and also the medial prefrontal cortex (Lindstrom *et al.* 1999), which was normalized after treatment with neuroleptics drugs (Gefvert *et al.* 2003). Increased FDOPA influx to the striatum correlated with reduced activation of the prefrontal cortex during performance of a cognitive task in an fMRI study of schizophrenia (Meyer-Lindenberg *et al.* 2002). In first-degree relatives of patients with schizophrenia, FDOPA was elevated in the caudate nucleus by about 23%, and to a lesser extent in the putamen (Huttunen *et al.* 2008). In addition to elevated synthesis, the turnover of [^{18}F]fluorodopamine formed in the striatum was elevated in patients with schizophrenia (Kumakura *et al.* 2007b). Even in the presence of somewhat elevated FDOPA influx to the brain, this elevated turnover resulted in a reduction in the steady-state FDOPA V_d in the brain of the patients (Figure 5.7), a circumstance which has been described as "poverty in the midst of plenty."

The above studies show that increased dopamine synthesis capacity is one of the best-established PET findings in schizophrenia. However, this neurochemical abnormality cannot be pathognomonic of schizophrenia, since there is frequent overlap in the tracer influx rates between the clinical groups and the normal control subjects. FDOPA influx was normal in untreated patients with non-psychotic mania, but treatment with the mood stabilizer divalproex sodium significantly reduced this influx to below normal values (Yatham *et al.* 2002b).

There is evidence for gender difference in the handling of FDOPA in human brain. Specifically, the FDOPA influx (K_{in}^{app}) was greater in the caudate nucleus of women than in men, a difference possibly related to greater age-related declines in the male group (Laakso *et al.* 2002). The magnitude of K_{in}^{app} was 30% greater in the caudate nucleus of smokers than in non-smoking control subjects (Salokangas *et al.* 2000). It remains uncertain whether this reflects a pharmacological action of tobacco smoke, or an underlying personality trait disposing toward addiction. However, the finding that acute treatment with nicotine increased the utilization of β-[^{11}C]DOPA in striatum of awake monkeys (Tsukada *et al.* 2005) suggests a direct causal link. In this respect, it is interesting that the magnitude of FDOPA K_{in}^{app} was entirely normal in the striatum of a group of alcoholics, but nonetheless correlated inversely with craving and risk of relapse (Heinz *et al.* 2005). This result implies that the symptom of craving expresses itself through a dopamine innervation that is essentially normal. However, this top-down model still implies an uncertain sequence of causality, since it cannot be known a priori if the presynaptic innervation measured with FDOPA is determined by the craving, or vice versa.

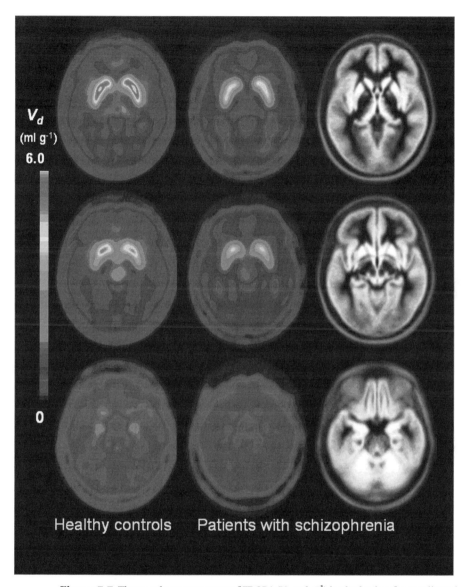

Figure 5.7 The steady-state storage of FDOPA (V_{d}, ml g^{-1}) in the brain of unmedicated patients with schizophrenia and healthy age-matched control subjects. Reproduced with permission from Kumakura *et al.* (2007b). (For color version, see plate section.)

5.7. Personality and cognition

Psychological test batteries can be used to assess scores on distinct traits and propensities, and their relationship between results of PET studies. One of the more widely used personality tests is the Tridimensional Personality Questionnaire of Cloninger. The results of this test provide scores on three distinct axes, known as reward dependence, novelty seeking, and harm avoidance, to which is sometimes added the additional dimension of persistence. Analogous ratings of personality traits can be assessed using the Karolinska Scales of Personality (KSP) and other instruments.

In a study of personality traits, high scores in ratings of anxiety and aggressivity correlated with low influx of FDOPA in the caudate nucleus of normal young subjects (Laakso *et al.* 2003). FDOPA uptake in the caudate of Parkinson's disease patients correlated positively with the novelty-seeking (Menza *et al.* 1995) and harm-avoidance scores (Kaasinen *et al.* 2001b). These results lend support to the usual clinical assessment that Parkinson's disease patients tend to be withdrawn, and lacking in adventurousness. However, there was no corresponding relationship between FDOPA influx and harm-avoidance scores in healthy elderly controls (Kaasinen *et al.* 2002b).

In an FDOPA study employing principal component analysis, impaired FDOPA utilization segregated with motor symptoms, but not cognitive function and mood of Parkinson's patients without diagnosis of major depression (Broussolle *et al.* 1999). This would seem to exclude important contributions of nigrostriatal degeneration per se to cognitive function and mood disorders. Others have reported that impaired FDOPA influx to caudate (but not putamen) of Parkinson's disease patients was predictive of poor performance of the Stroop interference task (Rinne *et al.* 2000). In this test of executive function of the frontal cortex, the subject is required to suppress the tendency to conflate a color word such as red or blue, and the color of the font. Other tasks implicating executive function include performance of tests for digit span, verbal fluency, and other indicators of working memory. In a PET study of normal subjects, working memory as measured by listening span, correlated with the uptake of FMT in striatum (Cools *et al.* 2008). We have seen that FDOPA influx in the frontal cortex is likely a mixed indicator of noradrenaline and dopamine innervations, either of which might contribute to cognitive function. Thus, the FDOPA influx specifically in the frontal cortex, where it was reduced to 45% of control values, correlated with impaired performance of Parkinson's disease patients (Rinne *et al.* 2000) which may be related to degeneration of nonadrenergic fibres innervating the cerebral cortex. In a subsequent FDOPA study of cognition in Parkinson's disease patients, there was a very high correlation between impaired FDOPA uptake in the caudate nucleus and putamen with scores in an item known as "concentration difficulties" (Koerts *et al.* 2007). However, this finding need not necessarily indicate a causal link, since the decline in striatum FDOPA metabolism might be a surrogate marker for some concomitant neurochemical changes more directly impinging on cognitive function.

The score in the Stroop test correlated with FDOPA K_{in}^{app} throughout the striatum of a group of healthy volunteers (Vernaleken *et al.* 2007a). In another dual-modality imaging study, the magnitude of activation of the BOLD signal evoked in the frontal cortex by emotionally positive visual stimuli correlated with FDOPA K_{in}^{app} in the ventral striatum (Siessmeier *et al.* 2006). These findings seem to be in contrast to the results of the relationship between prefrontal BOLD signal and FDOPA influx in patients with schizophrenia, cited above, in which impaired prefrontal activity predicted especially elevated FDOPA uptake; the normal relationship between cortical and subcortical function is subverted in schizophrenia.

6

Conjugation and sulfonation of dopamine and its metabolites

6.1.   Biochemistry of COMT

COMT catalyzes the transfer of active methyl from S-adenosylmethionine (SAM) to dopamine and other catechols (Axelrod & Tomchick 1958). The methylation is preferentially directed to the *p*-hydroxyl group of most substrates. In the brain, the enzyme exists in two distinct molecular forms: a soluble form with low affinity for catecholamine substrates, and a membrane-bound form with μM affinity with respect to dopamine (Jeffery & Roth 1984). The membrane-bound form can be solubilized with strong detergent, suggesting that it is an integral membrane protein. The activity of both forms is dependent on the presence of Mg^{2+}, and is maximal at pH greater than 7. Mechanistic studies of the membrane-bound form suggest that catalysis is initiated with binding of the co-substrate SAM, followed by the formation of a ternary complex with dopamine. The reaction is inhibited by low concentrations of the end-product S-adenosylhomocysteine (Rivett & Roth 1982). Some biochemical properties of COMT are summarized in Table 6.1.

The membrane-bound form of COMT differs from the soluble form in having an extra 50-residue hydrophobic sequence at the N-terminus (Ulmanen *et al.* 1997). When expressed in transfected mammalian cells, the membrane-bound COMT is associated with the endoplasmic reticulum and nuclear membranes, but not in the plasma membrane – an indication that its substrates must be present in the cytosol rather than on the external plasma membrane, as was once believed. COMT has its highest activity in the liver and kidney, where more than 99% occurs as the soluble form (Rivett, Francis, & Roth 1983). Both forms are coded by a single gene, but different promoters regulate the tissue-specific expression of the long and short transcripts (Tenhunen *et al.* 1994). In human

Table 6.1. *Some kinetic properties of catechol-O-methyltransferase (COMT) and arylsulfotransferase*

COMT		
Affinity for dopamine, membrane-bound COMT from human brain	$3\,\mu M$	Jeffery & Roth 1984
Soluble enzyme from human brain	$280\,\mu M$	
Affinity for dopamine, membrane-bound COMT from human brain	$4\,\mu M$	Rivett & Roth 1982
Affinity for SAM	$3\,\mu M$	
End-product inhibition by S-adenosylhomocysteine	$1\,\mu M$	
Affinity for Mg^{2+}, membrane-bound COMT from human brain	$1.6\,\mu M$	Jeffery & Roth 1987
V_{max} for dopamine, soluble enzyme from rat striatum	$27\,nmol\,g^{-1}\,min^{-1}$	Rivett, Francis, & Roth 1983
V_{max} for membrane-bound enzyme*	$1.6\,nmol\,g^{-1}\,min^{-1}$	
Concentration of SAM in whole rat brain	$15\,\mu M$	Yassin *et al.* 1998
Arylsulfotransferase		
Affinity of rat brain enzyme for dopamine	$130\,\mu M$	Rivett *et al.* 1984
Activity for dopamine in rat		
Hypothalamus*	$680\,pmol\,g^{-1}\,min^{-1}$	
Striatum*	$340\,pmol\,g^{-1}\,min^{-1}$	
Cerebellum*	$40\,pmol\,g^{-1}\,min^{-1}$	
Affinity for dopamine, soluble fraction from human brain	$3\,\mu M$	Baran & Jellinger 1992
Activity in temporal cortex	$129\,pmol\,g^{-1}\,min^{-1}$	
Enzyme purified from human brain, affinity for dopamine	$5\,\mu M$	Renskers, Feor, & Roth 1980
Affinity for PAPS	$250\,nM$	
End-product inhibition by PAP	$70\,nM$	Whittemore, Pearce, & Roth 1985
Molecular weight, expressed human brain enzyme	34 196	Veronese *et al.* 1994
Molecular weight, enzyme purified 300-fold from human cortex	62 000	Yu, Rozdilsky, & Boulton 1985
Homospecific activity, human enzyme expressed in *E. coli*	$0.8\ dopamine\ min^{-1}\ enzyme^{-1}$	Sakakibara *et al.* 1998
pH optimum, human brain cortex	7.9	Yu, Rozdilsky, & Boulton 1985

Note: Abbreviations: SAM, S-adenosylmethionine; PAPS, 3′-phosphoadenosine-5′-phosphosulfate, PAP, 3′-phosphoadenosine-5′-phosphate.
*Calculated as 10% protein by weight.

brain, the long transcript is expressed ubiquitously, but substantial amounts of the soluble form of the enzyme may be formed from incomplete transcription of the long message (Hong *et al.* 1998).

In the brain, the presence of COMT can be detected with specific antibodies in neurons and glial cells, and also in ventricular ependymal cells (Karhunen *et al.* 1995). The COMT immunoreactivity was particularly associated with post-synaptic neurons, but is also found in the cytosol of astrocytes. COMT is detected in microglia proliferating in the striatum after infusion of a glial toxin (Reenila *et al.* 1997). Lesion studies with kainic acid suggest that the membrane-bound form is localized mainly in neurons, while the soluble form occurs in astroglia (Rivett, Francis, & Roth 1983). Large increases in the activity of the soluble form were apparent in homogenates from lesioned rat striatum, presumably indicating proliferation and activation of astrocytes. However, the concentration of the dopamine metabolite 3MT in cerebral microdialysates decreased after striatal lesions, even though the extracellular dopamine concentration increased. Therefore, the membrane-bound COMT relevant to metabolism of released dopamine seems to occur in neuronal elements post-synaptic to the dopamine fibers (Naudon *et al.* 1992).

The tissue uptake of the competitive COMT inhibitor [^{18}F]Ro 41–0960 has been tested in living baboon using PET. The net clearance of this tracer to the liver was reversibly blocked by pretreatment with the cold inhibitor (Ding *et al.* 1998). However, no uptake to brain was detected, in spite of the structural similarity of the tracer to tolcapone, a centrally acting COMT inhibitor in the rat (Cumming *et al.* 1992).

6.2.   Behavioral correlates of COMT activity

COMT first became a target for therapeutics in the context of DOPA therapy for Parkinson's disease, in which the metabolite OMD can interfere with or limit clinical response (Rao *et al.* 1972). The prototypic COMT inhibitor U-0521 enhanced the behavioral effects of DOPA (Nuutila, Kaakkola, & Mannisto 1987), and potentiated the brain uptake of FDOPA in rats, by increasing the area under the plasma input curve (Cumming *et al.* 1987b). More effective and less toxic COMT inhibitors are now routinely used as adjunct treatment for Parkinson's disease; the COMT inhibitor entacapone prolongs the clinical response to DOPA, and may be especially useful in the adjunct treatment of Parkinson's disease with motor fluctuations (Rinne *et al.* 1998).

In the absence of abundant dopamine transporters, COMT is a major factor in the regulation of interstitial dopamine concentration in the rat cerebral cortex

(Karoum, Chrapusta, & Egan 1994; Karoum, Neff, & Wyatt 1977). Nonetheless, the centrally acting COMT inhibitor tolcapone did not enhance extracellular dopamine concentrations in rat frontal cortex at baseline, but did potentiate the depolarization-evoked release (Tunbridge *et al.* 2004). Thus, specifically phasic dopamine signaling in the cortex may be shaped by the action of COMT. This property predicts a possible role for COMT in aspects of cognitive and psychiatric disorders, in spite of its small contribution to striatal dopamine catabolism.

Valine–methionine substitution at codon 158 imparts heat lability and relatively lower catalytic activity to COMT (Lotta *et al.* 1995), and has been associated with the incidence of bipolar disorder in a Han Chinese population (Li *et al.* 1997). However, in a meta-analysis, there was only a slight trend toward over-representation of the more active valine allele in Asian patients with schizophrenia (Fan *et al.* 2005), although the valine allele seems to predict worse cognitive deterioration in patients with schizophrenia (Mata *et al.* 2006), and imparted particular risk for development of schizophrenia in adolescent users of cannabis (Caspi *et al.* 2005). Indeed, transcriptional regulation of COMT may be a risk factor for psychosis; hypomethylation of the COMT promoter sequence in post mortem specimens of frontal cortex was linked to low expression of COMT, and had an association with psychosis (Abdolmaleky *et al.* 2006). Furthermore, an abnormal laminar distribution of COMT expression in the cerebral cortex has been reported in patients with schizophrenia (Matsumoto *et al.* 2003).

Catecholestrogens are substrates for COMT, which can modulate turnover of catecholamines in the hypothalamus (Parvizi & Wuttke 1983). Indeed, low activity of COMT has been identified as a risk factor for development of post-menopausal carcinoma of the breast (Lavigne *et al.* 1997), consistent with an elevated lifetime exposure to estrogenic compounds. It is not known whether prolonged COMT inhibition can increase the risk of estrogen-sensitive tumors.

6.3.   Arylsulfotransferase

Dopamine and other phenolic compounds can be sulfo-conjugated in extracts of the brain (Meek & Neff 1973) by the enzyme phenolsulfotransferase, in the presence of the sulfate donor 3′-phosphoadenosine-5′-phosphosulfate (PAPS). With respect to the exogenous substrate *p*-nitrophenol, two distinct activities are present in rat brain, but only one activity is present with respect to dopamine substrate (Rivett *et al.* 1984). The enzyme purified from human liver consists of a homodimer of subunits weighing about 32 000 (Falany *et al.* 1990;

Veronese *et al.* 1994). Likewise, two cDNAs cloned from human liver and brain expression libraries predict molecular weights close to 34 000, and possessed considerable sequence homology. A very short amino acid sequence is critical for substrate specificity of the two forms of the arylsulfotransferase enzyme (Sakakibara *et al.* 1998). Whereas the hepatic enzyme is probably involved in the metabolism of xenobiotic substances, dopamine is the preferred substrate for brain metabolism. After lesions with the neurotoxin kainic acid, the arylsulfotransferase activity declined substantially in rat striatum, suggesting a predominantly neuronal localization for the brain enzyme (Rivett, Francis, Whittemore, & Roth 1984).

Some kinetic properties of arylsulfotransferase are summarized in the lower part of Table 6.1. The enzyme purified from the brain has very high affinity for PAPS and for dopamine, but is inhibited by dopamine at concentrations above 20 μM. Among the other monoamine substrates for brain arylsulfotransferase are 3MT, tyramine, and norepinephrine (Renskers, Feor, & Roth 1980). The relatively low capacity of the enzyme in brain may limit its contribution to dopamine metabolism in brain. In addition, a phosphatase in brain may greatly restrict the availability of PAPS for dopamine sulfation (Whittemore & Roth 1985). Nonetheless, the concentration of dopamine sulfate in human CSF exceeds that of the free dopamine (Tyce *et al.* 1986), but at least some of the dopamine sulfate may cross into the CSF from peripheral tissues. Therefore, the absolute rate of sulfation of brain dopamine remains unknown, although kinetic rate constants predict that as much as 15% of brain dopamine could be conjugated (Rivett, Eddy, & Roth 1982). Arylsulfotransferase is a major enzyme in the handling of the acidic dopamine metabolites DOPAC and HVA. One half of these compounds are sulfated prior to diffusion from the brain to the CSF (Dedek *et al.* 1979).

7

Dopamine synthesis and metabolism rates

7.1.   Steady-state and the epistemology of dopamine metabolism

The steady-state is defined as the condition of equilibrium between the rates of formation and elimination of a substance in a particular compartment. This occurs when the chickens in Figure 3.3 reach a constant size. In the strict sense, the steady-state is necessarily a hypothetical condition, since the concentration of any substance in the brain can fluctuate with time. The rate of increase in the concentration of DOPA after blockade of AAADC was introduced as an approach to calculating steady-state dopamine synthesis, but subject to the caveats that decarboxylation is not the unique fate of DOPA formed in the brain, and that the pharmacological treatment can itself perturb the steady-state. The trace amines tyramine and phenylethylamine present another instance of steady-state calculations; the lack of a secure storage compartment for these compounds results in very rapid metabolism by MAO, such that the steady-state concentrations in rat brain are very low relative to the amount of dopamine. However, there is a linear and substantial increase in their concentrations during several hours after blockade of MAO with pargyline (Durden & Philips 1980). That this process remains linear with time suggests that their accumulation does not modulate their own rate of synthesis. In contrast, the accumulation of dopamine in the brain is linear only for the initial 15 min after blockade of MAO, reflecting the more responsive feedback mechanisms in neurotransmitter synthesis (Venero, Machado, & Cano 1991).

The branched pathway for dopamine catabolism (Figure 1.1) results in the formation of the acid metabolite HVA via the intermediates of 3MT or DOPAC. The steady-state concentration of 3MT in rat striatum is low in comparison to that of the pooled acidic metabolites, which total to one third of the whole tissue concentration of dopamine. It seems intuitively obvious that concentrations of the acidic metabolites can serve as an index of the net rate of dopamine consumption. However, it is uncertain that DOPAC and HVA are adequate surrogate indicators of *dopamine turnover*, a somewhat vague term referring to the dynamics of dopamine metabolism. More specifically, it is possible to conceive of circumstances wherein dopamine neurons are quiescent, but nonetheless constantly consuming dopamine, in which case the concentrations of acidic metabolites would be uninformative about the rate of dopamine release (Commissiong 1985).

More definitive associations between dopamine turnover and metabolite levels can be obtained on the basis of radiotracer studies ex vivo. Analysis of temporal changes in the concentrations of [^{3}H]DOPA and FDOPA metabolites formed in rat striatum suggests that the rate of dopamine catabolism is determined in effect by its transit time through the insecure cytoplasmic compartment (Deep *et al.* 1997; Deep, Gjedde, & Cumming 1997). This argument furthermore suggests that newly formed dopamine is particularly at risk for catabolism, since it must run the gauntlet of MAO before finding refuge in vesicles. Thus, DOPAC, and by extension HVA, may properly be considered as indicators of the partitioning of dopamine between the vesicular and the cytosolic compartments, rather than as indicators of dopamine synthesis or utilization per se.

7.2.   Turnover of dopamine

The results of various steady-state estimates of dopamine kinetics are summarized in Table 7.1. The slope of the initial accumulation of dopamine in rat striatum after MAO treatment suggests a synthesis rate close to 1 nmol g^{-1} min^{-1} (Venero, Machado, & Cano 1991). The magnitude of this estimate exceeds the rate of accumulation of DOPA after NSD 1015 treatment, likely due to the failure of the latter method to correct for the diffusion of DOPA from brain. Turnover can also be calculated by monitoring the disappearance of dopamine after blockade of synthesis. During the several hours following blockade of TH with high doses of AMPT or its methyl ester (200 mg kg^{-1}, i.p.), the concentration of dopamine in rat brain undergoes a mono-exponential decline, with half-lives ranging from 30 to 150 min (Brodie *et al.* 1966). The rate constant for dopamine consumption after AMPT treatment was not identical in all brain regions; relative to the half-life in the striatum, turnover of dopamine was faster in the prefrontal cortex and slower in the olfactory tubercle (Galloway, Wolf, & Roth 1986). In this latter report, the product of the observed turnover rate constant and the steady-state dopamine concentration in the striatum predicts steady-state turnover of

Table 7.1. *Turnover of dopamine, its acidic metabolites, and some trace amines in rodent brain*

Measure	Rate constant (min^{-1})	Rate (nmol g^{-1} min^{-1})	Reference
Accumulation of dopamine after pargyline	0.005	330	Westerink & Spaan 1982a
Initial accumulation of dopamine after pargyline	0.015	950	Westerink, Bosker, & Wirix 1984
Clearance of DOPAC after pargyline	0.0048	310	
Formation of DOPA after NSD 1015	–	250	
Accumulation of dopamine after pargyline	0.017	1250	Venero, Machado, & Cano 1991
Accumulation of acidic metabolites after probenecid	–	190	Sarna, Hutson, & Curzon 1984
Accumulation of dopamine after pargyline 17-day-old rat	0.028	750	Crawford, McDougall, &
In the adult rat	0.019	850	Bardo 1994*
Disappearance of dopamine pool 1 after AMPT	0.077	1200	Doteuchi, Wang, & Costa 1974
Disappearance of dopamine pool 2 after AMPT	0.0056	270	
Disappearance of dopamine after AMPT	0.0055	300	Brodie *et al.* 1966
Disappearance of dopamine after AMPT	0.0057	440	Mignot & Laude 1985
Disappearance of dopamine after AMPT			
From striatum	0.0043	267	Nissbrandt, Pileblad,
From substantia nigra	0.023	120	& Carlsson 1985
Disappearance after AMPT of dopamine in perfusates	0.014	–	Leviel, Gobert, & Guibert 1989
Disappearance after AMPT of [^{3}H]dopamine formed from perfused [^{3}H]tyrosine	0.024	–	
Formation of [^{18}F]DOPAC from [^{18}F]dopamine formed after intravenous [^{18}F]DOPA	0.055	–	Cumming, Kuwabara, & Gjedde 1994
Formation of [^{3}H]DOPAC from tissue [^{3}H]dopamine after intravenous [^{3}H]DOPA	0.013	–	Cumming *et al.* 1995b
Formation of [^{3}H]DOPAC from [^{3}H]dopamine			Cumming *et al.* 1997a
Baseline	0.025	–	
After acute flupenthixol	0.10	–	
After acute apomorphine	0.003	–	
Formation of [^{3}H]DOPAC from [^{3}H]dopamine			Reith, Cumming, &
Baseline	0.043	–	Gjedde 1998
After dizocilpine	0.69	–	

Table 7.1. (*cont.*)

Measure	Rate constant (min^1)	Rate (nmol g^1 min^1)	Reference
Disappearance of noradrenaline in whole mouse brain after synthesis inhibition	0.095	30	Li, Warsh, & Godse 1984
Accumulation of phenylethylamine in whole rat brain after pargyline	1.7	25	Durden & Philips 1980
Accumulation of tyramine in whole rat brain after pargyline	2.5	4	

Note: Results were calculated by measuring the accumulation of substances after blockade of catabolism with the MAO inhibitor pargyline, or the declining concentrations of dopamine after blockade of synthesis with AMPT. Where possible, rate fraction constants are presented along with steady-state turnover estimates. In radiotracer studies, fractional rate constants were calculated from the product–precursor relationship. Unless otherwise indicated, results are per gram of whole rat striatum.
*Calculated as 10% protein by weight.

300–500 pmol g^{-1} min^{-1}, safely within the range of most estimates obtained by the several other methods for measuring dopamine turnover in the striatum.

When striatal dopamine concentrations were measured at brief intervals after TH inhibition with AMPT, a bi-exponential decline in dopamine concentration was evident in the striatum (Spector, Sjoerdsma, & Udenfriend 1965). This observation was interpreted to indicate the presence of two distinct pools of dopamine: a small pool comprising one quarter of the tissue dopamine with rapid turnover (half-life = 9 min), and a larger pool with much slower turnover (half-life = 124 min) (Javoy & Glowinski 1971). However, as usual for steady-state estimates, these results may be complicated by several factors, namely the caveats to the NSD 1015 method. Specifically, it cannot be assumed that TH inhibition in the brain is instantaneous and complete, because a high concentration of AMPT (95 μM) did not occur in the striatum until 40 min after AMPT treatment. Furthermore, substantial amounts of the sympathomimetic metabolites p-hydroxyamphetamine and p-hydroxynorephedrine are formed by the decarboxylation of AMPT in the striatum, an occurrence which seems likely to perturb dopamine turnover (Doteuchi, Wang, & Costa 1974).

Notwithstanding these reservations about the AMPT method, a large pool of dopamine with rapid turnover and a smaller pool with very slow turnover were observed in the substantia nigra, but were absent from the striatum of the same group of animals (Nissbrandt et al. 1989; Nissbrandt & Carlsson 1987). Thus, the claim of two storage compartments for dopamine is not consistently demonstrated in the striatum, but may be true in other brain regions. The available evidence is more consistent with the presence of a cytosolic/extracellular dopamine pool, which suffers a high rate of metabolism, and a non-labile vesicular compartment. In this scenario, the turnover of bulk dopamine is normally determined by the rate of transfer from the vesicular to the unbound pools, or by the transit of dopamine through the cytosol.

The lack of responsiveness of the DOPA synthesis rate in the substantia nigra to autoreceptor regulation has been noted above. Consistent with AAADC inhibition studies, the rate of decline in dopamine concentrations in the substantia nigra after AMPT treatment is not reduced by apomorphine, an autoreceptor agonist, nor is it accelerated by haloperidol, an antagonist (Nissbrandt *et al.* 1989).

7.3.   Turnover of the acidic metabolites

7.3.1.   *Transport mechanisms*

The dopamine acidic metabolites DOPAC and HVA (and the sole serotonin metabolite 5-hydroxyindoleacetic acid, 5-HIAA), if formed within neurons, must travel across neuronal membranes in order to enter the interstitial space. Because these compounds are highly charged at physiological pH, they are unlikely to cross membranes by simple diffusion. Depolarization of neurons with potassium ion greatly stimulates the release of dopamine in cat striatum, but decreases the extracellular concentrations of DOPAC and HVA to near zero. This finding suggests that the acidic dopamine metabolites are normally transported across the cell membrane in a manner driven by the resting membrane potential (Miyamoto, Uezu, & Terashima 1991), as has also been noted with 5-HIAA (Miyamoto *et al.* 1990). Addition of an inhibitor of the vacuolar H(+)-ATPase to the perfusion medium reduced the interstitial concentrations of the acidic metabolites in cat putamen (Miyamoto *et al.* 1993), also suggesting the occurrence of a transport mechanism.

On entering into the interstitial space, the acidic metabolites can diffuse into the CSF, and thence be carried to the choroid plexus for export into the blood, or can be transported directly across the blood–brain barrier. Efflux of these compounds into blood is mediated by the organic anion transporter type 3, which is located in the abluminal membrane of brain capillaries (Ohtsuki 2004). Probenecid is the prototypic inhibitor of transporters for organic anions in various tissues, and was formerly used to potentiate the action of penicillin by interfering with the otherwise rapid renal elimination. Transport of acidic neurotransmitter metabolites from the CSF is also inhibited by probenecid

(Sharman 1967). Indeed, there are considerable similarities in the pharmacology of acidic metabolite transport in the choroid plexus and kidney cortex (Huang & Wajda 1977).

A steroid metabolite has been found to be a substrate for the probenecid-sensitive transporter of organic anions and also for the multi-drug resistance associated protein in the choroid plexus (Nishino *et al.* 1999), suggesting that both processes are mediated by a common mechanism. Haloperidol and other antipsychotic drugs are among the many non-specific inhibitors of the efflux of the dopamine acidic metabolites from brain. Indeed, several antipsychotic compounds are potent inhibitors of the multi-drug resistance pump of tumor cells and the blood–brain barrier, which is mediated by a well-described glycoprotein (Szabo *et al.* 1999).

In principle, the turnover of dopamine acidic metabolites might be calculated from the rate of increase in their tissue concentrations after probenecid treatment, which blocks their efflux from the brain. However, probenecid was without great effect on the concentration of free DOPAC in the CSF (Elghozi, Mignot, & Le Quan-Bui 1983), the striatum (Dedek *et al.* 1979), or the interstitial fluid of the rat striatum (Cumming *et al.* 1992). This lack of effect of probenecid is due to the presence of alternate pathways for DOPAC elimination, i.e. conjugation and COMT. In contrast, interstitial 5-HIAA concentrations increased substantially after probenecid treatment, since there is no other route for disposal of 5-HIAA.

7.3.2.   *Efflux of acidic metabolites from brain*

A number of steady-state estimates for the clearance of the acidic dopamine metabolites are presented in Table 7.2. The concentrations of DOPAC and HVA both decline in brain tissue and in CSF after blockade of TH with AMPT (Mignot & Laude 1985). Assuming first-order kinetics, the linear regression slope of a semilog plot of the time–concentration series should give an estimate of the rate constant for elimination of these metabolites from the brain. However, due to the presence of a substantial reservoir of dopamine, the response of acidic metabolite concentrations to AMPT treatment is not immediate, but becomes evident after a delay of about 30 min. Consequently, DOPAC and HVA efflux rates estimated from the initial efflux occurring after blockade of dopamine synthesis with AMPT tend to underestimate the true rate.

There is a progressive decrease in the concentration of DOPAC (and HVA) in brain tissue and in the interstitial fluid following blockade of MAO with pargyline. Plotting the semilog plot of the DOPAC concentration as a function of time reveals the net rate constant of the first-order processes by which DOPAC is cleared from the brain in the steady-state, assuming that pargyline is without intrinsic effect on the rate of this clearance (Figure 7.1A, B). There is some evidence of an initial

Table 7.2. *Kinetics of DOPAC turnover in rat striatum*

Measure	Rate constant (min^{-1})	Rate (pmol g^{-1} min^{-1})	Reference
Clearance of DOPAC after AMPT	0.0054	35	Mignot & Laude 1985
Clearance of DOPAC after pargyline	0.10	600	Karoum, Neff, & Wyatt 1977
Clearance after pargyline	0.061	425	Westerink & Spaan 1982a
From olfactory tubercle	0.090	633	
From frontal cortex	0.041	13	
Clearance of free DOPAC	0.0015	10	Dedek *et al.* 1979
0-methylation of DOPAC	0.038	225	
Sulfoconjugation of DOPAC	0.016	95	
Elimination of DOPAC sulfate	0.027	93	
Total clearance			
Baseline	0.075	770	Nissbrandt & Carlsson 1987
After COMT inhibition	0.036	370	
Total clearance			
Young adult rat	0.052	475	Venero, Machado, & Cano 1991
Aged rat	0.055	352	
Total clearance			
17-day-old rat	0.084	–	Crawford, McDougall, & Bardo 1994
Young adult rat	0.095	–	
Total clearance from interstitial fluid	0.062	–	Cumming *et al.* 1992
After COMT inhibition	0.036	–	
Clearance from interstitial fluid	0.039	–	Data from Tuomainen, Tornwall, & Mannisto 1996
After pargyline and COMT inhibition	0.025	–	
Clearance rate constant of [^{3}H]DOPAC formed from [^{3}H]dopamine	0.052	–	Lippens *et al.* 1988
Formation rate constant of [^{3}H]HVA from [^{3}H]DOPAC	0.019	–	

Note: Declining concentrations of DOPAC in brain extracts or in microdialysates after pharmacological blockade of synthesis were used to estimate the rate constant and steady-state turnover of DOPAC. In some cases, simultaneous blockade of DOPAC synthesis with pargyline and blockade of metabolism with COMT inhibitors was used to separate the fractions of the several pathways for DOPAC elimination. Alternately, the temporal changes in the concentrations of radiolabeled metabolites formed in brain were used to estimate the rate constants.

rapid phase of DOPAC clearance after pargyline, suggesting that DOPAC may occur in distinct brain compartments (Francis *et al.* 1980). However, for most purposes, brain DOPAC is assumed to occupy a single compartment, such that whole brain and interstitial DOPAC concentrations are roughly similar. After pargyline treatment, the onset of declining HVA concentration measured in brain extracts was delayed by 30 min due the presence of a significant precursor pool of DOPAC in the brain (Westerink & Spaan 1982a), as can also be seen in striatal microdialysates after pargyline treatment (Figure 7.1A).

The rate constant for the tissue clearance of HVA was two-fold higher in rat limbic brain regions than in the cerebral cortex (Westerink & Spaan 1982a), indicating that the carrier for the acid metabolites is not uniformly distributed in the brain. This presents a further complication in the physiological interpretation of acid metabolite concentrations, since HVA levels at steady-state must reflect the composite effects of dopamine turnover, and also the inherent clearance properties of a particular brain region. As noted above, the rate constant for the elimination of DOPAC from the brain can be sensitive to drug treatments. Specifically, acute haloperidol ($1\,\text{mg}\,\text{kg}^{-1}$) decreased the rate constant for clearance of DOPAC from rat striatum and other brain regions by 40% (Westerink, Bosker, & Wirix 1984). Other treatments reducing the rate constant for the elimination of DOPAC from the basal ganglia include yohimbine, chloral hydrate, and cocaine (Westerink & Kikkert 1986), while reserpine increased the rate of DOPAC clearance from the CSF (Mignot, Laude, & Elghozi 1984). Consequently, it must be considered that pharmacological perturbation of metabolite clearance can sometimes change metabolite concentrations in a manner unrelated to the rate of dopamine synthesis or turnover per se.

What fraction of brain DOPAC is metabolized by COMT? The net rate of DOPAC clearance in extracts from striatum or substantia nigra was reduced by half when COMT was blocked with tropolone (Nissbrandt & Carlsson 1987; Westerink & Korf 1976). Similarly, the rate constant of the elimination of interstitial DOPAC after pargyline treatment was reduced by 50% in animals with concomitant COMT inhibition (Figure 7.1D) (Cumming *et al.* 1992). Thus, one half of DOPAC in rat striatum is normally directed to HVA synthesis, and the balance is conjugated to DOPAC-sulfate and/or eliminated directly from the brain by a probenecid-sensitive process (Figure 7.1B), although the magnitude of this latter process is probably low.

7.3.3.   *Conjugation of acidic metabolites*

The efflux of sulfoconjugated metabolites of DOPAC and HVA from the brain is also sensitive to probenecid (Sarna, Hutson, & Curzon 1984). Consequently, a laborious assay of free and conjugated acid metabolites would be necessary in

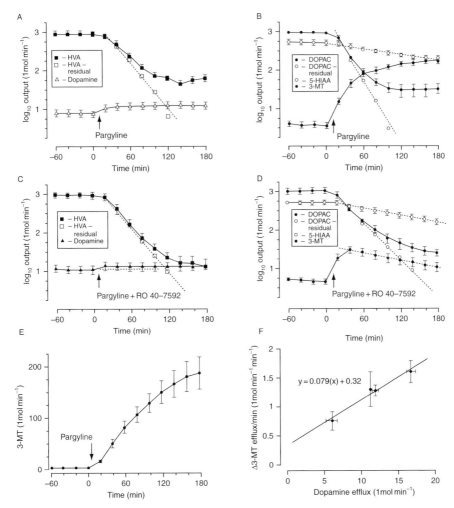

Figure 7.1 The effects of MAO and COMT inhibition on interstitial dopamine metabolite concentrations. Pargyline treatment results in exponential decline with time in the concentrations of (A) HVA and (B) DOPAC. Concomitant treatment with pargyline and a COMT inhibitor (C) does not alter the rate of HVA clearance, but (D) reduces DOPAC clearance by half, indicating the branching ratio for the metabolic fates of interstitial DOPAC. After MAO inhibition, there is (E) an initially linear increase with time in the 3MT concentration, which is (F) proportional to the individual interstitial dopamine concentration, indicating first-order kinetics for the activity of COMT with respect to dopamine. Redrafted from figures in Cumming *et al.* (1992).

order to account fully for the rate of acidic metabolite accumulation after probenecid treatment. In routine HPLC fractionation of brain extracts, the sulfate conjugates are not resolved from the solvent front, and so are only quantified if brain extracts are first hydrolyzed in hot sulfuric acid, releasing the free DOPAC and HVA. Due to this technical requirement, the importance of conjugation pathways for elimination of DOPAC and HVA from the brain has often been overlooked.

In experiments with probenecid treatment and COMT inhibition, the temporal changes in the concentrations of free and conjugated acidic metabolites can reveal the rate constants for each possible step of the pathway (Dedek, Gomeni, & Korf 1979; Dedek et al. 1979). These results indicate that almost one half of DOPAC and HVA are conjugated prior to elimination from the brain. In general, assays of the accumulation of HVA in the striatum after probenecid predict a dopamine turnover rate at the lower end of the range of estimates obtained by other methods (Table 7.1). However, the inhibition by probenecid of the efflux of acidic metabolites need not be instantaneous and complete (Karoum, Neff, & Wyatt 1977). After treatment with probenecid, the concentrations of conjugates in rat CSF increased twice as fast as did the concentrations of the free acidic compounds (Curzon et al. 1985), suggesting that the rate of elimination of the sulfates is more rapid than for the free acids. Thus, low steady-state concentrations of conjugates in the brain need not indicate low flux of dopamine and its metabolites through the conjugation pathway. It must also be considered that probenecid treatment can perturb the system by increasing exposure of the acidic metabolites to the arylsulfotransferase (Curzon et al. 1986). However, in the case of the serotonin acidic metabolite 5-HIAA, the rate of accumulation in rat striatum after probenecid was identical to the rate of disappearance after pargyline, indicating a single pathway for elimination of unconjugated metabolite (Cumming et al. 1992; Neff & Tozer 1968).

7.3.4.   Cerebrospinal fluid metabolites

The assay of acid metabolites in the CSF was formerly an important method for obtaining insight into the integrity of dopamine transmission in the brain of living humans. Thus, for example, the concentration of HVA was elevated in CSF collected from patients with psychosis as compared to healthy control subjects (Bowers, Heninger, & Gerbode 1969), providing early evidence for enhanced dopamine transmission in schizophrenia. There was a general concordance between the concentration of dopamine and HVA in CSF from the lateral ventrical and the concentrations in the striatum from the same post mortem human specimens (Wester et al. 1990). Human CSF is generally sampled by lumbar puncture, i.e. spatially removed from the site of formation in the brain. Whereas there was no effect of age on CSF HVA levels in a large sample of neurologically normal subjects, there was an inverse correlation between height and the HVA levels (Blennow et al. 1993). This phenomenon presumably reflects the longer diffusion path from the source in the telencephalon to the point of sampling. In support of this proposal, the presence of a rostral-caudal gradient in the concentrations of DOPAC and HVA has been formally demonstrated in canine CSF (Vaughn *et al.* 1988).

The concentrations of DOPAC and HVA in rat CSF respond in predictable ways to a pharmacological challenge (haloperidol) stimulating dopamine metabolism (Mignot, Laude, & Elghozi 1984), suggesting that CSF can indeed provide a surrogate marker for the activity of central dopamine neurons. Nonetheless, lumbar CSF from patients with Parkinson's disease did not reveal a decline in HVA levels (Gonzalez-Quevedo *et al.* 1993), consistent perhaps with the elevated turnover of residual dopamine in that condition. However, results of a study in rats show that HVA levels in cisternal CSF reflects the whole brain metabolism of dopamine, rather than exclusively the contribution of the nigrostriatal system (Hutson & Curzon 1986).

7.4.   3-Methoxytyramine

7.4.1.   *General aspects of 3MT*

In the interstitial fluid, the 3MT concentration is tightly coupled to the prevailing concentration of interstitial dopamine. Specifically, concentrations of DA and 3MT increase in parallel after stimulation of dopamine release with haloperidol or amphetamine, and decline after inhibition of dopamine release with γ-butyrolactone or tetrodotoxin (Brown *et al.* 1991). These results show that the majority of interstitial 3MT in the striatum is formed from dopamine upon its release from nigrostriatal fibers. The concentration of 3MT in rat striatum is normally much lower than that of DOPAC and HVA. Even so, the effects of post mortem metabolism can lead to substantial overestimation of the steady-state 3MT concentration in tissue, unless rapid microwave fixation is used (Westerink & Spaan 1982b). Indeed, the concentration of 3MT in human brain increases linearly with the post mortem interval, such that its concentration could in principle be used forensically to help determine the time of death (Sparks, Slevin, & Hunsaker, 1986).

7.4.2.   *Blockade of 3MT synthesis and metabolism*

It was originally supposed that catechol substrates were metabolized by COMT within the extracellular milieu (Axelrod & Tomchick 1958), but this need not be the case if there is rapid exchange of dopamine and 3MT between the cellular site of metabolism and the interstitial fluid. When COMT is blocked with potent inhibitors, the concentrations of 3MT in extracts from the striatum (Westerink & Spaan 1982a), and in the interstitial fluid (Cumming *et al.* 1992),

Table 7.3. *Turnover of 3MT in rat brain*

Measure	Rate constant (min^{-1})	Rate (pmol g^{-1} min^{-1})	Reference
Formation from dopamine in the striatum after pargyline	0.0018	125	Westerink & Spaan 1982b
Formation from dopamine after pargyline			
In striatum	0.0011	103	Nissbrandt & Carlsson
In substantia nigra	0.0074	503	1987
Accumulation in striatum after pargyline		133	Nissbrandt *et al.* 1989
+ haloperidol treatment		400	
+ GBL pretreatment		0	
Accumulation during the first 2.5 min after pargyline		296	Di Giulio *et al.* 1978
The first 10 min		114	
The first 60 min		85	
Disappearance during initial 5 min after COMT inhibition	0.30	32	Westerink & Spaan 1982b
Formation of [^{3}H]3MT from [^{3}H]dopamine			
In tissue	0.0029		Lippens *et al.* 1988
Or interstitial space	0.056		
Formation from interstitial dopamine after pargyline	0.079		Cumming *et al.* 1992
Elimination from interstitial fluid after COMT inhibition	0.0075		

Note: Unless otherwise indicated, results were obtained from whole tissue concentrations measured in striatum.

decline to undetectable amounts within minutes, presumably due to the action of MAO in some post-synaptic compartment. Conversely, there is a time-dependant increase in the concentration of 3MT in interstitial fluid of the rat striatum (Figure 7.1B) and in whole tissue extracts following MAO inhibition.

Some estimates of the turnover of 3MT in brain extracts and microdialysates are presented in Table 7.3. The rate of accumulation of interstitial 3MT after inhibition of MAO-A with the relatively selective inhibitor clorgyline was somewhat less than that observed after pargyline treatment, indicating that interstitial 3MT is a substrate for both forms of MAO (Segal, Kuczenski, & Okuda 1992). However, 1 h after treatment with clorgyline, the interstitial concentrations of DOPAC and HVA in rat striatum had declined to nearly zero, indicating that MAO-B does not normally contribute to the bulk of dopamine catabolism, at least in the rodent. The interstitial 3MT which had accumulated after pargyline treatment declined slowly when further synthesis was blocked by COMT inhibition, reflecting a minor diffusion or conjugation process contributing to the establishment of steady-state extracellular 3MT concentrations (Cumming *et al.* 1992).

In accordance with the principles of steady-state kinetics, the accumulation of 3MT after pargyline treatment can be used to calculate the kinetics of 3MT turnover. The apparent rate of this accumulation declines progressively with increasing duration of MAO inhibition, consistent with the rapid onset of feedback inhibition of dopamine synthesis (Di Giulio *et al.* 1978). Nonetheless, steady-state turnover of 3MT has been estimated from the accumulation during 30 min after pargyline treatment (Westerink & Spaan 1982b). This procedure may likely have resulted in underestimation of the basal 3MT synthesis rate if feedback inhibition of dopamine synthesis and release had indeed already occurred, as is suggested by close examination of Figure 7.1B, in which the slope declines at late times after MAO inhibition.

The rate of 3MT accumulation in striatal microdialysates during the initial 30 min after pargyline treatment occurred as a first-order process (0.08 min^{-1}; Figure 7.1F) relative to the interstitial dopamine concentration (Cumming *et al.* 1992). Nearly identical results were obtained for the rate constant of interstitial [^{3}H]3MT formation relative to the interstitial [^{3}H]dopamine concentrations (Lippens *et al.* 1988). However, the magnitude of this rate constant was much higher than when calculated relative to the total tissue [^{3}H]dopamine concentration, further emphasizing the importance of compartmentation of dopamine with respect to the formation of 3MT.

The initial accumulation of 3MT measured in extracts of rat striatum after pargyline treatment is approximately one third of the total rate of DOPAC turnover. It follows that the 3MT pathway should account for about one third of the total dopamine consumption in the striatum (Westerink & Spaan 1982b). However, results of a microdialysis study with MAO and COMT inhibition suggest that formation of 3MT accounts for only 5% of the total metabolite turnover (Cumming *et al.* 1992). This discrepancy is doubtless due to the relative contributions of COMT to dopamine metabolism in intracellular and interstitial compartments. Ignoring the contribution of dopamine sulfation, the total dopamine turnover in the striatum should equal the sum of the rates of turnover for DOPAC and 3MT (approximately 600 pmol g^{-1} min^{-1}), a figure which corresponds well with diverse other estimates of dopamine turnover in the striatum.

The rate of accumulation of 3MT after pargyline treatment is greater in the *substantia nigra* than in the striatum (Nissbrandt, Pileblad, & Carlsson 1985), perhaps reflecting the relatively weak dependence of local dopamine release upon depolarization. Results of dopamine depletion studies with AMPT reveal that 3MT formation is a major route for dopamine catabolism in the *substantia nigra*. However, the coupling between amphetamine-evoked dopamine release and increased interstitial 3MT concentrations was much less evident in the *substantia nigra* than in the striatum (Elverfors *et al.* 1997). These findings suggest that 3MT is indeed formed inside dendrites and soma of the dopamine neurons, in contrast to the terminal fields, where 3MT seems to be formed after dopamine release.

Pharmacological blockade of COMT is without great effect on the interstitial concentration of dopamine in rat striatum under baseline conditions (Cumming *et al.* 1992). However, the elevation in dopamine overflow in the rat striatum following blockade of dopamine reuptake is clearly potentiated by co-administration of tolcapone, a COMT inhibitor acting on the central nervous system (Budygin *et al.* 1999). Thus, COMT subserves a default pathway for striatal dopamine catabolism, attaining a particular importance in the handling of phasic increases in dopamine release. Electrochemistry studies in COMT knockout mice show that 50% of dopamine in prefrontal cortex is normally cleared by COMT (Yavich *et al.* 2007). Based on its particular importance in the regulation of cortical dopamine, COMT is emerging as a molecular target for treatment of cognitive dysfunction in patients with schizophrenia (Apud & Weinberger 2007).

8

MAO activity in the brain

8.1. Enzymology

The oxidative deamination of dopamine and other monoamines is catalyzed by two distinct forms of MAO with high sequence homology (MAO-A, MAO-B), the genes of which have both been localized to nearby bands on the X-chromosome (Kochersperger *et al.* 1986). The deduced amino acid sequences for the enzymes expressed in human liver predict molecular weights close to 59 000 for both forms, and contain a C-terminus alpha helix which is the likely site of fixation in membranes (Bach *et al.* 1988). The two genes share considerable homology and have the same intron–exon structure, suggesting an ancient duplication event of the ancestral gene (Grimsby *et al.* 1991). Consistent with their ancient origin, the amino acid sequences have considerable homology across species, especially in the domain containing the cystein residue which binds the prosthetic flavin adenine dinucleotide (FAD) (Kwan, Bergeron, & Abell 1992). The pure enzyme is devoid of iron or other transition metal ions. The catalytic cycle for MAO involves the successive binding of the amine substrate and oxygen, followed by liberation of the aldehyde product and equimolar amounts of ammonia and hydrogen peroxide. In general, the aldehyde produced by MAO is immediately oxidized further by non-specific enzymes, yielding a carboxylic acid, hence the acidic metabolites of dopamine. The production of (toxic) hydrogen peroxide may be problematic under certain circumstances, especially given the location of MAO in the outer mitochondrial membrane. Thus, for example, the oxidation deamination of tyramine can cause oxidative damage to mitochondrial DNA in vitro (Hauptmann *et al.* 1996).

The acetylenic drugs clorgyline, deprenyl, and pargyline constitute an important class of irreversible inhibitors of MAO. Whereas low concentrations of clorgyline are largely specific for MAO-A, low concentrations of deprenyl preferentially block MAO-B. The selectivities of acetylinic compounds are derived from the dissociation kinetics of the reversible substrate–enzyme complex. Consequently, under saturating conditions in vitro, substrate specificity is not absolute (Tipton & Mantle 1981). Although pargyline has a certain preference for MAO-B, high concentrations completely and irreversibly block both isozymes. Although there is a reversible phase of binding (as in the case of organophosphate insecticides binding to acetylcholinerterase), these MAO suicide substrates subsequently form reactive imine products, which ultimately form a covalent, irreversible adduct to a flavin ring-nitrogen (Singer & Salach 1981) thus killing the enzyme. Inhibition of MAO is complete and permanent with the incorporation of isomolar amounts of the suicide substrates.

The two types of MAO have been distinguished on the basis of substrate preferences (Schoepp & Azzaro 1981b). Serotonin and noradrenaline are the preferred substrates for MAO-A, but the trace amine phenylethylamine is the preferred substrate for MAO-B (Yang & Neff 1973), at least under non-saturating conditions (Table 8.1). The catabolism of dopamine and tyramine

Table 8.1. *Some kinetic properties of MAO in vitro*

MAO-A		MAO-B		
V_{max} ($\mu mol\,g^{-1}\,min^{-1}$)	K_d (μM)	V_{max} ($\mu mol\,g^{-1}\,min^{-1}$)	K_d (μM)	Reference
				Synaptosome preparation, with dopamine substrate (Azzaro *et al.* 1985)
2	120	0.6	300	Rat striatum
0.9	390	2.3	400	Guinea pig striatum
0.6	160	1.7	180	Human caudate
				Synaptosome preparation, with rat striatum (Schoepp & Azzaro 1981b)
0.4	78	1.1	5.6	Phenylethylamine substrate
2.0	120	0.6	300	Dopamine substrate
2.1	66	1.1	160	Tyramine substrate
130	120	30	340	Rat forebrain homogenate, with dopamine substrate* (Fowler & Benedetti 1983)
70	180	10	1200	Rat brain homogenate, with serotonin substrate (Fowler & Tipton 1982)
170		50		Homogenate, young rat striatum*
120		60		Homogenate, aged rat striatum* (Leung *et al.*, 1981)

Note: *Velocity calculated assuming 10 % protein wet weight.

is catalyzed equally by both MAO isozymes. However, the activities of MAO type A and B with respect to dopamine can be assayed separately after selective inhibition of one isozyme or another, when measured in the presence of appropriate concentrations of clorgyline or deprenyl.

The preponderant activity with respect to dopamine is MAO-A in the rat brain, but is MAO-B in striatum from human or guinea pig (Azzaro *et al.* 1985). The majority of type A and B activities are present outside of dopamine neurons (Demarest, Smith, & Azzaro 1980), which need not indicate that dopamine catabolism occurs only after release. Indeed, the selective inhibition of MAO-A with clorgyline decreases the rate of dopamine synthesis in slices of rat striatum, whereas similar concentrations of deprenyl are without effect (Schoepp & Azzaro 1981a). This suggests that MAO-A within dopamine neurons is the major factor in the regulation of intraneuronal dopamine concentration. However, the post-synaptic metabolism of [^{3}H]dopamine by both types of the enzyme becomes more important under conditions of augmented dopamine release in striatal slices (Schoepp & Azzaro 1982). Furthermore, lesion studies with kainic acid indicate that HVA is formed in post-synaptic neurons, while the greater part of DOPAC formation occurs within the dopamine fibers.

The greater activity of MAO-B in human brain has often been taken to indicate that dopamine metabolism must be catalyzed mainly by this enzyme. However, enzyme activities are usually measured in homogenates in which the normal compartmentation of brain dopamine is absent. Thus, it is not proven that MAO-B isozyme is more important for striatal dopamine metabolism in humans than in rats. Indeed, the CSF concentration of HVA was reduced by 30% in humans treated with clorgyline and by 65% in patients treated with pargyline, suggesting that both MAO forms normally contribute to dopamine metabolism (Major *et al.* 1979).

8.2.   Neurochemical anatomy of MAO

Selective antisera recognize MAO-B within serotonin neurons and astroglia of rat brain (Levitt, Pintar, & Breakefield 1982). The cellular distribution of MAO in brain can also be demonstrated by a histochemical procedure in which the hydrogen peroxide produced by oxidative deamination of a substrate is coupled to the reduction of a dye (Graham & Karnovsky 1965). Using tyramine as a substrate, specific groups of cell bodies are then labeled, specifically the hypothalamic magnocellular histamine neurons, the noradrenergic locus coeruleus and other adrenergic or noradrenergic cell groups of the pons and medulla, and in mesencephalic serotonin neurons, but not in the *substantia nigra* (Arai, Kimura, & Maeda 1986). Using MPTP as an MAO-B selective substrate, intense histochemical staining was restricted to the magnocellular histamine neurons of the hypothalamus, and serotonin neurons of the dorsal raphe nucleus, but staining of dopamine neurons was notably absent (Vincent 1989). Analgous techniques have detected MAO-A in the dopamine neurons (Demarest, Smith, & Azzaro 1980). Generally consistent with the histological methods, in situ hybridization techniques have detected the mRNA for MAO-A in the locus ceruleus and other monoaminergic cells of the brainstem and the substantia nigra, while high concentrations of MAO-B expression had more restricted distribution in the serotonin neurons of the dorsal raphe (Jahng *et al.* 1997).

The ultrastructural distribution of MAO-B has been examined by electron microscopy in transgenic mice lacking MAO-A. Fibers histologically stained for MAO-B formed axodendritic synapses, which were notably concentrated in the shell of the nucleus accumbens (Ikemoto *et al.* 1997). Injection of kainic acid to the striatum destroys the resident interneurons and projection neurons, while relatively sparing glia and afferent fibers. Several days after this lesion, the oxidation deamination of [^{3}H]dopamine by both forms of MAO in brain slices declined, indicating that post-synaptic neuronal metabolism can indeed occur. Following proliferation of glia after kainic acid lesions, the activity of MAO-B increased in the lesioned tissue (Schoepp & Azzaro 1983), suggesting the glia are the likely site for generation of the toxic MPTP metabolite MPP+.

8.3.   Effects of MAO inhibition and knockout on dopamine transmission

Blockade of MAO-A with clorgyline did not alter the baseline or cocaine-evoked increases in interstitial dopamine concentration in the rat nucleus accumbens, although basal noradrenaline levels were increased (Pepper *et al.* 2001). However, blockade of MAO-A with the competitive inhibitor harmine greatly potentiated the amphetamine-evoked dopamine release in rat striatum (Iurlo *et al.* 2001). Mice not expressing MAO-B and wild-type mice had similar concentrations of dopamine in microdialysis samples of the extracellular space in striatum (Chen *et al.* 1999), and the effects of cocaine or DOPA treatment on interstitial dopamine levels were similar in the two strains (Fornai *et al.* 1999). Thus, MAO-B does not normally contribute to the catabolism of dopamine formed from exogenous DOPA in normal mouse striatum.

The β-carboline harmine selectively inhibits MAO-A at nM concentrations. Harmine has a long history in the context of ethnopharmacology, being one of the key active constituents of *ayahuasca*, an infusion of plants containing primarily *N,N*-dimethyl-tryptamine (DMT) from *Psychotria sp.*, and harmine from *Banisteriopsis caapi* (Riba *et al.* 2003), which is employed in Amerindian visionary rituals. Potentiation of the weak hallucinogenic action of methyltryptamines by concomitant MAO inhibition has been attributed to blockade of extensive first-pass metabolism of DMT by MAO in the gut (McKenna, Towers, & Abbott 1984).

8.4.   Disorders of MAO and knockouts

Constitutive absence of MAO has consequences for post-synaptic aspects of dopamine transmission. Thus, the concentration of dopamine D_2 receptors was elevated in striatum of MAO-B knockout, while D_1 density was unchanged (Chen *et al.* 1999). However, the induction of *c-fos* expression in nucleus accumbens by the dopamine D_1 agonist SKF 38 393 was greatly enhanced in the MAO-B knockouts. The authors suggested that altered sensitivity of dopamine receptors could be responses to the psychostimulant trace amine phenylethylamine, which is greatly elevated in MAO-B deficient mice (Grimsby *et al.* 1997).

The activity of MAO-A in rat brain decreases with aging, whereas MAO-B activity was unchanged (Leung *et al.* 1981). In contrast, MAO-B activity is generally increased in post mortem brain of aged humans (see, e.g., Ballesteros *et al.* 2008), which presumably reflects proliferation of astrocytes. Mice with targeted overexpression of MAO-B activity specifically induced in astrocytes had a progressive loss of dopamine neurons and revealed several indicators of oxidative stress (Mallajosyula *et al.* 2008). Despite the obvious association with MPTP-toxicity, cerebral MAO-B activity in idiopathic Parkinson's disease remains poorly documented.

The two MAO genes map to the same region of the X-chromosome as Norrie disease, an uncommon recessive disorder characterized by retinal blindness (Lan *et al.* 1989). The complex phenotype of Norrie disease can include mental retardation, and severe behavioral disorders. Psychiatric disorders and reduced MAO activity have been noted in female carriers of the Norrie deletion without presenting mental retardation (Collins *et al.* 1992). Although the absent Norrie protein causes the phenotype of blindness, a concomitant MAO deficiency may contribute to the behavioral syndrome of Norrie disease. MAO-B knockout mice are behaviorally normal in contrast to MAO-A knockout mice, which are highly aggressive (Shih, Chen, & Ridd 1999). Similarly, humans with deletion of MAO-B are clinically nearly normal (except for high urinary levels of phenylethylamine), whereas deficiency of MAO-A results in cognitive disfunction and poor impulse control (Lenders *et al.* 1996). A GT repeat polymorphism in the second intron of MAO-B was strongly associated with the Parkinson's disease phenotype (odds ratio 4.6) in a cohort of 200 Australians (Mellick *et al.* 1999), but genetic associations were more compex and subtle in a subsequent polymorphism study (Kang *et al.* 2006).

8.5.   MAO activity in vivo

8.5.1.   *Irreversible MAO ligands*

The first molecular imaging studies of MAO made use of the irreversible ligand [^{11}C]deprenyl. Ignoring the presence of labeled metabolites entering from the blood, the concentration of radioactivity in brain tissue measured by PET consists of the free [^{11}C]deprenyl which reversibly diffuses across the capillary epithelium, and the pool of tracer which has irreversibly bound to the enzyme, at a rate determined by the rate constant k_3. Thus, [^{11}C]deprenyl kinetics in living brain closely resemble the circumstances described earlier for [^{11}C]tyrosine. Consequently, the net clearance of [^{11}C]deprenyl from blood to brain (K_{in}^{app}, ml g^{-1} min^{-1}) can be calculated as a function of the metabolite-corrected arterial input using a linear graphical analysis. [^{11}C]Deprenyl is rapidy metabolized in peripheral tissues, so the untranformed fraction in plasma extracts must be determined in plasma extracts collected at intervals during the PET recording. An intermediate in the plasma metabolism of [^{11}C]deprenyl is [^{11}C]methamphetamine (Cumming *et al.* 1999), the entry of which into the brain may conceivably bias the calculation of MAO-B activity in PET studies of living brain.

As noted above, the covalent binding of [^{11}C]deprenyl to MAO-B in the brain is catalyzed by the enzyme itself. Consequently, the rate of association of free [^{11}C] deprenyl to specific binding sites in the brain (k_3) is proportional to the enzyme activity with respect to the labeled substrate (V_{max}). In principle, a two-compartment model could be fitted to the [^{11}C]deprenyl time–activity curve in the brain, in order to obtain separate estimates of the reversible blood–brain clearance (K_1), the efflux from the brain (k_2), and the rate constant for irreversible binding in the brain (k_3, min^{-1}). However, the magnitude of K_1 for [^{11}C]deprenyl is close to 0.3 ml g^{-1} min^{-1} in the anesthetized baboon (Arnett *et al.* 1987), and in whole human brain (Lammertsma *et al.* 1991); relative to the magnitude of cerebral blood flow (0.5 ml g^{-1} min^{-1}), this corresponds to an extraction fraction of 60%. Thus, unlike the cases of the amino acids [^{11}C] tyrosine and FDOPA, which have extraction fractions less than 10%, the magnitude of the cerebral blood flow (0.5 ml g^{-1} min^{-1}) the majority of [^{11}C]deprenyl entering the cerebral circulation is deposited in the brain. Compartmental modeling of [^{11}C]deprenyl uptake gave estimates of k_3 ranging in magnitude from 0.22 min^{-1} in cerebral cortex to

$0.53\,\mathrm{min}^{-1}$ in the basal ganglia (Lammertsma *et al.* 1991), i.e. ten-fold faster than corresponding estimates of AAADC activity with respect to FDOPA.

In spite of its pharmacological specificity, [^{11}C]deprenyl resembles a perfect blood flow tracer, since most of the tracer entering the brain is irreversibly trapped by MAO-B, which is nearly ubiquitous. Its rapid unidirectional blood–brain clearance and its very rapid binding in the brain makes it very difficult to estimate k_3, the parameter specifically related to MAO-B activity in the brain. Consequently, changes in the net blood–brain clearance of [^{11}C]deprenyl could indicate altered cerebral blood flow or altered MAO-B activity. The apparent magnitude of the [^{11}C]deprenyl V_e (i.e. K_1/k_2) increased by 50% after pargyline treatment (Bench *et al.* 1991). It is unlikely that the pargyline treatment could itself have altered the partitioning of [^{11}C]deprenyl between brain and blood. Instead, this result suggests that, in the unblocked condition, the rate of clearance of tracer from the brain (k_2) was over-estimated at the expense of under-estimation of the true rate of binding in the brain (k_3). This presents an example of the problem of over-specification of a kinetic model, especially exacerbated due to the nearly complete trapping of [^{11}C]deprenyl in living brain.

For the above kinetic reasons, it would be very difficult to detect increases in MAO activity with [^{11}C]deprenyl-PET. However, the effects of MAO inhibition are easy to detect. Pretreatment of the baboons or humans with a single dose of non-radioactive deprenyl decreased the magnitudes of $K_{in}{}^{app}$ and k_3 by as much as 90%. The competition in vivo against the uptake of [^{11}C]deprenyl can thus be used to test the potency of new MAO inhibitors. By this means, the dose–response relationship of the reversible MAO inhibitor Ro 19-6327 was measured in the brain of normal volunteers (Bench *et al.* 1991) and in patients with Parkinson's disease (Fowler *et al.* 1993).

In principle, the precision of the estimate of the [^{11}C]deprenyl k_3 might be improved by constraining the magnitude of K_1/k_2 to the value measured after complete blockade of MAO. However, this procedure would require conducting two complete PET studies in each subject. Use of a [^{11}C]deprenyl derivative with an inherently lower k_3 could provide a more practical method than the approach employing serial radiotracer injections, in the blocked and unblocked conditions. Substitution of deuterium for hydrogen in the α-carbon of deprenyl results in an isotope effect, which substantially lowers the catalytic rate of covalent bond formation between the substrate and enzyme (Fowler *et al.* 1988). The high initial uptake of deuterated [^{11}C]deprenyl in the brain is followed by a partial washout phase due to the much slower irreversible association with MAO (Bergstrom *et al.* 1998). As a consequence, net blood–brain clearance of this tracer in different brain regions maps the MAO-B distribution in brain, without undue weighting to the local cerebral perfusion rate.

Suicide substrates irreversibly poison MAO. The gradual return of MAO activity following irreversible inhibition requires de novo synthesis of the enzyme, and is thus an indicator of the turnover for the enzyme in vivo. Thus, the MAO activity with respect to tyramine in homogenates from rat striatum returns to normal levels with a half-life of 13 days following irreversible blockade (Goridis & Neff 1971). Sequential PET scanning of baboons with [^{11}C]deprenyl over a period of months after deprenyl intoxication indicated a half-life for MAO-B of 30 days (Arnett *et al.* 1987). In humans, treatment with the irreversible MAO-B blocker rasagiline likewise resulted in a complete blockade of the specific binding of [^{11}C]deprenyl, which had returned half-way to baseline levels at two weeks after cessation of the treatment (Freedman *et al.* 2005). The half-life of MAO in catfish hypothalamus decreased from 22 to 12 days during spawning (Senthilkumaran & Joy 1995), indicating a seasonal and steroidal regulation of MAO expression, at least in bony fish.

[^{11}C]Clorgyline has been employed for PET studies of MAO-A (Fowler *et al.* 1987); its irreversible binding in human brain, like that of [^{11}C]deprenyl, was blocked by pretreatment with the non-specific MAO inhibitor phenelzine. [^{11}C]Clorgyline and [^{11}C]deprenyl PET were used to test for possible action of a *Ginko biloba* extract at MAO in human brain (Fowler *et al.* 2000), but the treatment was without effect on either form of MAO. Based upon the experience with [^{11}C]deprenyl, a deuterated form of [^{11}C]clorgyline has also be prepared and tested (Fowler *et al.* 2001). As expected, the deuterium substitution reduced the rate of association to MAO-A, but this effect was most noticeable in gray matter of human brain. A non-MAO-binding component in the white matter of the brain seemed resistant to the effect of deuterium substitution. Due to concerns about its specificity, [^{11}C]clorgyline has not found wide use in PET studies.

8.5.2.   Reversible MAO ligands

As an alternative to the irreversible ligands, β-carbolines such as harman are potent, reversible inhibitors of MAO-A in rat brain (May, Rommelspacher, & Pawlik 1991). [^{11}C]Harmine binds to rat brain cryostat sections with an apparent affinity of 2 nM, and in a manner inhibited by other selective MAO-A inhibitors. Likewise, the net influx of this tracer to normal baboon was substantially reduced by pretreatment with selective MAO inhibitors (Bergstrom, Westerberg, & Langstrom 1997). Competitive PET binding studies with [^{11}C]harmine have been used to test the efficacy of single doses of novel MAO-A inhibitors in healthy volunteers (Bergstrom *et al.* 1997).

[^{11}C]Harmine is metabolized very rapidly in plasma of living pig, such that only 10% of the plasma radioactivity is untransformed tracer at times after 30 min (Figure 8.1A). The [^{11}C]harmine V_d at equilibrium can be calculated using linear analysis with the Logan arterial input plot (Figure 8.1B), which shows the

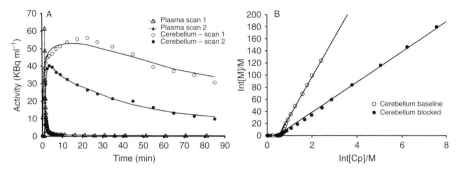

Figure 8.1 Plasma and cerebral kinetics of [^{11}C]harmine in the pig. (A) The concentration of untransformed [^{11}C]harmine in plasma declines very rapidly due to metabolism and distribution, whereas there is a substantial accumulation in the cerebellum, only partially blocked by MAO inhibition (scan 2). Imperfect fitting to the data measured at baseline is likely due to imprecision in the vanishing small arterial input of untransformed tracer. (B) Replotting of the same data by the arterial input Logan method shows that the condition of equilibrium binding is obtained in the blocked and unblocked conditions, and that the linearization procedure can accommodate the vanishing arterial input, as indicated by the linear fitting.

rapid occurrence of a linear phase indicating a state of equilibrium binding. However, the magnitude of the estimate of equilibrium V_d is vulnerable to imprecision in the arterial input. This rapid plasma metabolism requires particular attention to the HPLC analysis of plasma extracts collected during the PET recording. Mean voxel-wise parametric maps of [^{11}C]harmine equilibrium V_e in a group of five pigs are illustrated in Figure 8.2. The brain concentration relative to that plasma is high throughout brain, but reveals "hot spots" of high MAO-A binding in specific structures, such as the ventral forebrain and the thalamus. Blocking MAO with pargyline shows that substantial specific [^{11}C]harmine binding is present throughout the brain, consistent with the known ubiquity of MAO-A.

Due to the presence of substantial MAO-A activity throughout the brain, reference tissue methods are unsuited for the quantitation of [^{11}C]harmine binding. However, the magnitude of equilibrium V_d in the blocked condition can be used to calculate the specific binding in the unblocked condition. The sum of the non-specific and specific equilibrium V_d for any reversibly binding ligand is defined as $[K_1/k_2 (1 + k_3/k_4)]$, where k_3 is the association rate constant to the binding site, and k_4 the dissociation rate constant. When k_3 is blocked with pargyline, the [^{11}C]harmine V_e then declines to K_1/k_2. If assumed to be constant throughout brain, and if the pargyline treatment did not otherwise perturb the partitioning of the tracer between blood and brain, the observation of equilibrium V_d in the blocked condition can be used to calculate the magnitude of k_3/k_4

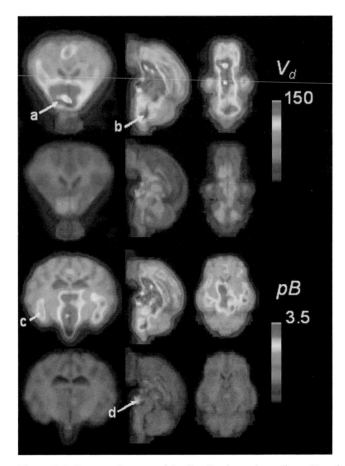

Figure 8.2 Parametric maps of the distribution volume (here, V_d, $ml\,g^{-1}$) and binding potential (pB) for $[^{11}C]$harmine in the brain of Göttingen minipigs. Each image is the mean of five separate determinations in the untreated condition and after acute pargyline treatment, co-registered to the common stereotaxic MR coordinates (grey scale). Relative to the V_d maps [$X=0$, $Y=-15$, $Z=20$], the pB maps [$X=0$, $Y=-5$, $Z=7$] are shown in planes 13 mm posterior and 10 mm ventral. Zones of particular interest are indicated as follows: (a) the ventral forebrain, (b) vicinity of the locus coeruleus, (c) the amygdala and hippocampal formation, and (d) the pituitary gland. Reproduced with permission from Jensen *et al.* (2006). (For color version, see plate section.)

in the unblocked condition, i.e the specific binding. This unitless parameter, commonly known as the binding potential (pB), is in the present context an index of the total number of MAO molecules, relative to the affinity of MAO for the ligand,

$$pB = \frac{k_3}{k_4} = \frac{B_{max}[C]}{K_d + [C]}$$

where B_{max} and K_d are the Michaelis–Menten saturation binding parameters, and [C] is the concentration of the ligand in the brain. In most PET studies, this ligand concentration is vanishingly small, so the measured pB approaches the simple ratio of B_{max}/K_d. In the case of [^{11}C]harmine, the k_3 is proportional to the *number* of MAO binding sites, as distinct from the case of [^{11}C]deprenyl, where it is the enzyme catalytic activity which determines the magnitude of k_3 (enzyme number and activity need not be related in a simple manner). Parametric maps of [^{11}C]harmine pB so calculated are shown in Figure 8.2. They contain the same information as do the original equilibrium V_e maps, but have effectively removed the non-specific binding component from the picture.

As an alternative to [^{11}C]harmine, the selective and reversible ligand [^{11}C]befloxatine has been developed for PET studies MAO-A. The great majority of the uptake of [^{11}C]befloxatine in brain of living baboon could be blocked by pretreatment with excess non-radioactive befloxatine (Bottlaender *et al.* 2003). Yet another possibility is presented by the MAO-A ligand [^{11}C]ROMAO, which has slow plasma metabolism and favourable kinetics in brain of living pigs (Jensen *et al.* 2008). As yet, no reversible ligand specific for MAO-B has been identified for PET studies.

8.6.   Clinical PET studies of MAO

The promoter region for human MAO-A contains a polymorphism thought to regulate gene expression. Nonetheless, PET with [^{11}C]clorgyline did not reveal a difference in the activity of MAO-A in brain of non-smoking healthy subjects with genotypes predicting high and low activity (Fowler *et al.* 2007). Sclerotic hippocampus from patients treated for intractable epilepsy had elevated binding of [^{3}H]deprenyl (presumably in astrocytes), and also the microglia tracer [^{3}H]PK11195 (Kumlien *et al.* 1992). In human PET studies with deuterated [^{11}C]deprenyl, elevated binding could be seen within the mesial temporal lobes, in which epileptic foci had been detected using EEG (Kumlien *et al.* 1995). Diffuse astrocytosis has also been detected with deuterated [^{11}C]deprenyl in patients suffering from amyotrophic lateral sclerosis (Johansson *et al.* 2007).

In PET studies with [^{11}C]clorgyline or [^{11}C]deprenyl, a substantial inhibition of both forms of MAO has been detected in brain of smokers (Fowler *et al.* 1996, 1998b). These effects of smoking are not restricted to the central nervous system; a single exposure to tobacco smoke reduced the uptake of the reversible MAO-A tracer [^{11}C]beflaxatone into the myocardium of baboon (Valette *et al.* 2005), even though central effects on [^{11}C]deprenyl uptake were not obtained in humans smoking a single cigarette (Fowler *et al.* 1999). The constituents of tobacco smoke responsible for MAO inhibition have not been identified with certainty, but harmine-like β-carboline alkaloids are distinct candidates (Herraiz & Chaparro 2005).

The inhibition of MAO in brain and throughout the body of smokers has attracted considerable interest, given the substantial protection against idiopathic Parkinson's disease which is imparted by smoking (Checkoway *et al.* 2002), and the role of MAO-B in MPTP toxicity. However, it should be recalled that deprenyl treatment delayed only slightly the progression of Parkinson's disease in the multi-center DATATOP study. It has been argued that such clinical benefits as are obtained from deprenyl and other propargylamine compounds in the treatment of Parkinson's disease are mediated by attenuation of apoptotic pathways rather than by MAO-B inhibition *per se* (Olanow 2006). In spite of the reported linkage between MAO polymorphism and Parkinson's disease, there seems to have been no clinical imaging studies of MAO activity in neurodegenerative disorders.

In a clinical PET study, the $[^{11}C]$harmine V_e was increased by an average of 34% throughout the brain of patients with major depression, relative to a group of non-smoking healthy control subjects (Meyer *et al.* 2006a). This finding was discussed in the context of a revised theory of the biology of depression, in which elevated MAO-A activity results in depletion of monoamine substrates in the brain. However, the in vitro binding kinetics of harmine and MAO substrates suggest that competition from endogenous substrates may occur in living brain. This could imply the opposite interpretation of the clinical PET study, that a prior reduction in endogenous monoamine concentrations increased the availability of MAO-A sites in the brain of depressed subjects. This possibility might be tested by blockade of catecholamine synthesis with AMPT, which should result in increased availability of $[^{11}C]$harmine binding sites if substantial competition indeed occurs in the living brain.

In another $[^{11}C]$clorgyline PET study, cerebral MAO-A activity was lower in healthy subjects self-reporting high trait aggression (Alia-Klein *et al.* 2008), a finding consistent with behavioral observations in knockout mice. Thus, the associations of lower MAO-A activity with depression and also with aggression suggests that the two traits may be differential manifestations of a common underlying biochemical predisposition.

9

Vesicular storage of dopamine

9.1.   Biochemistry of vesicular monoamine transporters

Two vesicular monoamine transporters of adrenal chromaffin cells (VMAT1) and catecholamine neurons (VMAT2) belong to a family of vaculolar-type proton-ATPase proteins, which are related to the bacterial antibiotic resistance transporters. Both vesicular monoamine transporters accumulate monoamines within vesicles, employing an intrinsic ATPase activity to generate the proton gradient that establishes and maintains the accumulation of monoamine substrates; in a sense, vesicles behave as inside-out mitochondria. The genetic sequence for VMAT1 was isolated on the basis of its ability to and impart resistance to MPP+, the neurotoxic metabolite of MPTP (Liu *et al.* 1992), apparently by sequestering the toxic metabolite out of harm's way. Indeed, the reserpine-sensitive uptake of MPP+ by chromaffin and brain synaptic vesicles could produce 100-fold concentration gradients in the presence of ATP (Moriyama, Amakatsu, & Futai 1993).

Around the same time as the cloning of VMAT1, a sequence encoding VMAT2 was cloned from the human cDNA library on the basis of its ability to impart serotonin uptake to organelles in permeabilized cells (Erickson, Eiden, & Hoffman 1992). The sequence of the VMAT2 gene predicts a 512 amino acid protein with 12α-helical membrane spanning domains, both termini and several potential phosphorylation sites being present on the cytoplasmic side. In situ hybridization signal for VMAT2 is present in the dopamine, serotonin, noradrenaline, and adrenaline neurons of the brain, all of which biogenic amines are good substrates for vesicular uptake. Tyramine is another good substrate, but high concentrations are not attained with vesicles because of permeation of the uncharged amine back into the cytoplasm (Knoth *et al.* 1984). This accounts for the trace levels of tyramine and related compounds, which are rapidly consumed by MAO.

Heterozygous knockout mice expressing half the normal level of VMAT2 are similar in behavior to wild-type mice. However, the locomotor stimulant effects of amphetamine were enhanced in these mice, whereas the conditioned place preference for amphetamine, an index of rewarding properties, was reduced (Takahashi *et al.* 1997). Reducing the expression of VMAT2 may enhance the pool of amphetamine-releasable cyctosolic dopamine subserving the psychomotor stimulant effects of amphetamine. In contrast, the conditioned properties of amphetamines would seem to be more dependent upon the presence of a vesicular pool of dopamine, the release of which is impulse-dependent.

9.2.   Chromaffin granules

9.2.1.   *Biochemical properties*

The biophysics of catecholamine release has been extensively studied in adrenal chromaffin cells, which contain vesicles much larger than those found in mammalian dopamine neurons. Because of their great abundance and size, chromaffin granules are easier to study than are catecholamine vesicles. Using intracellular recording techniques it is possible to measure stepwise increases in electrical capacitance of the plasma membrane of chromaffin cells (Moser & Neher 1997), indicating the fusion of individual chromaffin granules to the plasma membrane. The initial increase in membrane capacitance after a single depolarization is not highly calcium-dependent, but trains of depolarization seem to be followed by exoctyosis when a sufficient threshold of calcium entry has occurred (Seward & Nowycky 1996). While the voltage-dependent entry of Ca^{2+} into the cell requires membrane depolarization, activation of nicotinic receptors on hyperpolarized chromaffin cells can evoke enough influx to activate exocytosis (Mollard, Seward, & Nowycky 1995). Furthermore, using the technique of flash photolysis of caged Ca^{2+}, rapid increases in the intracellular free calcium concentration can be obtained in living chromaffin cells, in a manner independent of depolarization. Flash photolysis evokes a rapid increase in plasma membrane capacitance, not always followed by increased catecholamine release as measured by voltammetry (Oberhauser, Robinson, & Fernandez 1996). This reinforces the claim that vesicular fusion and exocytosis are not perfectly coupled.

Several sequential steps must be involved in exocytosis from chromaffin cells. The granular fusion is reversible in the time course of catecholamine extrusion, such that the entire contents of a granule are not committed to release following fusion (Travis & Wightman 1998). This observation would seem to argue against the notion of "quantal release" of catecholamines. Not all granules in chromaffin cells are equally prepared for release. While ATP is required for sustained exocytosis, Ca^{2+} alone could induce exocytosis of granules already docked with the plasma membrane. Here, a few release events occur within milliseconds, but most events require a more prolonged calcium stimulus (Parsons *et al.* 1995). The rapid recruitment of individual granules for exocytosis is limited by a network of actin filaments, which can be disrupted by treatment of phorbol esters (Vitale, Seward, & Trifaro 1995).

It is generally assumed that similar mechanisms underlie the release of monoamine neurotransmitters from chromaffin cells and nerve terminals. Indeed, the exocytoic release of dopamine from nerve terminals is initiated by entry of Ca^{2+} into the cytosol. Activation of cytosolic Ca^{2+}/calmodulin-dependent protein kinase (type II) results in phosphorylation of several intracellular substrates, including synapsin, which mobilize fusion of vesicles with the inner plasma membrane. The PC12 chromaffin tumor cells become morphologically more neuron-like when cultured in the presence of nerve growth factor. Whereas untransformed chromaffin cells release catecholamines directly from the cell body, differentiated cells release catecholamines from varicose neurites (Zerby & Ewing 1996). Furthermore, the range of vesicular content of monoamines is reduced upon differentiation, as the cells become more like neurons.

High concentrations ($0.6\,\mu M$) of catecholamines can occur within chromaffin granules due to the stabilizing effect of a complex formed with intragranular ATP (Winkler & Westhead 1980). As with VMAT1, the VMAT2 drives catecholamines into the vesicle against this extraordinarily high concentration gradient via a proton gradient established at the expense of the catalytic hydrolysis of magnesium-ATP in the cytosol. In the normal chromaffin granule, the proton gradient results in acidification of the granule interior by nearly two pH units. The same proton gradient is responsible for excluding Mg^{2+} from the interior of the granule, where it would otherwise destabilize the complex between catecholamines and ATP within the organelle (Fiedler & Daniels 1984). This gradient cannot be measured directly with microelectrodes, but can be calculated from the observed distribution of charged molecules such as $[^{14}C]$methylamine between the vesicle and incubation medium. Pharmacological inactivation of the membrane-bound ATPase inhibits catecholamine uptake by chromaffin granules, but uptake can be transiently reinstated by imposing a pH gradient through exposure of acidified vesicles to a basic medium (Schuldiner, Fishkes, & Kanner 1978). Although catecholamine uptake is not directly coupled to proton exchange, the main driving force is extrusion of one or two protons. The exact stoichiometry of transport has been uncertain because of the unknown charge of the ionic species which is transported (Johnson, Carty, & Scarpa 1981, 1982). Given that the quaternary amine MPP+ and catecholamines are taken up by chromaffin granules with similar kinetics, the substrate for transport must certainly be a cation (Daniels & Reinhard 1988).

9.2.2.   *Reserpine alkaloids*

Vesicles are poisoned by reserpine, an indole alkaloid first isolated from *Rauwolfia serpentina*, the Indian snakeroot. Preparations of this plant were used in Ayurvedic medicine for the treatment of snakebite (hence the name), and also as a sedative for what would now be called psychiatric disorders. The inhibition of reserpine binding by various compounds agrees very closely with the inhibition of dopamine uptake into vesicles (Near & Mahler 1983). However, the reserpine binding and catecholamine uptake sites seem not to be identical. Mutants of the VMAT2 have been identified that are unable to bind the usual substrates, but retain high affinity for reserpine binding, which is itself dependent upon the integrity of the proton gradient (Merickel *et al.* 1995). Low concentrations of reserpine block catecholamine uptake into normal vesicles, without interrupting the proton gradient, indicating a specific inhibition of catecholamine translocation, while much higher reserpine concentrations are required to block the proton pump itself (Zallakian *et al.* 1982). [^{3}H]Reserpine binds to vesicles and inhibits the uptake of dopamine at nanomolar concentrations. Tetrabenazine, a closely related compound, also blocks dopamine uptake at nM concentrations, but its binding is not sensitive to the pH gradient (Henry & Scherman 1989).

Amphetamine inhibits the uptake of dopamine into vesicles ($K_i = 5\,\mu M$) (Philippu & Beyer 1973) with greater potency than it inhibits the binding of tetrabenazine to vesicular transporters from rat striatum (IC$_{50} = 40\,\mu M$) (Teng, Crooks, & Dwoskin 1998), consistent with the functional distinction between substrate transport and alkaloid binding sites. In contrast, methamphetamine may block dopamine uptake into vesicles (IC$_{50} = 400\,nM$) (Peter *et al.* 1994) by interacting with the reserpine binding site, rather than by competing directly against biogenic amine transport.

9.3.   Regulating and knocking out VMAT2

The non-hydrolizable GTP analogs, which non-specifically activate the G-proteins, and also the purified GαO$_2$ subunit, both inhibited the uptake of noradrenaline in chromaffin granules, and interfered with the calcium-dependent release of noradrenaline from chromaffin cells (Ahnert-Hilger *et al.* 1998). Using electron microscopy and specific antisera, the VMAT2 was found to be closely associated with GaO_2 in monoaminergic terminals of rat cerebral cortex (Holtje *et al.* 2000), suggesting a mechanism for the regulation of vesicular content. Furthermore, VMAT2 expressed in hamster cells is constitutively phosphorylated at specific serine residue, apparently via casein kinase II (Krantz *et al.* 1997). Whereas VMAT2 is not a substrate for protein kinase A, expression of this enzyme is necessary for the correct trafficking of the transporters into vesicles of PC12 cells (Yao, Erickson, & Hersh 2004). Thus, intracellular second messengers can modulate the vesicular uptake and release of neurotransmitters by several mechanisms.

There is little evidence that the expression of monoamine transporters can itself be modulated. Chronic treatment with deprenyl reduced the density of post-synaptic dopamine D_2 receptors by 20% and also reduced the concentration of dopamine uptake sites measured in rat striatum by autoradiography. However, this treatment was without effect on the binding of methoxytetrabenazine to vesicular transporters (Vander Borght *et al.* 1995). In contrast, the concentration of VMAT1 in bovine adrenal chromaffin cells was substantially increased by prolonged and continuous depolarization with potassium (Desnos *et al.* 1995). It is unknown if similar adaptive mechanisms can regulate the expression of VMAT2 in the brain.

9.4.   Ligands and tracers for VMAT2

Some in vitro kinetic properties of vesicular monoamine transporters are presented in Table 9.1. The VMA2 has high affinity for substrates such as dopamine, serotonin, and also for inhibitors such as amphetamine. As noted above, reserpine alkaloids bind ambivalently to monoaminergic vesicles within terminals of dopamine, serotonin, adrenaline, and noradrenalin fibers. Therefore, the specific reserpine binding in the brain must reveal the composite of these several monoaminergic innervations. Monoamine vesicles in rat brain sections can be selectively labelled with 7-amino-8-[125I]iodoketanserin, when its binding to serotonin receptors is blocked with selective antagonists (Darchen *et al.* 1989). However, the non-specificity of this tracer makes its use in vivo difficult. [3H]Dihydrotetrabenazine ([3H]DTBZ) binds with high affinity (2–5 nM) to a single class of binding sites in rat brain sections and in the synaptic vesicle fraction prepared from bovine striatum (Near 1986). A second binding component was of greater abundance in bovine striatum, but its affinity was

Table 9.1. *Some kinetic properties of the vesicular monoamine transporter (VMAT2) measured in vitro, and corresponding results obtained in PET studies with [^{11}C]DTBZ*

Vesicles from pig caudate		
K_m for dopamine	1.5 μM	Philippu & Beyer 1973
K_i for amphetamine	2.7 μM	
Cloned human VMAT2		
K_m for serotonin	1.3 μM	Erickson & Eiden 1993
K_i of dopamine against serotonin	0.8 μM	
K_i of reserpine against serotonin	34 nM	
K_i of tetrabenazine against serotonin	78 nM	
VMAT2 from transformed COS cells		
K_m for serotonin	190 nM	Peter et al. 1994
K_m for dopamine	320 nM	
K_m for MPP+	1.6 μM	
Bovine synaptic vesicles		
K_m for [^{3}H]DTBZ	8 nM	Meshgin-Azarian et al. 1988
Mouse striatal vesicles, K_i displacement of		
[^{3}H]MPP$^+$ by dopamine or tyramine	6 nM	Del Zompo et al. 1992
Amphetamine	22 nM	
Reserpine	130 nM	
Serotonin transport per [^{3}H]DTBZ site	0.5 sec^{-1}	Peter et al. 1994
[^{3}H]methoxytetrabenazine B_{max} (K_D) in autoradiograms of rat striatum*	120 pmol g^{-1} (4 nM)	Vander Borght et al. 1995b
[^{3}H]tetrabenazine B_{max} in substantia nigra		
Normal controls ($n=6$)	187 ± 11 pmol g^{-1}	Thibaut et al. 1995
Parkinson's disease ($n=4$)	84 ± 14 pmol g^{-1}	
[^{3}H]DTBZ B_{max}, dorsal putamen, normal		
controls ($n=6$)	43 ± 8 pmol g^{-1}	Lehericy et al. 1994
Parkinson's disease ($n=4$)	7 ± 4 pmol g^{-1}	
Alzheimer's disease ($n=4$)	35 ± 6 pmol g^{-1}	
(+)-[^{11}C]DTBZ V_d, normal human ($n=7$)		
Caudate	11.3 ± 2.3 ml g^{-1}	Koeppe et al. 1996
Frontal cortex	3.7 ± 0.8 ml g^{-1}	
Cerebellum	3.8 ± 0.6 ml g^{-1}	
(+)-[^{11}C]DTBZ pB (k_3/k_4), normal human ($n=7$)		
Caudate	6.4 ± 4.8	
Frontal cortex	0.9 ± 0.2	
Cerebellum	0.8 ± 0.3	
(+)-[^{11}C]DTBZ pB (k_3/k_4), caudate		
Normal human ($n=7$)	2.7 ± 0.3	Gilman et al. 1999
Multiple system atrophy ($n=8$)	1.5 ± 0.2	
Olivopontocerebellar atrophy ($n=6$)	2.3 ± 0.2	

Table 9.1. (*cont.*)

(+)-[^{11}C]DTBZ reference tissue *pB*, putamen		
Normal control (*n* = 7)	3.9 ± 0.3	Gilman *et al.* 1998
Alcoholics (*n* = 7)	3.5 ± 0.3	
(±)-[^{11}C]DTBZ *pB* in putamen		
Normal control subjects (*n* = 16)	0.96 ± 0.09	Lee *et al.* 2000
Early Parkinson's disease (*n* = 13)	0.36 ± 0.19	
Advanced Parkinson's disease (*n* = 22)	0.26 ± 0.06	
(+)-[^{11}C]DTBZ *pB* in putamen		
Healthy young monkey (*n* = 6)	1.43 ± 0.14	Doudet *et al.* 2006
Healthy aged monkey (*n* = 4)	1.20 ± 0.16	
(+)-[^{11}C]DTBZ B_{max} ($K_D{}^{app}$) by PET	178 ± 32 pmol g^{-1}	Sossi *et al.* 2007
Normal rat striatum (*n* = 6)	(48 ± 9 nM)	
6-OHDA lesioned striatum (*n* = 6)	31 ± 6 pmol g^{-1}	
	(43 ± 15 nM)	

Note: *Calculated as 10% protein by wet weight. PET studies were carried out using either (±) the racemic mixture or (+) the active enantiomer.

two orders of magnitude lower (Meshgin-Azarian *et al.* 1988). In gel electrophoresis studies, the high-affinity binding component migrated along with the vesicular marker synaptophysin. The concentration of this binding site is very low in the brain of neonate rats, but approaches the adult levels by postnatal day 20 (Leroux-Nicollet *et al.* 1990).

The pattern of uptake of labeled methoxytetrabenazine in living rodent brain matched the distribution of monoamine neurotransmitters, but 20% of the radioactivity extracted from rodent brain was labeled metabolites (Vander Borght *et al.* 1995a). This is an unfavorable property for a prospective PET tracer, due to the difficulties in kinetic modeling presented by brain-penetrating plasma metabolites (namely the cases of FDOPA and [^{11}C]depre-nyl). Similarly, the PET tracer [^{11}C]tetrabenazine accumulates progressively in human striatum, but this uptake reflects the composite of the parent compound and its major metabolite [^{11}C]DTBZ (Kilbourn *et al.* 1993). Due to these complications, the use of the more biochemically stable [^{11}C]DTBZ has come to predominate in PET studies of VMAT2. There is rapid initial influx of [^{11}C]DTBZ in living human brain, with an approximate extraction fraction of 50%, meaning that one half of the tracer in blood is deposited during its passage through the brain. Due to the short physical half-life of [^{11}C], routine use of [^{11}C]DTBZ is restricted to PET centers equipped with a cyclotron and radiochemistry facility. In order to overcome this limitation, [^{18}F]fluoropropyl-DTBZ has been proposed as an alternate tracer (Kung *et al.* 2007). Studies in mice confirm that this ligand has excellent properties for the detection of VMAT2 in living brain. MicroPET studies showed the resolved active enantiomer (+)-[^{18}F]fluoropropyl-DTBZ proved it had superior specific binding at equilibrium in rat striatum than did (+)-[^{11}C]DTBZ or the [^{18}F]fluoroethyl derivative (Kilbourn *et al.* 2007).

In the case of [^{11}C]DTBZ, stable estimates of the equilibrium V_d relative to the arterial input could be obtained in striatum of healthy volunteers, using a one-compartment (K_1/k_2) model; attempts to fit a two-compartment (k_3/k_4) model to the data resulted in rather high variance in the magnitude of the estimates (Koeppe *et al.* 1996), as is typical of over-specified models. Indeed, it is very seldom that four parameters can be independently estimated in PET studies with reversible ligands, without risk of considerable bias favoring one kinetic parameter or another. As an alternate to over-specified compartmental analysis, the [^{11}C]DTBZ equilibrium V_d can be measured under steady-state conditions obtained with continuous tracer infusion. In this design, one half of the dose is administered as a single bolus, followed by a constant infusion of the remaining dose over a period of about 1 h (Koeppe *et al.* 1997). Under these conditions, the arterial concentration of untransformed tracer is essentially clamped, resulting in a rapid approach to equilibrium binding in brain. The bolus and equilibrium infusion methods have been compared using [^{3}H]DTBZ in the living rat (Kilbourn & Sherman 1997). Both methods gave regional values of equilibrium V_d which correlated well with known monoamine vesicle concentrations, although the single bolus method appeared to introduce a small positive bias in some regions.

The abundance of VMAT2 is very low in cerebellum, such that the time–radioactivity curve in that tissue can be used for reference tissue calculation of the magnitude of *pB* using the linear graphical analysis of Logan (Chan *et al.* 1999). However, displacement studies with reserpine revealed the presence of a small [^{3}H]DTBZ binding component in cerebellum of the rat (Kilbourn & Sherman 1997). Thus, the reference tissue method must slightly underestimate the true *pB* of this ligand. Significant binding of [^{11}C]DTBZ could be seen in mesencephalon of healthy humans, whereas the cortical binding constituted 5% of the striatal binding (Koeppe *et al.* 1999). Parametric maps of *pB* calculated by the Logan reference tissue method in brain of rhesus monkeys (Figure 9.1) show a similarly heterogenous binding. In this study, the extrastriatal binding was largely, but not entirely, resistant to MPTP-poisoning (Doudet *et al.* 2006), although small reductions in [^{11}C]DTBZ *pB* in the frontal cortex suggested vulnerability of cortical catecholamine innervations to the neurotoxin. However, the precision of the method is necessarily low in regions of low specific binding. Comparison of representative molecular imaging results (Table 9.1) shows that specific binding of the active enantiomer (+)-[^{11}C]DTBZ consistently exceeds that of the racemic mixture.

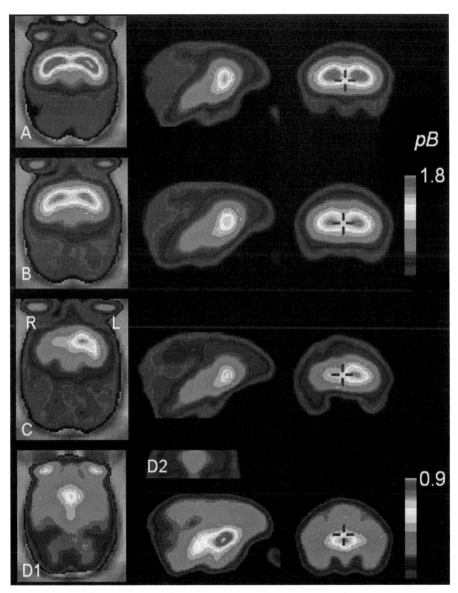

Figure 9.1 The binding potential (pB) of (+)[^{11}C]dihydrotetrabenazine (+[^{11}C]DTBZ) for monoamine vesicles in the brain of monkeys. Mean parametric maps were calculated in (A) normal young ($n=7$), (B) normal aged ($n=4$) rhesus monkeys, (C) aged monkeys with unilateral intracarotid infusion of MPTP ($n=3$), and (D) monkeys of intermediate age with systemic MPTP administration (N=6). Mean parametric maps are co-registered to the MR template, shown as gray-scale in the horizontal plane images. A sector containing the striatum in the horizontal plane from the MPTP group (D2) is presented with identical intensity scaling as in the intact animals. The cursor in the coronal plane images indicates the position (0,10,10) in the MR coordinate system. Reproduced with permission from Doudet *et al.* (2006). (For color version, see plate section.)

9.5.   Clinical PET studies of VAT2

Using an equilibrium infusion method, the [^{11}C]DTBZ pB was measured in a large group of healthy subjects over an extended range of ages. There was no significant difference between male and female subjects, and both gender groups experienced a 5% reduction of striatal binding with each decade of life (Bohnen *et al.* 2006). Similarly, the [^{11}C]DTBZ pB declined by 15% between groups of 8-year-old and 22-year-old rhesus monkeys (Doudet *et al.* 2006). In the putamen of patients with early, unilateral Parkinson's disease, the [^{11}C]DTBZ pB was reduced by 50% on the asymptomatic side and by 60% on the symptomatic side (Lee *et al.* 2000), as also seen in the subsequent study of Bohnen *et al.* (2006). [^{11}C]DTBZ binding in putamen correlated with several aspects of the pharmaco-dynamic response to DOPA in patients with asymmetric Parkinson's disease (Kumar *et al.* 2003). Furthermore, there was already a 35% decline in [^{11}C]DTBZ binding in caudate nucleus on the least affected side of these patients (Martin *et al.* 2008). Based upon these results, [^{11}C]DTBZ-PET may be the most sensitive assay for age-related reductions in striatal dopamine innervations, and seems also to be the most sensitive available indicator of the pathophsysiology of early Parkinson's disease.

A number of other neurological disorders have been investigated in PET studies with [^{11}C]DTBZ. In patients with multiple system atrophy, the [^{11}C]DTBZ pB in striatum was reduced to a greater extent in those patients presenting mainly with parkinsonism rather than cerebellar signs (Gilman *et al.* 1999). Partial declines in pB were found in patients with olivopontocere-bellar atrophy (Gilman *et al.* 1996), in agreement with the declines in post mortem brain concentrations seen in that disease (Kish *et al.* 1992a). Thus, the concentration of synaptic vesicles in striatum may be directly proportional to the dopamine concentration in brain tissue. An extraordinary exception to this rule is presented in patients with DOPA-responsive dystonia, in whom the abundance of "empty vesicles" was actually elevated (de la Fuente-Fernandez *et al.* 2003); this increase in [^{11}C]DTBZ pB could reflect a compensatory response to chronic deficiency of dopamine, or might indeed be related to decreased competition of endogenous dopamine for ligand binding sites. In support of the latter proposition, the binding of (+)-[^{11}C]DTBZ in rat striatum was increased by 14% after AMPT and decreased by 20% after DOPA treatment (Tong *et al.* 2008).

[^{11}C]DTBZ can be used for the discriminative diagnosis of dementia with Lewy bodies, where striatal binding was reduced, and Alzheimer's disease, where vesicular binding in striatum was nearly normal (Gilman *et al.* 2004). The [^{11}C]DTBZ pB was decreased in the posterior putamen of patients with Huntington's disease, especially those with the rigid-akinetic form of the disease (Bohnen *et al.* 2000). Here, atrophy of the basal ganglia may have exacerbated the partial volume effects, leading to biased underestimation of *pB*. However, the decreased tracer uptake remained after correcting for the volume loss of the regions of interest.

In other clinical PET studies, the presence of large defects in vesicular density of patients with familial paroxysmal dystonic choreoathetosis has been excluded (Bohnen *et al.* 1999). Similarly, the binding of [^{11}C]DTBZ in the basal ganglia was identical in a group of eight patients with Tourette's syndrome and in age-matched healthy volunteers (Meyer *et al.* 1999), although results of a more recent voxel-wise study from the same group indicated an increase in binding specifically in the ventral striatum (Albin *et al.* 2003). In patients with schizophrenia, there was no apparent abnormality in [^{11}C]DTBZ binding, nor was the age-related decline different in these patients than in a healthy control group (Taylor *et al.* 2000).

The striatal binding of [^{3}H]DTBZ was normal in autoradiograms from patients dying with alcoholism (Tupala *et al.* 2008) but was 50% reduced in baboons treated 3 weeks earlier with a neurotoxic dose of methamphetamine (Villemagne *et al.* 1998). In general, effects of drugs of abuse on vesicular transporters have scarcely been investigated with [^{11}C]DTBZ-PET.

Dopamine release: from vesicles to behavior

10.1. Methods for measuring dopamine release

10.1.1. *HPLC with electrochemical detection*

Biological samples are mixtures of many compounds. The assay of biological samples usually begins with separation of the mixture into its components. Classically, dopamine and its metabolites have been separated from tissue samples by extraction into organic solvents or by ion exchange. During the past 25 years, the preferred method of separation of dopamine and its metabolites has been HPLC. Using this technique, dopamine, its acidic metabolites, and its amino acid precursors can be separated from extracts of brain tissue, or in samples of extracellular fluid acquired by cerebral microdialysis. Once this separation has been obtained, the separate analytes must be detected by some means, either due to the presence of a radioactive label, or on the basis of some other inherent property.

The chemical structure of dopamine is based upon catechol, an aromatic ring in which two adjacent ring protons are replaced with hydroxyl groups. The catechol structure imparts critical properties related to the interactions between dopamine and its receptors, but also reduces the chemical stability of molecules bearing it. The catechol group is highly oxidizable, meaning that electrons are readily withdrawn by other molecules or by catalytic surfaces. Exposure of a catechol to an electric field with a potential difference of one volt causes an oxidation reaction in which four electrons are transferred to the surface of the electrode, with the production of an oxidized quinone molecule. The loss of the electrons produces an electrical current in proportion to the number of molecules oxidized with time. When the outflow of an HPLC separation is passed through an electrochemical detector, concentrations of DOPA, dopamine and its metabolites can be quantified with great precision and sensitivity.

10.1.2.   Synaptosomes and slices

Dopamine and associated enzymes can be isolated from brain tissue extracts, but the complex machinery regulating dopamine release is destroyed in the extraction process. However, aspects of biological function can be retained in other biological preparations. Special techniques can be used to isolate from the brain a *synaptosome* fraction, which is enriched in functioning fragments of dopamine terminals, and remains vital for several hours. When suspended in an appropriate medium, synaptosomes from the striatum can be used to study the uptake and vesicular release of dopamine.

Slices prepared from fresh striatum provide a more intact model for studying the mechanisms of dopamine release. These slices can be maintained for several hours in an oxygenated medium containing glucose. Although dopamine fibers in the slices are devoid of axonal action potentials, they nonetheless retain other functional properties of the intact innervation. Most importantly, the dopamine fibers can take up [^{3}H]dopamine from the incubation medium, and store it in synaptic vesicles. However, [^{3}H]dopamine in rat brain slices "leaks" into the medium at a fairly constant rate over a period of several hours. Brief episodes of elevated [^{3}H]dopamine release can be evoked by increasing the potassium concentration in the medium, but this release is dependent upon the presence of calcium (Barnes *et al.* 1990). Slices retain some properties of the regulated release of dopamine in living brain, particularly the modulation by autoreceptor agonists and antagonists.

10.1.3.   Cerebral microdialysis

The cerebral microdialysis technique permits sampling of the brain interstitial fluid of living animals, whilst minimally perturbing the environment from which the fluid is sampled. In this technique, a cylindrical dialysis membrane is surgically implanted in the brain, often using stereotaxic surgery in order to allow precise anatomical localization of the probe. An artificial CSF is then pumped through the tube, sampling by diffusion the small molecules present in the interstitial fluid of the brain. The outflow of the microdialysis medium is collected for assay by HPLC with electrochemical detection, or by other means. An advantage of the microdialysis is that dopamine release can be monitored in awake, freely moving rats.

The transit of small molecules across the microdialysis membrane is bidirectional, such that the interstitial environment around the probe can be altered by the introduction of a drug or specific ions into the microdialysis fluid. For example, addition of tetrodotoxin to the dialysis medium results in very rapid

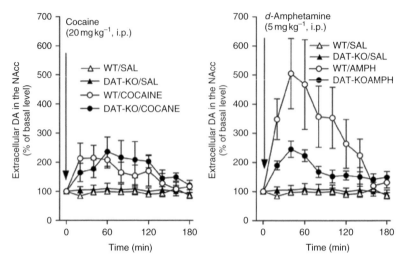

Figure 10.1 Effects of acute treatment with cocaine (left) and amphetamine (right) on the interstitial dopamine concentrations in the mouse nucleus accumbens. The sensitivity to psychostimulant challenge is compared in groups of wild-type animals, and in mice with knockout (KO) of the dopamine transporter (DAT). Reproduced with permission from Sotnikova *et al.* (2006).

disappearance of dopamine outflow in striatal microdialysis (Brown *et al.* 1991), indicating that the signal reflects a sodium-dependent pool of released dopamine. The calculation of absolute dopamine concentrations by microdialysis is difficult, being determined by the length of the diffusion path (the tortuosity factor) in the brain, and the extracellular volume fraction occupied by the analyte (Benveniste, Hansen, & Ottosen 1989). These factors can be calculated in artificial media such as suspensions of red blood cells, but cannot readily be quantified in the brain. Consequently, most microdialysis studies are used to measure the effect of treatment or condition on the dopamine efflux relative to that in a baseline condition (Figure 10.1). An advantage of microdialysis is that efflux of dopamine and its acidic metabolites can be measured in the same sample, although the temporal resolution of the method is generally about 10 min.

The bidirectional diffusion of substances across the microdialysis membrane can be exploited to calculate the endogenous concentration of analytes in the interstitial fluid. If dopamine or its metabolites are introduced into the microdialysis medium at a range of concentrations, there can be found some condition at which the net flux across the membrane is equal to zero. Using this zero net flux method, the interstitial concentration of dopamine was 4 nM in the rat nucleus accumbens, while the concentration of DOPAC was 6 μM, more than 1000-fold higher (Parsons & Justice 1992). In extracts of whole striatum, the total dopamine concentration is 70 μM, versus a DOPAC concentration of 10 μM. Thus, there is little or no gradient for DOPAC concentrations between parenchyma and interstitium, while the dopamine gradient normally comprises about four orders of magnitude. It is this gradient that is permissive to signaling via the controlled release of dopamine.

The efflux of dopamine is highly sensitive to the concentration of Ca^{2+} in the perfusion medium. In the interstitial fluid, the mean Ca^{2+} concentration is 1.2 mM (Moghaddam & Bunney 1989); increasing the Ca^{2+} concentration in the perfusion medium to 3.4 mM, a concentration typical of commercially manufactured Ringer's solution, resulted in a two-fold increase in the basal dopamine efflux. Altering the Ca^{2+} concentration within this range had effects on the interstitial dopamine concentration calculated by the zero net flux method (Chen, Lai, & Pan 1997), indicating that results can be very sensitive to experimental conditions.

In striatum ipsilateral to a 6-OHDA lesion, the interstitial concentration of dopamine (8 nM) was identical to that in unlesioned control animals, although the in vivo recovery was lower in the lesioned group (Parsons, Smith, & Justice 1991). This finding presents a problem for understanding the behavioral consequences of the dopamine depletion: how can the extracellular dopamine be normal in the lesioned hemiparkinsonian animals? One interpretation is that microdialysis samples the tonic interstitial dopamine, as distinct from the more spatially and temporally distinct phasic release events that characterize normal dopamine transmission. The dopamine sampled by microdialysis lies at the end of the gauntlet of metabolism, diffusion, facilitated uptake, and subsequent vesicular storage, all of which might conceal the spatial and temporal pattern of dopamine release relevant to neurotransmission. Thus, for example, stimulation of dopamine synthesis with DOPA has little effect on the interstitial dopamine concentrations in intact rats (Wachtel & Abercrombie 1994), but evoked 20-fold increases in rats with 6-OHDA lesions. Reuptake mechanisms must be intact in order to "buffer" alterations in the the interstitial dopamine concentrations following a pharmacological challenge with DOPA.

10.1.4.   In vivo electrochemistry

The oxidation of dopamine and other electroactive species in solution produces an electrical current, which can be amplified and recorded. Consequently, an electrode placed in the brain parenchyma can, upon application of a potential difference, produce an electrical current indicative of all the oxidizable species near the electrode surface. However, interstitial concentrations of DOPAC in rat striatum are normally 1000 times greater than that of dopamine itself. In contrast to HPLC with electrical detection, all the oxidizable species are mixed together in the interstitial fluid. The problem of selectivity is compounded by the presence in the brain of high concentrations of ascorbic acid and uric acid, which are also oxidizable. Modifications of the electrode surface with the addition of an anionic detergent can be used to exclude the majority of DOPAC and other anions from oxidation, thus isolating the dopamine signal. Another approach is to apply the voltage as a ramp so as to oxidize species in succession according to their individual redox potentials (cyclic voltammetry). Alternately, the voltage can be applied as a pulse, with gating of the transient capacitance current in order to isolate (ostensibly) the current due specifically to dopamine oxidation, a technique known as chronoamperometry.

Electrochemistry techniques in vivo can approach the ultimate sensitivity, which is the detection of all dopamine molecules present. With cyclic voltametry it is thus possible to detect "quanta" of calcium-dependent catecholamine release from isolated adrenal chromaffin cells (Wightman *et al.* 1991). The episodic oxidation currents were consistent with the release of a few million catecholamine molecules with each event. Individual release events have not yet been detected in the central nervous system, in part because of the much smaller size of the vesicles in dopamine terminals. However, electrochemical detection has the distinct advantage of high temporal resolution; the waveform of dopamine release and reuptake can be sampled at intervals of a fraction of a second (Figure 10.2).

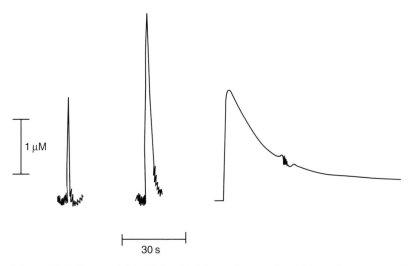

Figure 10.2 The reuptake of interstitial dopamine in mice striatum slices measured with electrochemistry. Changes in the dopamine clearance measured after multiple intravenous administrations of cocaine and complete genetic deletion of the dopamine transporter. Electrically evoked (1 s, 60 Hz, 300 µA) dopamine signals detected by fast-scan cyclic voltammetry in the nucleus accumbens of an anesthetized rat before and 5 min after cocaine (3 mg kg^{-1}, i.v.) injection (the first two traces), and in the nucleus accumbens of an anesthetized dopamine transporter knockout mouse (the right most trace). Figure generously provided by Prof. Evgeny Budykin, Wake Forest University.

10.2.   Concentration gradients for dopamine across the plasma membrane

The dynamics of the stimulated release of a population of dopamine vesicles can be recorded with cyclic voltammetry in living striatum. Electrical stimulation of the medial forebrain bundle transiently increases the electrochemical signal measured in the striatum due to interstitial dopamine (Wiedemann *et al.* 1992). The rate of decline in the oxidation current during the seconds after cessation of the electrical stimulation can be used to calculate the Michaelis–Menten constants, i.e. the maximal dopamine uptake at very high stimulus frequency (V_{max}), and the affinity of DAT for dopamine (K_m) (Wiedemann *et al.* 1992). These mechanistic studies show that most interstitial dopamine is cleared within seconds of release, at least in the striatum.

The impermeability of plasma membranes normally presents a barrier to the diffusion of dopamine between the cytosolic and extracellular compartments. However, DAT facilitates the transfer of dopamine and some other molecules across the plasma membrane, utilizing the inward sodium gradient as a driving force. DAT would thus, in the absence of other factors, establish equilibrium between intracellular and extracellular dopamine as a function of resting membrane potential, and according to the Nernst equation. A more correct description of the transmembrane distribution of dopamine accommodates the co-transport of Na^+ and the gradient for Cl^- across the polarized membrane (Stein 1986). The equation predicts an equilibrium ratio for dopamine of 100 000 across the membrane (Jones *et al.* 1999). This theoretical concentration gradient is permissive to the dopamine-releasing action of amphetamine and other sympathomimetic amines via facilitated exchange diffusion, to be discussed in detail below. Superfusion of slices of rat striatum with potassium depolarizes the membranes, and produces a substantial depletion of the amphetamine-releasable dopamine, which is probably synonymous with the cytoplasmic dopamine (Caviness & Wightman 1982).

The zero net flux microdialysis studies suggest an interstitial dopamine concentration of about 5 nM, but what is the cytosolic concentration? The intracellular free dopamine cannot be measured directly in mammalian neurons because of the large size of carbon fiber electrodes. However, in the cytosol of a land snail's giant dopamine neuron, the dopamine concentration is approximately 1 μM (Chien, Wallingford, & Ewing 1990). While this concentration is only 200 times greater than interstitial dopamine, it evidently subserves the amphetamine-evoked dopamine release. The active storage of dopamine within cytosolic vesicles doubtless reduces cytosolic dopamine concentration below the 100 000-fold gradient that might be expected on the basis of the Nernst equation.

10.3.   The action of psychostimulants

10.3.1.   *Amphetamines*

Amphetamine and other sympathomimetic amines have the capacity to release dopamine from nigrostriatal fibres by a mechanism of facilitated exchange diffusion (Liang & Rutledge 1982). The amphetamine-evoked dopamine release is blocked with cocaine, indicating that amphetamine transport into the cell is essential, not binding to the uptake site per se (Fischer & Cho 1979), as also suggested by the results of a thermodynamic study (Liang & Rutledge 1982). Unlike dopamine, cytosolic amphetamine is not subsequently stored in synaptic vesicles, but remains in the cytosol. Each amphetamine molecule entering the cytosol of a polarized dopamine neuron is normally able to displace a single dopamine molecule, irrespective of the state of neuronal activity. As such, the release of dopamine by amphetamines circumvents the usual process of calcium- and impulse-dependent release of vesicular neurotransmitter. For example, the dopamine receptor agonist apomorphine (Anden *et al.* 1967) reduces the firing rate of nigrostriatal neurons (Bunney, Aghajanian, & Roth 1973), but does not interfere with the efflux of dopamine in microdialysates evoked by amphetamine (Kuczenski, Segal, & Manley 1990).

The release of dopamine evoked in microdialysates of rat striatum by local application of potassium ion was not greatly reduced by pretreatment with reserpine, except when animals were also treated with nomifensine, a dopamine re-uptake inhibitor. This indicates that potassium-induced depolarization is permissive to dopamine efflux via the uptake sites, i.e. reverse transport, rather than vesicular release. After inhibition of TH with AMPT, the potassium-induced dopamine release was reduced, and was further reduced after prolonged TH inhibition (Fairbrother *et al.* 1990). While this observation might indicate the presence of pools of dopamine, it also shows that the magnitude of quantal release declines with prolonged inhibition of dopamine synthesis.

The theory of quantal release assumes that each vesicle is normally loaded with a fixed amount of dopamine. Indeed, the concentration of dopamine in a vesicular fraction from rat striatum was only slightly increased by DOPA treatment, which nonetheless trebled the brain concentration of dopamine (Buu 1989). This result suggests that dopamine vesicles are normally nearly saturated, or loaded with as much dopamine as they can contain. However, inhibiting impulse flow with γ-butyrolactone nearly doubles the concentration of dopamine in rat striatum, but this increase is abolished by pretreatment with reserpine (McMillen & Shore 1980). This observation indicates that accumulation of unused dopamine requires an intact vesicular compartment, and furthermore suggests that the vesicular compartment is normally only 50% saturated; in this scenario, additional dopamine synthesis does not increase tissue concentrations when the vesicular storage compartment is saturated, because of rapid MAO-catabolism of dopamine overflow in the cytosol.

As noted above, the vesicular content of chromaffin granules can be highly variable, but neuronal vesicles may be more uniform in size. The magnitude of single dopamine release events has been studied in giant dopamine neurons from the *Planorbus* snail. An electrode placed adjacent to the cell body can record the entire oxidation current following the exocytosis of a single vesicle. In this snail, the dopamine release had a bimodal distribution, indicating two types of vesicles. Treatment with amphetamine resulted in the appearance of a third vesicles type with reduced dopamine content (Chen & Ewing 1995).

Dopamine release evoked by the trace amine, tyramine, was largely blocked by nomifensine or reserpine, but was not immediately reduced by AMPT treatment, and was not altered by depletion of extracellular calcium (Fairbrother *et al.* 1990). Thus, the more immediate sympathomimetic effects of tyramine depend upon liberation of unbound dopamine from the cytosol, possibly by interfering with vesicular storage. While vesicular storage of dopamine normally keeps the cytosolic dopamine concentration low, reserpine alkaloids reduce the spontaneous release of dopamine from slices, without altering the release which could be evoked by amphetamine (Niddam *et al.* 1985), and without notably increasing the extracellular dopamine concentration (Jones *et al.* 1999). By default, MAO appears to have the final say in setting cytosolic dopamine levels, and by extension, dopamine release.

In microdialysis studies of living striatum, amphetamine treatment increased the interstitial dopamine signal five-fold in striatum of wild-type mice, but evoked only a transient two-fold increase in mice with knockout of DAT (Budygin *et al.* 2004) (Figure 10.1). Using the in vivo electrochemistry method, the extracellular concentration of dopamine in slices from striatum DAT-knockout mice was only slightly increased by acute amphetamine treatment, but the electrically evoked release of dopamine was gradually reduced by amphetamine, just as in slices from normal mice (Jones *et al.* 1998b). Thus, the first phase of amphetamine-induced dopamine release is mediated by facilitated exchange diffusion of cytosolic dopamine, which is disabled in DAT knockouts. Presumably, amphetamine slowly enters dopamine neurons by a non-carrier-mediated process, ultimately obtaining a concentration sufficient to interfere with vesicular storage. The uptake of dopamine into vesicles is reduced in transgenic mice with "knocked down" expression of VMAT2 (Takahashi *et al.* 1997). These mice had enhanced locomotor response to amphetamine, consistent with potentiation of the amphetamine-releasable cytosolic dopamine pool.

10.3.2.   Cocaine

Local application of cocaine rapidly evokes a calcium-dependent release of dopamine into microdialysates from striatum, which returns to basal levels within 30 min. The cocaine-evoked dopamine release was of lower magnitude than that evoked by amphetamine (Hurd & Ungerstedt 1989), but can nonetheless last several hours after peripheral administration of cocaine (Figure 10.1). The temporal pattern of cocaine-evoked changes in interstitial dopamine has been tested by microdialysis with sampling every minute (Newton & Justice 1994). Upon addition of cocaine (20 μM) to the perfusion medium, there was a ten-fold increase in the dopamine concentration, peaking in the third minute after arrival of cocaine to the brain. Indeed, the reinforcing properties of cocaine may be related to its particularly rapid onset of action in vivo. During sustained exposure to cocaine, the interstitial dopamine levels tend to decline slightly; following a washout interval of 15 min, a second exposure to cocaine evoked a peak response which is reduced by about 40%. Increased occupation of autoreceptors by dopamine may mediate an acute desensitization to the effects of cocaine, which may in turn account for the brevity of the psychostimulant effects of cocaine.

10.3.3.   Nicotine

The mesolimbic dopamine innervation is of particular importance in sustaining the reinforcing properties of nicotine. Self-administration of nicotine is greatly decreased during the weeks after dopamine depletion in the nucleus accumbens (Corrigall *et al.* 1992). With respect to the rewarding properties of nicotine, it is notable that high concentrations of nicotine binding sites are located on the soma and terminals of the nigrostriatal neurons and the neurons projecting from the VTA to the nucleus accumbens (Clarke & Pert 1985). The nicotinic receptor is a ligand-gated cation channel with a high permeability for calcium. Its occupation by nicotine or other agonists consequently increases the firing rate of the dopamine neurons, and facilitates spontaneous dopamine release at the nerve terminals.

10.3.4.   Other pharmacological factors

Heroin, amphetamine, nicotine, and other widely abused drugs increased the concentration of dopamine in microdialysates from rat dorsal striatum, but the effects were especially great in the nucleus accumbens (Di Chiara & Imperato 1988). Indeed, the potentiation of dopamine transmission in the ventral striatum is particularly linked to the reinforcing properties of psychostimulants. The responsiveness of dopamine neurons to pharmacological challenge with amphetamine can be altered by previous exposure to psychoactive compounds. Thus, the large increases in dopamine release evoked in the rat nucleus accumbens by psychoactive drugs was blunted by pretreatment with γ-vinyl GABA, a drug which potentiates inhibitory neurotransmission (Gerasimov *et al.* 1999). Conversely, prolonged treatment of rats with nicotine sensitizes the behavioral stimulation produced by nicotine, and also potentiated the nicotine-induced increase in dopamine outflow in the ventral striatum (Benwell & Balfour 1992). Repeated treatment with nicotine also sensitized the behavioral response to amphetamine, without potentiating the amphetamine-induced dopamine release (Birrell & Balfour 1998), suggesting post-synaptic factors in behavioral sensitization.

Haloperidol and other blockers of autoreceptors acutely stimulate dopamine synthesis and release. In rats treated chronically with haloperidol, a challenge dose of haloperidol following a period of withdrawal evoked a supernormal dopamine release in electrically stimulated striatum (Wiedemann *et al.* 1992). Furthermore, the magnitude of the electrically stimulated dopamine release was elevated after chronic haloperidol treatment (Dugast *et al.* 1997). Conversely, chronic cocaine treatment reduced the inhibitory effect of a directly acting dopamine agonist on dopamine release in the nucleus accumbens (Pierce, Duffy, & Kalivas 1995). These results indicate that chronic drug treatment can modulate the sensitivity of autoreceptors.

10.4.   Behavioral correlates of dopamine release

10.4.1.   *Ordinary movement*

What is the relationship between movement and dopamine metabolism? Does an individual voluntary movement in some sense consume extra dopamine? These questions have been addressed in a number of studies in which changes in dopamine metabolism in rat brain were measured during periods of forced locomotor activity. Running on a treadmill at moderate or high speed increased the concentration of dopamine in microdialysates from striatum by about 25%, whereas running at low speed was without effect (Hattori, Naoi, & Nishino 1994). The elevated dopamine concentration returned to baseline about 1 h after a bout of running lasting 20 min. The concentrations of both HVA and DOPAC were elevated by 20% for several hours after running at moderate speed, and by 40% after high-speed running. The authors concluded that accelerated dopamine metabolism was induced only by running at speeds greater than some threshold. In the same study, a bout of running increased TH activity in striatal homogenates for several hours, suggesting a stimulation of dopamine synthesis consistent with the period of elevated extracellular dopamine metabolites. Taken together, these results suggest that effortful running utilizes extra dopamine; upon cessation of the effortful running, this excess dopamine production and metabolism continue for an extended period.

Rats are nocturnal animals. Their rate of light-beam crossings, rearing, and head movements greatly increase in the dark. Thus, circadian behavioral changes provide an opportunity for testing the role of dopamine in voluntary movement. The concentration of dopamine in microdialysates from the rat caudate nucleus increases by 30% in the dark, correlating highly with the increased movement (Paulson & Robinson 1994). In contrast, interstitial dopamine in the nucleus accumbens did not increase in the dark, although the acidic dopamine metabolites were elevated in that region.

10.4.2. Turning

The unilateral destruction of nigrostriatal fibres with 6-OHDA infusion in the rat medial forebrain bundle results in a syndrome of hemiparkinsonism, manifesting in rotational behavior known as "turning" (Ungerstedt & Arbuthnott 1970). Several weeks after an extensive unilateral 6-OHDA lesion, an indirect agonist such as amphetamine produces rotation toward the denervated side (ipsiversion). Receptor supersensitivity on the denervated side is made evident by administration of dopamine agonists, acting directly upon dopamine receptors. In these animals, rotation is toward the intact side (contraversion). During the first few days after a unilateral 6-OHDA lesion, a single administration of amphetamine can produce a "paradoxical" contraversion in rats. However, the amphetamine-releasable dopamine pool is rapidly exhausted on the lesioned side (Robinson *et al.* 1994). The transient contraversion seems to reflect the early development of behavioral supersensitivity in the presence of a small pool of amphetamine-releasable dopamine, even though the dopamine depletion may already be nearly complete.

Contraversion following stimulation of dopamine release in the intact striatum suggests that dopamine release preferentially activates motor behavior on the same side of the animal's body. This notion does not immediately seem consistent with the anatomical relationship between the basal ganglia and the ipsilateral motor and sensory cortices; one might expect that facilitation of dopamine transmission should increase contralateral motor activity, resulting in ipsiversion. However, contraversion, as in the turning of a tractor, could occur either by increased "breaking" of muscles on one side of the body, or by increased power transmission to the other side. Whereas dopamine depletion results in increased tonus of the skeletal muscles contralateral to the lesion, stimulation of dopamine transmission should reduce tonus in the contralateral side. The biomechanics of turning is further complicated by the imbalance between flexor and extensor tone occurring in hemi-parkinsonism. Thus, turning can be understood as movement toward the side of least muscular resistance, more in the manner of a mud-bound motor vehicle slipping toward the side with wheels spinning.

Spontaneous turning preferences occur in intact rats, suggesting a functional asymmetry of striatal dopamine innervations. However, there was no simple relationship between the bias in turning preference and the rate of dopamine uptake by synaptosomes prepared separately from the left and right striata (Shapiro, Glick, & Hough 1986). In contrast, a strain of rat with hereditary spontaneous turning has reduced concentrations of dopamine and its metabolites in the basal ganglia ipsilateral to the spontaneous turning, analogous to a partial dopamine depletion (Richter *et al.* 1999). The density of DAT was lower in the striatum contralateral to spontaneous turning (Gordon, Rehavi, & Mintz 1994), as if asymmetry in the release and clearance of interstitial dopamine could subserve turning bias. However, male and female rats tended to have opposite relationships between asymmetry of DAT activity and spontaneous turning bias (Shapiro, Glick, & Hough 1986); there were subgroups of animals that turned toward or away from the striatal side with the highest dopamine uptake capacity, a finding which requires the conclusion that spontaneous turning bias must have several main causes.

Scanning behavior in these rats in an open field appeared to favor the whiskers on the side of the face opposite to the stimulation and the dopamine release. The concentrations of dopamine and its acidic metabolites were unchanged in extracts from striatum of rats trained to turn by water reinforcement (Szostak *et al.* 1986). Nonetheless, rats trained to run in a circle for a sucrose reward had a substantial increase in specific radioactivity of [^{3}H]dopamine in striatum contralateral to the direction of turning (Bennett & Freed 1986), and increased rate of DOPA synthesis (Morgan, Yamamoto, & Freed 1984). If the trained turning activity were dependent only on newly synthesized dopamine, one might expect a concomitant increase in the specific activity of dopamine metabolites. However, the specific activity of [^{3}H]DOPAC failed to increase to the same extent as that of [^{3}H]dopamine (Bennett & Freed 1986), suggesting that turning behavior was sustained by a substantial recruitment of (non-radioactive) dopamine in a granular storage pool. Since the specific activity of [^{3}H]DOPAC reflects the transit time of newly synthesized [^{3}H]dopamine through the labile cytosolic compartment, this result may indicate that trained turning behavior asymmetrically increased the coupling between dopamine synthesis and vesicular storage.

Inherently asymmetric dopamine function is not the only factor in spontaneous turning bias. For example, the noradrenergic innervation from the locus ceruleus to the ipsilateral substantia nigra had a facilitatory effect on dopamine transmission;

its destruction facilitates dopamine agonist-induced contraversion (Donaldson *et al.* 1976). Cholinergic stimulation of the caudal substantia nigra with carbachol increased dopamine release in the striatum, and increased contralateral turning (Hernandez-Lopez *et al.* 1994). The rate of spontaneous turning after unilateral dopamine depletions is partially sensitive to ablation of the overlying cortices (Crossman *et al.* 1977), such that cortical ablation or indeed pharmacological blockade of excitatory cortical striatal input reduced the asymmetric behavioral response to amphetamine (Lopez-Martin *et al.* 1998). Tactile stimulation to the vibrissae on one side of the rat's face increased dopamine concentration in microdialysates from rat striatum ipsilateral to the stimulation (Adams *et al.* 1991), supporting the notion that sensorimotor input might influence turning. Lesions of the rat subthalamic nucleus result in transient spontaneous ipsiversion, i.e. turning away from the side of the lesion (Kafetzopoulos & Papadopoulos 1983). The spontensous turning subsided several weeks after the lesion, but administration of a dopamine agonist persistently evoked contraversion. Taken together, these results suggest that spontaneous turning preferences in rats reflect the net result of idiosyncratic biases in cortical inputs, and in specific components of the basal ganglia and its output structures.

Continuous video monitoring of normal humans has revealed preferential turning, more marked in women than in men, which might be an expression of an underlying asymmetry of dopaminergic transmission (Bracha *et al.* 1987). It was initially reported that left-prone circling occurs predominantly in unmedicated patients with schizophrenia, whereas normal subjects were equally divided between left circlers and right circlers, but this finding was not subsequently replicated in a larger series of patients (Levine *et al.* 1997). It seems possible that an amphetamine challenge might unmask subtle predisposition for circling in humans, perhaps relevant to the preclinical detection of Parkinson's disease. As will be discussed in greater detail below, meta analyses of several imaging studies has revealed a slightly greater (5%) abundance of D_2 receptors in the right striatum of normal humans (Larisch *et al.* 1998), an asymmetry which might subserve spontaneous turning bias.

10.4.3. *Appetitive behaviors*

The concentration of dopamine in microdialysates from the nucleus accumbens (but not striatum) of male rats increased by 20% upon presentation of a receptive female, and was doubled during about 1 h following copulation (Pfaus *et al.* 1990). Visual presentation of a male rat produces a very slight increase in the extracellular dopamine in nucleus accumbens of sexually receptive female rats; copulation increased the signal by as much as 20% above baseline in nucleus accumbens, and 10% in the striatum (Pfaus *et al.*

1995). The release of dopamine in the nucleus accumbens during copulation is unconditioned in male rats (Wenkstern, Pfaus, & Fibiger 1993); the dopamine release was elevated upon the first presentation of receptive female rats.

Rats having an innate preference for eating sugar are more sensitive to the locomotor stimulant effects of amphetamine and have a greater amphetamine-stimulated efflux of dopamine in the nucleus accumbens (Sills, Onalaja, & Crawley 1998). Sugar-preference did not predict increased sensitivity to directly acting agonists, suggesting that the trait was related to presynaptic factors. The dopamine concentration in microdialysates from the rat amygdala is elevated several-fold during feeding, as are the concentrations of the acid metabolites. Increased dopamine efflux in amygdala could be evoked by glucose injections, whereas insulin decreased the dopamine efflux by 50% (Hajnal & Lenard 1997).

10.4.4. Stress

Exposure to electrical shocks is a stressor which increases the utilization of dopamine in the frontal cortex of rats, as measured by the extent of depletion of dopamine at 1 h after treatment with AMPT (Thierry *et al.* 1976). The shock stress also slightly increased dopamine turnover in nucleus accumbens, but not in the dorsal striatum. Another model of stress is obtained by introducing rats to the home cage of an aggressive male; the new rats are frequently attacked until they assume a submissive posture. This social defeat is associated with a 60% increase in the concentration of dopamine in microdialysates from the nucleus accumbens and the medial prefrontal cortex, whereas dopamine and its metabolites were unaffected in the dorsal striatum (Tidey & Miczek 1996). Thus, the stress-induced dopamine release is most notable in limbic cortical regions.

Immobility conditioned by previous exposure to electrical shocks is associated with reduced dopamine concentration in microdialysates from rat striatum (Katoh *et al.* 1996). The dopamine release in accumbens following footshock can be classically conditioned by association with a tone stimulus, itself inadequate to alter dopamine release (Young, Joseph, & Gray 1993). The conditioned release of dopamine was subject to latent inhibition, i.e. the dopamine release could be abolished by repeated exposure to the conditioned stimulus. Involuntary restraint is itself a potent stressor for rats, resulting in transient increases in dopamine in microdialysates from the nucleus accumbens. Interestingly, release from restraint stress also results in an increase in dopamine and its metabolites during the 30 min following release from restraint (Imperato *et al.* 1992).

In spite of the association between self-administered drugs and dopamine release in the ventral striatum, it is clear that dopamine release in the nucleus accumbens is not rewarding intrinsically and without qualification. Rather, dopamine release is an indicator of increased arousal produced by any change, for better or for worse, in the rat's environment. Furthermore, the conditioned anticipation or expectation of imminent stress or reward evokes the same dopamine release as the stressor itself. Whereas the dopamine release evoked by restraint declines after repeated tests, the release-evoked dopamine release persists for at least a week (Imperato *et al.* 1992), indicating that the rewarding and aversive changes in dopamine release can be separately regulated.

This common pathway of stimulant- and and stress-evoked dopamine release in ventral striatum suggests the possibility of cross-sensitization, such that stresses experienced by an animal could alter the responsiveness of mesolimbic dopamine fibers to subsequent exposure to psychostimulants. This would provide a heuristically useful mechanism underlying the predisposition to drug-seeking behavior. In support of this model, previous electrical shock treatment potentiates the cocaine-induced dopamine release in the rat nucleus accumbens (Sorg & Kalivas 1993). Furthermore, adult rats which had been exposed to maternal separation, a powerful stressor of neonate rats, were supersensitive to the stimulant effects of cocaine, and had increased dopamine release in response to a mild stress (Brake *et al.* 2004). Thus, the responsiveness of the dopamine system bears the mark of previous experience.

The plasma membrane dopamine transporter

11.1. Molecular biology of DAT and regulation of expression

The DAT gene cloned from a rat brain expression library codes for 620 amino acids, with a sequence predicting 12 transmembrane domains (Giros *et al.* 1991). Its expression in various cell lines confers vulnerability to the toxin MPP+ (Pifl, Giros, & Caron 1993), in addition to conferring the ability to transport dopamine. The uptake of dopamine in striatal slices and synaptosomes has a saturable component with high affinity, and apparently also a high-capacity, low-affinity site (Mireylees, Brammer, & Buckley 1986). It is the saturable component that is characterized by sensitivity to cocaine and related compounds. Thus, the potency of many drugs displacing [^{3}H]cocaine from striatal membranes is highly correlated with the inhibition of [^{3}H]dopamine uptake in slices or synaptosome preparations (Madras *et al.* 1989).

The intracellular domain of DAT presents several potential sites for phosphorylation by protein kinases C and A (Giros *et al.* 1992). Treatment with phorbol esters, which activate PKC directly, reduced the maximal velocity of [^{3}H]dopamine uptake by synaptosomes from rat striatum (Copeland *et al.* 1996), and also reduced the velocity of dopamine uptake in frog oocytes expressing human DAT (Zhu *et al.* 1997). This latter reduction in velocity was associated with reduced [^{3}H]mazindol binding to intact cells, without any concomitant change in the ligand binding to homogenates, which indicates that the treatment altered the association of functional transporters with the plasma membrane. Activation of PKC also potentiates the reverse transport of dopamine, whereas DAT inhibitors blocked the amphetamine-induced efflux of dopamine (Cowell *et al.* 2000). Thus, phosphorylation of DAT may differentially alter the bidirectional transport of dopamine across the plasma membrane. In this regard, it is interesting that a rare human allele of DAT identified in two children with ADHD supported exaggerated dopamine efflux at depolarized potentials (Mazei-Robison *et al.* 2008).

In normal prenatal development, nigrostriatal neurons begin to express the DAT gene several days after TH or VMAT2. In culture, embryonic day 13 dopamine neurons are induced to express DAT when allowed to make contact with striatal neurons (Perrone-Capano *et al.* 1996). As shown by the experiments with phorbol esters, the availability of DAT at the plasma membrane seems to be subject to rapid regulation. In order to investigate this regulation, the population of cell-surface proteins in synaptosomes can be labeled with a biotinylated reagent. Using this technique, acute amphetamine treatment substantially but transiently increased the DAT surface expression within less than 1 min, which apparently reflected increased delivery of DAT to the plasma membrane (Johnson *et al.* 2005). However, more prolonged amphetamine treatment of cultured cells expressing human DAT protein, reduced the dopamine uptake capacity, and evoked translocation of the transporters into an intracellular compartment (Kahlig, Javitch, & Galli 2004). This translocation process could be disabled in cell lines expressing a mutation of dynamin, an enzyme involved in clathrin-mediated endocytosis (Saunders *et al.* 2000).

11.2.   Functional aspects of DAT, and how to live without it

In autoradiographic studies of rats with incomplete unilateral 6-OHDA lesions, there was a linear relationship between the extent of the lesion, as indicated by [^{3}H]mazindol binding in vitro, and the rotational behavior evoked by challenge with apomorphine or amphetamine; the rate of rotation only became significant with greater than 60% depletions (Przedborski *et al.* 1995). In a similar study, there was a hyperbolic relationship between the rotation behaviors after a challenge with methamphetamine, and the availability of DAT was measured with the tropane ligand [^{11}C]PE21 in conjunction with microPET; the rate of rotation was substantial only in rats with more than 80% loss of DAT in the lesioned striatum, and declined rapidly with less extensive lesions (Inaji *et al.* 2005a). Both studies, however, indicate a rather sharp threshold for behaviorally significant dopamine lesions in the otherwise intact rat.

The amount of hybridization signal for the plasma membrane DAT per surviving nigrostriatal neuron was reduced in post mortem brain from patients with long-standing Parkinson's disease (Harrington *et al.* 1996). While this may indicate a non-specific pathology of ailing cells, it is also consistent with an adaptive downregulation of the dopamine clearance mechanism in the partially denervated striatum. In support of this proposal, the density of DAT in aged rats was reduced by almost 50%, whereas the concentration of [^{3}H]DTBZ binding sites was reduced by less than 25% (Leroux-Nicollet & Costentin 1994). After a prolonged depletion of dopamine with AMPT, the density of DAT declined by 50% in the striatum of young rats. Quinpirole, a dopamine agonist, had similar effect on the expression of DAT (Han, Rowell, & Carr 1999), indicating that activation of dopamine autoreceptors can modulate DAT expression so as to maintain interstitial dopamine concentration in the presence of declining pre-synaptic elements.

The functional state of DAT sites may also be regulated independently of gene expression. Transgenic mice lacking the dopamine D_2 receptor have normal basal extracellular dopamine concentrations and normal concentrations of DAT by autoradiography. Nonetheless, the uptake of extracellular dopamine is greatly impaired in these animals (Dickinson *et al.* 1999).

Using fast scan cyclic voltammetry, after transient depolarization, the apparent affinity of DAT dopamine is in the range of 0.2–0.6 μM in rat brain slices. However, the calculated capacity or maximal transport rate varied considerably in different brain regions, with higher V_{max} for DAT in the caudate nucleus than in the amygdala (Jones *et al.* 1995). This observation reiterates the concept of volume transmission, since the volume of tissue affected by electrically released dopamine must be greater in the amygdala than in the striatum, where the process of reuptake is much more efficient. In other electrochemical studies, the rate of dopamine clearance, and the vulnerability of this clearance to cocaine treatment, was highly sensitive to the local concentration of DAT in divisions of the rat striatum. However, these reponses seemed insensitive to the position of the electrode with respect to the strisome/matrix compartment (Cline *et al.* 1995).

Mice with knockout of the expression of DAT were behaviorally hyperactive when presented to a novel environment (Sotnikova *et al.* 2006). As might be predicted, absence of DAT has diverse consequences for the dynamics of dopamine signaling. Whereas the amount of evoked dopamine release was somewhat reduced, the content of the dopamine storage pool is only 5% of that in wild-type mice. Knockout of DAT was nonetheless associated with a five-fold increase in interstitial dopamine levels, measured by the zero net flux micro-dialysis method (Jones *et al.* 1998a). In striatal slices from DAT-knockout mice, the clearance of interstitital dopamine is greatly impaired (Figure 10.2); the rate constant in these mice was 0.04 s^{-1} to be compared with 8 s^{-1} in wild-type mice, and to 0.3 s^{-1}, in the presence of cocaine (10 μM) (Budygin *et al.* 2002). Thus, cocaine emulates the DAT-knockout condition by disabling the clearance mechanism, and consequently allowing for more prolonged action of released dopamine in a great volume of the brain.

If blockade of DAT mediates the reinforcing properties of cocaine, congenital lack of DAT should disable the behavioral and rewarding effects of cocaine. DAT-knockout mice have elevated spontaneous locomotor activity during both night and day. Surprisingly, peripheral administration of cocaine still increased interstitial dopamine in striatal microdialysates of DAT-knockout mice (Figure 10.1) (Sotnikova *et al.* 2006). Following electrically evoked dopamine release, the extracellular dopamine measured in striatal slices by electrochemistry was cleared 100-times slower than normal in brain of these mice (Giros *et al.* 1996), a circumstance that is emulated pharmacologically by cocaine (Figure 8.1B). These mice retain the ability to learn conditioned place preference after exposure to cocaine (Sora *et al.* 1998), suggesting that "drug-liking" need not be dependent on the action of cocaine at DAT per se. Mice without serotonin uptake sites could likewise establish conditioned place preference to cocaine. It may be that the post-natal development in the absence of DAT or serotonin uptake sites shifts the bias of cocaine responsiveness from one monoamine uptake site to the other. However, other studies in intact animals indicate that the full expression of the psychostimulant effects of cocaine are mediated by DAT in terminal regions, and by serotonin-mediated actions on the soma of dopamine neurons in the VTA (Mateo *et al.* 2004).

The contribution of other monoamine transporters to dopamine clearance in the striatum has been a matter of debate; pharmacological blockade of noradrenaline or serotonin transporters was without discernible effect on the kinetics of dopamine uptake in the DAT-knockout mice (Budygin *et al.* 2002). In contrast, studies employing synaptosome preparations from mouse brain showed that 20% of dopamine uptake in the striatum could be blocked with nisoxetine, an inhibitor of noradrenaline tranporters (Moron *et al.* 2002). Furthermore, the preponderance of dopamine uptake in the frontal cortex synaptosomes was blocked by nisoxetine, and was insensitive to DAT knockout. Thus, the noradrenaline transporter might more properly be designated the catecholamine transporter, which favors the uptake of dopamine in the cerebral cortex (Yamamoto & Novotney 1998). In brain regions of low DAT expression, COMT also plays a preferred role in the clearance of interstitial dopamine (Yavich *et al.* 2007).

Notwithstanding the alternate pathways, the relative indolence of dopamine clearance in the cerebral cortex results in surprisingly high interstitial dopamine concentrations. Using the zero net flux microdialysis method, the interstitial dopamine concentration in rat frontal cortex (1.5 nM) was only slightly less than in the striatum (Chen, Lai, & Pan 1997). This result may have consequences for receptor competition models, to be discussed at length in a later chapter.

11.3.   Ligands for the detection of DAT

11.3.1.   Tropanes

The prototypic ligand for DAT is cocaine, a tropane alkaloid extracted from the leaves of *Erythroxylum coca*, which has been cultivated for centuries for its psychostimulant properties. The inactive enantiomer (+)-[^{11}C]cocaine is hydrolyzed so rapidly in plasma that amounts detectable by PET do not enter the living brain (Gatley *et al*. 1990). However, the active enantiomer (−)-[^{11}C]cocaine is rapidly transferred to the brain and establishes reversible binding to DAT, a property which lends itself to linear graphical analysis relative to the metabolism-corrected arterial tracer input (Volkow *et al*. 1995b). Relative to its uptake in the cerebellum, a non-binding reference region, the (−)-[^{11}C]cocaine *pB* in human striatum was close to 0.6 when measured using a tracer dose of the ligand (20 μg); this specific binding was largely displaced by pretreatment with specific DAT inhibitors. However, pharmacologically active doses of the same tracer also bound to a high-capacity, low-affinity site that was not displaceable by monoamine uptake inhibitors. Thus, pharmacological effects of cocaine need not be restricted to blockade of monoamine uptake sites, as suggested also by the results of behavioral studies in rodents with DAT knockouts. However, [^{11}C]cocaine has the advantage for human studies in that it behaves kinetically exactly as the drug itself. Consequently, the half-live observed for the washout of [^{11}C]cocaine from the brain, which ranges from 20 to 30 min in humans, should have some bearing on the pharmacodynamics of cocaine abuse (Telang *et al*. 1999).

The chemical structure of cocaine has served as the point of departure for the development of diverse topane alkaloids used for DAT imaging studies. For example, the analog β-carbomethoxy-β-[4-iodophenyl]tropane (β-CIT, also known as RTI-55) and various related compounds such as fluoropropyl-β-CIT (FP-CIT, also known as DATSCAN), like cocaine itself, bind with high affinity to dopamine, serotonin, and also noradrenaline uptake sites. FP-CIT has a slight preference for DAT sites (3.5 nM) over SERT sites (10 nM), in contrast to β-CIT, which is entirely ambivalent (Abi-Dargham *et al*. 1996). Notwithstanding a certain lack of selectivity, members of this class of ligands have been prepared with [^{125}I] for autoradiographic studies in vitro, [^{123}I] for SPET studies, or [^{11}C] for PET studies.

This ambivalent nature of many tropane ligands is revealed by autoradiographic studies in vitro with [^{125}I]β-CIT, which binds exclusively to DAT in rat striatum in the presence of citalopram, or labels only serotonin transporters when a non-radioactive selective DAT ligand is added to the incubation medium (Figure 11.1). The figure also serves to show the relative ubiquity of serotonin

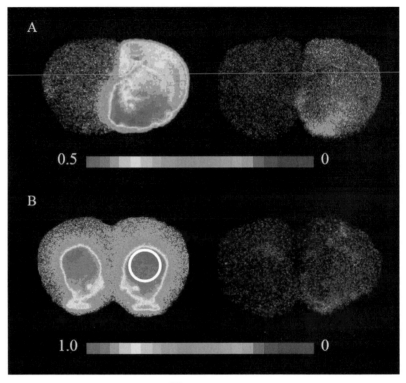

Figure 11.1 The ambivalence of [^{125}I]RTI-55 for transporters of dopamine and serotonin. Autoradiograms with [^{125}I]RTI-55 in coronal cryostat sections from a rat with unilateral destruction of the serotonin innervation. [^{125}I]RTI-55 (10 pM) was employed under conditions specific for SERT (A) and DAT (B). Total binding is shown to the left and non-specific binding to the right. The scale is in units of fmol mg^{-1} tissue. Figure courtesy of Dr. Søren Dinesen Østergaard, Aarhus University PET Centre (For color version, see plate section).

transporters, in contrast to the restricted distribution of DAT in the extended striatum. Whereas the great majority of [^{125}I]β-CIT binding sites in the amygdala and cerebral cortex could be displaced with citalopram, a selective serotonin uptake inhibitor, other displacement studies showed that 80% of the binding in striatum was to DAT (Staley *et al.* 1994). Likewise, the accumulation of [^{11}C]β-CIT in living thalamus and cortex was partially displaced with more selective inhibitors of serotonin or norepinephrine uptake; the binding in the striatum could only be displaced by treatment with a selective DAT ligand, GBR 12909 (Farde *et al.* 1994). In spite of the slight preference of [^{123}I]FP-CIT for DAT in vitro, a large proportion of its extrastriatal binding in human brain was displaced by acute treatment with the selective serotonin reuptake inhibitor paroxetine (Booij *et al.* 2007), whereas extrastriatal [^{123}I]β-CIT binding was displaced with citalopram (de Win *et al.* 2005), a treatment which furthermore isolates the specifically dopaminergic component of [^{123}I]β-CIT binding in human striatum (Ryding *et al.* 2004). In addition, kinetic differences in the rate of association of the ligand to dopamine and serotonin transporters could be used to distinguish the two main binding sites for [^{123}I]β-CIT, which could be a useful approach to analysis, given that pharmacological challenge paradigms are not always applicable in a clinical setting.

In dynamic SPET studies, the initial influx of [^{123}I]β-CIT and other tropanes to human brain is close to the limit established by cerebral perfusion, as seen previously for lipophilic tracers such as [^{11}C]deprenyl. The evolution of contrast between the striatum and the cerebellum, a reference region nearly devoid of mononamine uptake sites, is slow, due to the very slow washout of reversible binding [^{123}I]β-CIT from the reference regions. The dissociation rate of [^{123}I]β-CIT from DAT sites is also extremely slow in living brain. Specifically, the return of normal [^{11}C]cocaine binding in monkey striatum after a pharmacological dose of β-CIT suggested a dissociation rate constant close to 0.0002 min^{-1} (Volkow *et al.* 1995c). This represents the opposite extreme of washout to that represented by [^{11}C]cocaine itself. However slowly it is obtained, the eventual approach to constant binding for [^{123}I]β-CIT represents an equilibrium condition which is proportional to the density of specific binding sites (B_{max}) in the striatum (Laruelle *et al.* 1993). Slow approach to equilibrium can be a virtue in clinical studies with radioligands for single photon studies in that it may be convenient to perform the emission recording on the day following the [^{123}I]β-CIT administration.

As noted above, the lack of pharmacological specificity of most tropane derivatives is compensated by the heterogenous distribution of DAT in the striatum, such that the contributions of other binding sites can be safely ignored in that region. However, quantitative analysis of the binding of some tropane ligands in vivo still suffers from the disadvantage that equilibrium binding is not attained within 90 min, the practical limit of PET studies with [^{11}C]-labeled compounds. The 4-fluorophenyl analog of [^{11}C]β-CIT, [^{11}C]CFT (also known as [^{11}C]-WIN 35428), suffers from a similar failure to attain equilibrium binding within 90 min (Frost *et al.* 1993). This practical limitation is overcome with the use of [^{18}F]CFT (Laakso *et al.* 1998), or the fluoropropyl-labeled derivative [^{18}F]β-FP-CIT, both of which benefit from the longer physical half-life of [^{18}F], and attain equilibrium a few hours after tracer administration (Lundkvist *et al.* 1997).

Among the many tropane ligands for SPET studies, [^{123}I]PE21 is notable for its rapid kinetics in vivo, obtaining equilibrium within 3 h of injection (Pinborg *et al.* 2005), and for its high selectivity for DAT in preference to serotonin or noradrenaline transporters (Stepanov *et al.* 2007). [^{11}C]PE2I has proven to be a sensitive agent for the detection by microPET of dopamine neurons grafted in the striatum of rats with 6-OHDA lesions (Inaji *et al.* 2005b).

[^{125}I]Altropane (also known as [^{125}I]ACFT) binds with an affinity of 5 nM to a single site in membranes from human or rat striatum (Madras *et al.* 1998), and is reported to have 28-fold selectivity for DAT over serotonin transporters. It can also be prepared as [^{11}C]altropane for PET studies, and obtains equilibrium binding within the time limits imposed by the short-lived isotope; the binding potential was 3.5 in the striatum of healthy monkeys (Fischman *et al.* 2001). The tropane [^{11}C]NS2214 (brasofensine) was developed as a PET tracer on the basis of its high affinity and selectivity for DAT in vitro. However, this ligand failed to detect DAT in the brain of living pig, which proved to be a general peculiarity of the binding site in porcine brain, rather than a failing of the ligand itself (Minuzzi *et al.* 2006). A novel compound, [^{3}H]LBT-999 binds to DAT in rat striatal membranes with 9 nM affinity, and apparently 100-fold selectivity over serotonin and noradrenaline transporters (Chalon *et al.* 2006). In a PET study of baboon brain, [^{11}C]LBT-999 reached equilibrium in the putamen as early as 40 min, when the binding ratio relative to the cerebellum was impressively high (15:1). In general, higher specific binding ratios for a DAT ligand predict more sensitive detection of subtle pathological changes in dopamine innervations, so long as some kind of equilibrium state can be obtained.

The advent of [^{99m}Tc]TRODAT-1 has greatly facilitated the clinical assessment of DAT; no cyclotron is required for its synthesis, but instead the metastable technetium is generated on-site using a relatively inexpensive generator. It has 10 nM affinity for DAT, and assumes its peak concentration in rat striatum an hour after injection (Kung *et al.* 1997), although optimal discrimination of healthy and Parkinson's disease subjects occurred at 4 h after tracer injection (Kao *et al.* 2001). Like many other tropanes, [^{99m}Tc]TRODAT-1 also binds to serotonin transporters. Indeed, it can be used to quantify serotonin transporters in the midbrain, where they are most abundant (Dresel *et al.* 1999).

The saturation-binding parameters for various DAT ligands are summarized in Table 11.1. There is generally good concordance between the estimates obtained in membranes and by quantitative autoradiography. However, estimates of the B_{max} for [^{11}C]PE2I in monkey striatum were more than twice the corresponding estimates obtained in vitro with [^{125}I]PE2I (Poyot *et al.* 2001), a discrepancy for which there is no immediate explanation. Whereas some DAT ligands bind to a single site in the striatum, tropane derivatives can distinguish a high-affinity component constituting 25% of the total specific binding and a second site of lower affinity, which recalls the PET finding with (−)-[^{11}C]cocaine, cited above. The significance of heterogeneous binding remains unclear, but it seems certain that the high-affinity site corresponds to the functional DAT. The concentration of high-affinity sites in membranes from rat striatum is substantially higher when measured at the usual laboratory temperature (20 °C) than at

Table 11.1. *Binding parameters for ligands of the plasma membrane DAT in striatum of rat, monkey, and human*

		Reference
[³H]GBR 12783, B_{max}, autoradiography, striatum		Leroux-Nicollet &
Young rats	$420 \pm 19 \, \mathrm{pmol \, g^{-1}}$	Costentin 1994
Aged rats	$235 \pm 57 \, \mathrm{pmol \, g^{-1}}$	
[³H]GBR 12935, $B_{max}(K_D)$, membranes*, rat striatum ($n=4$)	$600 \pm 150 \, \mathrm{pmol \, g^{-1}}$ $(1.4 \pm 0.7 \, \mathrm{nM})$	Cline *et al.* 1995
[³H]mazindol B_{max}, autoradiography, rat,		Marshall *et al.* 1990
Dorsal striatum	$700 \, \mathrm{pmol \, g^{-1}}$	
Ventral striatum	$336 \, \mathrm{pmol \, g^{-1}}$	
[³H]dopamine uptake, V_{max}, synaptosomes, rat		
Dorsal striatum	$26 \, \mathrm{nmol \, g^{-1} \, min^{-1}}$	
Ventral striatum	$16 \, \mathrm{nmol \, g^{-1} \, min^{-1}}$	
[³H]mazindol (4 nM), autoradiography, rat ($n=8$)		Przedborski *et al.* 1995
Rostal striatum	$374 \pm 20 \, \mathrm{pmol \, g^{-1}}$	
Nucleus accumbens	$217 \pm 20 \, \mathrm{pmol \, g^{-1}}$	
[³H]mazindole (9.5 nM), autoradiography, rat ($n=8$)		Cline *et al.* 1995
Lateral striatum	$800 \pm 20 \, \mathrm{pmol \, g^{-1}}$	
Medial striatum	$650 \pm 20 \, \mathrm{pmol \, g^{-1}}$	
[¹²⁵I]altropane, B_{max} (K_D), membranes		Madras *et al.* 1998
Human putamen ($n=4$)	$212 \pm 41 \, \mathrm{pmol \, g^{-1}}$	
Monkey striatum ($n=4$)	$(5.0 \pm 0.4 \, \mathrm{nM})$	
	$301 \pm 17 \, \mathrm{pmol \, g^{-1}}$	
	$(5.3 \pm 0.6 \, \mathrm{nM})$	
[³H]cocaine B_{max} (K_D), membranes, monkey striatum		Madras *et al.* 1989
Site 1	$28 \, \mathrm{pmol \, g^{-1}}$ $(19 \, \mathrm{nM})$	
Site 2	$283 \, \mathrm{pmol \, g^{-1}}$ $(1.1 \, \mathrm{\mu M})$	
[¹²⁵I]RTI B_{max} (K_D), membranes, human striatum		Staley *et al.* 1994
Site 1	$52 \, \mathrm{pmol \, g^{-1}}$ $(100 \, \mathrm{pM})$	
Site 2	$134 \, \mathrm{pmol \, g^{-1}}$ $(1.8 \, \mathrm{nM})$	
[¹²⁵I]RTI B_{max} (K_D), membranes, human striatum		Staley *et al.* 1995
Site 1	$57 \, \mathrm{pmol \, g^{-1}}$ $(250 \, \mathrm{pM})$	
Site 2	$148 \, \mathrm{pmol \, g^{-1}}$ $(5 \, \mathrm{nM})$	
[¹²⁵I]β-CIT B_{max} (K_D), membranes, baboon, cerebral cortex	$48 \, \mathrm{pmol \, g^{-1}}$ $(1.5 \, \mathrm{nM})$	Laruelle *et al.* 1994
Striatum, Site 1	$22 \, \mathrm{pmol \, g^{-1}}$ $(380 \, \mathrm{pM})$	
Striatum, Site 2	$423 \, \mathrm{pmol \, g^{-1}}$ $(18 \, \mathrm{nM})$	

Table 11.1. (*cont.*)

		Reference
[^{125}I]β-CIT SPET, binding ratio at 24 h, control subjects ($n=6$)		Innis *et al.* 1993
Caudate	13±0.6	
Putamen	11±1.0	
Parkinson's disease ($n=5$)		
Caudate	5.4±0.5	
Putamen	2.6±0.5	
[^{11}C]CFT PET, B_{max} (K_D), normal monkey striatum ($n=3$)	113 pmol g^{-1} (33 nM)	Morris *et al.* 1996
MPTP-lesioned monkey ($n=1$)	10 pmol g^{-1}	
[^{11}C]methylphenidate *pB*, control ($n=16$), caudate	1.45±0.17	Lee *et al.* 2000
Putamen	1.30±0.22	
Parkinson's disease ($n=35$), caudate	0.82±0.20	
Putamen	0.37±0.10	
[^{11}C]methylphenidate *pB*, monkey caudate		Doudet *et al.* 2006
Young ($n=6$)	1.08±0.23	
Aged ($n=4$)	0.67±0.21	
MPTP-lesioned monkey putamen ($n=6$)	0.18±0.03	
Healthy young	1.30±0.23	
Healthy aged	0.75±0.27	
MPTP-lesioned	0.18±0.05	
Age-adjusted [^{11}C]-CFT *pB*, healthy humans ($n=10$)		McCann *et al.* 1998
Caudate	8.7±1.6	
Putamen	8.3±1.4	
Methamphetamine users ($n=6$)		
Caudate	7.0±1.2	
Putamen	6.7±0.9	
Parkinson's disease ($n=3$)		
Caudate	5.4±1.2	
Putamen	3.1±0.6	
[^{11}C]cocaine B_{max}, PET study of striatum of human cocaine users ($n=12$)	650±350 pmol g^{-1}	Logan *et al.* 1997
[^{11}C]PE2I B_{max} (K_D), PET, normal baboon	658±103 pmol g^{-1}	Poyot *et al.* 2001
Putamen ($n=3$)	(25±11 nM)	
MPTP-lesioned ($n=3$)	36±30 pmol g^{-1}	
	(57±47 nM)	
[^{125}I]PE2I B_{max} (K_D), in vitro, normal baboon	249±36 pmol g^{-1}	
Putamen ($n=3$)	(2.9±0.1 nM)	
MPTP-lesioned ($n=3$)	18±11 pmol g^{-1}	
	(9±9 nM)	

Note: Concentrations in vitro are reported per gram of tissue, assuming, where specified (•) 10% protein content. In some instances, saturation binding parameters were obtained by PET using multiple tracer injections at differing specific activities.

body temperature (37 °C) (Laruelle *et al.* 1994), which seems contrary to the finding of lower [^{125}I]PE2I binding in vitro, cited above.

Compartmental modeling of radioligand uptake and binding in living brain often requires independent estimation of the non-specific binding component. This was not feasible in the case of [^{11}C]harmine presented in an earlier chapter, due to the ubiquity of MAO-A in the brain. In the case of tropane derivatives, the cerebellum constitutes the most commonly used reference region for constraining the magnitude of non-specific binding in the striatum. Thus, the approach to the equilibrium V_d of [^{11}C]cocaine is revealed by linear graphical analysis relative to the arterial input, and the magnitude of pB in the striatum is then calculated relative to V_d in the cerebellum (Logan *et al.* 1990). Although the use of the cerebellum as a reference region here seems justified by its very low specific DAT binding, we cannot be certain that the distribution properties of ligands in the cerebellum and striatum are entirely identical. Ideally, one should measure the non-specific binding in the region of interest, as in the earlier cases of [^{11}C]harmine after MAO-blockade. However, this approach cannot always be safe in human studies, especially in studies with ligands that are themselves psychostimulants. Alternately, an inactive isomer of the tracer might provide an assay of the non-specific binding component. However, this approach does not work in the case of cocaine, due to the rapid metabolism of the inactive enantiomer, cited above. An inactive isomer of [^{123}I]β-CIT does enter the primate brain, where it is devoid of specific binding. Vexingly, the inactive isomer does not have identical non-specific binding, thus precluding its use for the constrained estimation of specific binding (Scanley *et al.* 1994).

11.3.2. *Other DAT ligands*

The concentration of catecholamine (dopamine and noradrenaline) uptake sites can be measured in vitro with [^{3}H]mazindol; the presence of desmethylimipramine in the incubation medium imparts selectivity for DAT (Marshall *et al.* 1990). Alternate DAT ligands for studies in vitro include [^{3}H]GBR 12783 (Leroux-Nicollet & Costentin 1994), and [^{3}H]GBR 12935 (Richfield 1991). The latter compound has a small piperazine binding component, which can be blocked by the addition of trans-flupentixol to the incubation medium. A representative autoradiogram obtained with [^{3}H]GBR 12935 at a concentration of 2 nM (Figure 11.2) reveals a considerable gradient for DAT in the rat striatum, with highest binding in the dorsal striatum, as seen also in the autoradiographic case of [^{125}I]β-CIT under DAT-specific conditions (Figure 11.1).

As an alternative to the tropanes, the antidepressant drug [^{11}C]nomifensine binds reversibly to catecholamine transporters in living human brain, with a pB close to unity in the case of the active enantiomer (Salmon *et al.* 1990). While this

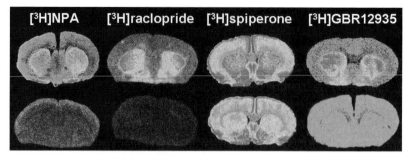

Figure 11.2 Autoradiograms of dopamine D$_2$ and DAT ligands in rat brain cryostat sections. Dopamine binding sites are labeled with the agonist [^{3}H]NPA, the benzamide antagonist [^{3}H]raclopride, and the butyrophenone antagonist [^{3}H] spiperone, in the presence of ketanserin. Also illustrated is the distribution of dopamine transporters labeled with [^{3}H]GBR 12935. All autoradiograms were obtained with ligand concentrations close to the affinities in vitro. The lower row shows the non-specific binding in the presence of butaclamol, in the case of receptor ligands. Figure courtesy of Dr. Luciano Minuzzi, Montreal Neurological Institute, McGill University. (For color version, see plate section.)

binding in the putamen is presumably largely specific for DAT, its substantial binding in the thalamus may reflect the high concentration of noradrenaline uptake sites in that structure. Similarly, the stimulant drug [^{11}C]methylphenidate, which also recognizes both types of catecholamine transporters, binds mainly to DAT in the striatum of living mouse, with a pB near unity (Gatley *et al.* 1995a). Whereas the binding of [^{3}H]WIN 35428 continued to increase in rodent striatum for at least 30 min, [^{11}C]methylphenidate concentration in the striatum eventually declined, indicating the greater reversibility of its binding in vivo. [^{11}C]methylphenidate, like [^{11}C]nomifensine, must be expected to label the ensemble of DAT and noradrenaline transporters. However, parametric maps show that [^{11}C]methylphenidate pB is most abundant in the striatum of normal monkeys, and is substantially depleted in MPTP-poisoned animals (Figure 11.2), as expected for a DAT tracer; the MPTP lesions may unmask the residual binding component of noradrenaline uptake sites, although it must be considered that MPTP is not entirely selective for dopamine neurons.

11.3.3.   Competition in living brain

In theory, competition from endogenous dopamine in the interstitial space might interfere in the binding of DAT ligands in living brain. However, the binding of [^{123}I]β-CIT in living monkey striatum was unaffected by acute treatment with a high dose of the indirect agonist, DOPA (Laruelle *et al.* 1993). Consequently, DOPA treatment need not be considered an interferant in the assay of DAT in clinical studies of Parkinson's disease. In contrast, amphetamine produced a partial displacement of striatal $[^{123}I]\beta$-CIT binding. It is unclear if this is due to competition from elevated interstitial dopamine, or a direct competition between amphetamine and the radioligand for binding to DAT. In other studies, treatment with drugs decreasing dopamine release increased the $[^{11}C]$cocaine pB by about 5% in living monkey striatum, consistent with the occurrence of some competition at DAT in living brain (Gatley *et al.* 1995b). In contrast, $[^{11}C]$methylphenidate binding was entirely insensitive to pharmacological-induced changes in dopamine tonus (Gatley *et al.* 1995a). In summary, competition from dopamine at DAT may bias the estimation of DAT abundance in vivo, but this effect seems not to be very great.

11.4.   Clinical DAT studies

11.4.1.   *Aging and genetics*

Rodent studies indicate age-related reductions in the abundance of DAT in the striatum (Table 11.1), which can also be seen in $[^{11}C]$methylphenidate pB maps from young and aged monkeys (Figure 11.3). Likewise, in populations of neurologically normal volunteers, the $[^{11}C]$methylphenidate pB in the caudate and putamen (Volkow *et al.* 1996a), and the $[^{123}I]\beta$-CIT binding in striatum (Pirker *et al.* 2000; van Dyck *et al.* 1995), both declined by 7–8% with each decade of healthy aging, as did the specific binding of $[^{123}I]$altropane (Fischman *et al.* 1998). In a SPET study of 55 healthy men and women, the age-related declines in $[^{99m}Tc]$-TRODAT-1 binding was clearly biphasic; the first half of life was characterized by DAT loss at a rate of 17% per decade, whereas later in life, the rate of loss declined to a rather more sedate 6% per decade (Mozley *et al.* 1999). This observation calls into question the general use of linear models, a topic considered earlier in the context of FDOPA and Parkinson's disease progression. Why indeed should DAT decline as a simple linear function of age, when other physiological indicators (cardiac output, bone mass) can have a more complex relationship with age?

By definition, non-pathological, age-related declines in DAT must have functional effects. For example, the simple reaction time measured in a neuropsychological study of the healthy elderly correlated positively with the striatal binding of $[^{123}I]\beta$-CIT, with and without correction for age within the aged cohort (van Dyck *et al.* 2008). Given that dopamine concentration measured post mortem in samples from neurologically normal subjects also decline by about 10% per decade (Kish *et al.* 1992b), there might be a simple relationship between DAT and dopamine content in the striatum. However, the elevated dopamine metabolite ratios in post mortem material, and the

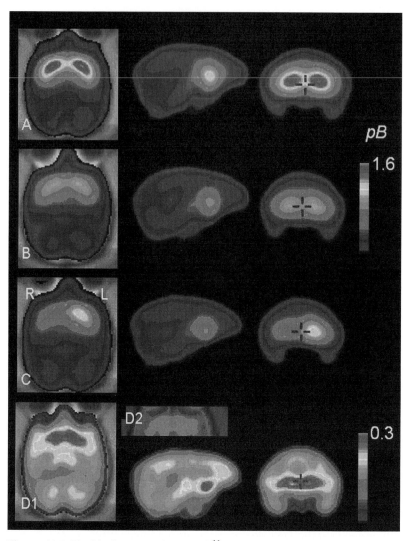

Figure 11.3 The binding potential (*pB*) of [^{11}C]methylphenidate for catecholamine uptake sites in the brain of monkeys. Images show the mean parametric maps in (A) normal young (*n* = 6), (B) normal aged (*n* = 4) rhesus monkeys, (C) aged monkeys with unilateral intracarotid infusion of MPTP (*n* = 3), and (D) monkeys of intermediate age with systemic MPTP administration (*n* = 6). Mean parametric maps are co-registered to the MR template, shown as gray-scale in the horizontal plane images. A sector containing the striatum in the horizontal plane from the MPTP group (D2) is presented with identical intensity scaling as in the intact animals. The cursor in the coronal plane images indicates the position (0,10,10) in the MR coordinate system. Reproduced with permission from Doudet *et al.* (2006). (For color version, see plate section.)

results of the FDOPA steady-state mapping studies cited in Chapter 5, suggest the occurrence of accelerated dopamine turnover in the elderly, which may itself be relevant to the age-related changes in the performance of cognitive and motor tasks. Declines in DAT expression predict that the temporal and spatial patterns of dopamine actions must be inherently different in aged subjects, characterized by a shift away from focal and discrete action toward a condition of volume transmission in the striatum.

The binding ratio of $[^{123}I]$FP-CIT in human striatum was higher in females than in males, but age-related declines did not show any gender effect (Lavalaye *et al.* 2000). Similarly, there was slightly greater $[^{123}I]\beta$-CIT binding in the striatum and other brain structures of females than in males (Staley *et al.* 2001). Others detected neither a gender difference in $[^{123}I]\beta$-CIT binding, nor any difference in binding between the luteal and follicular phase of menstruating females (Best *et al.* 2005). In a group of 18 normal subjects, there was a negative correlation between the availability of $[^{18}F]$CFT binding sites in the right putamen and the "detachment" score of a personality inventory (Laakso *et al.* 2000b). Insofar as DAT determines the rate of dopamine clearance from the interstitial space, this PET result suggests that a propensity for social withdrawal is associated with a more prolonged and spatially distributed action of dopamine at its post-synaptic receptors, as may also occur with normal aging.

The expression of DAT (or indeed any gene product) within a healthy population can be quite variable. To date, there have been lamentably few studies linking human genetics with DAT expression as measured by PET or SPET. In a study of polymorphism of the Taq1 A allele of the dopamine D_2 receptor gene, the A1 allele (which imparts risk for alcoholism) was associated with slightly higher $[^{123}I]\beta$-CIT binding in striatum (Laine *et al.* 2001). The DAT gene itself bears an unexpressed sequence of nine or ten tandem repeats, which has attracted considerable attention because of the allelic associations with several neuropsychiatric disorders. In a small group of normal subjets, heterozygocity of this sequence was associated with a 20% reduction in $[^{123}I]\beta$-CIT binding (Heinz *et al.* 2000), a finding which was not replicated in another study of a larger cohort (Martinez *et al.* 2001). In yet another study, this one involving 96 healthy Caucasians scanned with $[^{123}I]\beta$-CIT, the earlier association was replicated. Although the reduction in DAT binding for the ten-repeat homozygotes was only 10%, the effect was robust to age-correction (van Dyck *et al.* 2005). This history serves as an object lesson of the need for very large subject groups in order to detect relatively subtle genomic effects on entities such as DAT, especially when one considers the confounds due to age and numerous other variables.

11.4.2. Parkinson's disease

The normal attrition rate of DAT binding with healthy human aging suggests that a syndrome of parkinsonism may invariably emerge among healthy centenarians. However, the rate of loss of [^{123}I]FP-CIT binding in Parkinson's disease patients is ten times greater than is the rate of attrition of DAT with normal aging (Lokkegaard *et al.* 2007; Van Laere *et al.* 2004a; Winogrodzka *et al.* 2003), i.e. 8% per year in the putamen. Similar results were obtained in a longitudinal [^{18}F]CFT-PET study (Nurmi *et al.* 2003). Efforts have been made to establish the threshold for DAT loss resulting in clinical symptoms. The binding ratio of [^{123}I]β-CIT in the putamen to that in the cortex was reduced by approximately 80% in patients with early Parkinson's disease (Innis *et al.* 1993); lesser declines were seen in the caudate nucleus. Quite similarly, the [^{11}C]methylphenidate *pB* in the putamen could be reduced by more than 50% without contralateral signs of Parkinson's disease, but mild hemi-Parkinson's disease was associated with a 70% loss contralateral to the symptoms (Lee *et al.* 2000). Relative to the changes in FDOPA and [^{11}C]DTBZ seen in the same subject group, the reductions in [^{11}C]methylphenidate binding were greater, leading the authors to speculate that DAT is downregulated in early Parkinson's disease. Thus, there is a general agreement that symptomatic debut of Parkinson's disease occurs at a threshold DAT loss of more than 50%, with correction for the effects of normal aging (Booij *et al.* 2001). Perfomance of a complex motor task (the grooved peg board) correlated with [^{11}C]CFT binding to DAT only on the less-affected side, presumably due to the low specific signal remaining on the more-affected side (Bohnen *et al.* 2007). Results of these studies of threshold suggest that the suitable end point for future neuroprotective therapies might be to endeavor to protect the dopamine innervation on the less-affected side, rather than attempting to rescue the side on which DAT loss is already nearly complete at the time of diagnosis.

In a multi-tracer study of MPTP-lesioned monkeys (Figure 11.3) (Doudet *et al.* 2006), distinct reductions in [^{11}C]methylphenidate binding were evident in the striatum of healthy aged monkeys, whereas the FDOPA (Figure 5.3) and [^{11}C]DTBZ (Figure 9.1) indices were nearly normal. This observation supports the claim that compensatory down-regulation of DAT can occur, presumably serving to enhance the action of residual dopamine in the partially denervated striatum. In cynomolgus monkeys, repeated doses of MPTP resulted in the progressive loss of presynaptic dopamine markers, and the emergence of motor symptoms of acquired parkinsonism (Nagai *et al.* 2007). At an intermediate stage of symptom severity, [^{11}C]DOPA influx to the striatum was 50% preserved, whereas DAT labeled with [^{11}C]PE2I was already 80% decreased. Only

with continued MPTP-poisoning, eventually resulting in the emergence of tre-
mor, were both biomarkers reduced to the same extent. This discord implies
that there is some degree of nigrostriatal degeneration which DAT can function-
ally accommodate. However, this mechanism eventually fails as dopamine
depletions exceed approximately 80% of normal values. Interestingly, a series
of high-affinity DAT ligands was effective in the alleviation of motor symptoms
with severe MPTP-evoked parkinsonism when DAT loss had reached this threshold (Madras *et al.* 2006).

The possibility of DAT modulation can complicate the interpretation of
prospective studies of Parkinson's disease progression. In particular, the
Parkinson Study Group (2002) reports that $[^{123}I]\beta$-CIT binding in the putamen
declined by 5% per year in patients with early Parkinson's disease, i.e. five times
faster than the decline with normal aging. However, this rate of decline was
substantially lower in those patients treated with the direct agonist pramipexole than in those treated with the indirect agonist DOPA. It was noted that these
findings cannot discriminate between an actual protective effect of pramipexole against cell loss, or a modulatory action on the expression of DAT (Marek,
Jennings, & Seibyl 2002). Comparable studies of $[^{11}C]DTBZ$ binding, which seems
less subject to modulation, might serve to distinguish these possibilities, and
might thus serve as a more physiologically appropriate indicator of disease
progression.

In clinical imaging studies, an observation of normal DAT levels almost
excludes the diagnosis of degenerative Parkinson's disease. Thus, a normal
$[^{123}I]$ioflupane SPET scan can support the diagnosis of psychogenic parkinsonism (Gaig *et al.* 2006). In a follow-up study of 150 subjects with normal $[^{123}I]FP$-CIT
scans, only a very few showed a progressive loss of DAT, indicating that the
remainder suffered from non-degenerative parkinsonism (Marshall *et al.* 2006).
Vascular disease can result in sudden onset of parkinsonism, even in the
absence of discernible structural lesions to the basal ganglia. Diagnosis and
treatment of vascular parkinsonism can be assisted by $[^{123}I]FP$-CIT SPET
imaging and by identifying those patients with real nigrostriatal degeneration
(Lorberboym *et al.* 2004). Similarly, this approach can help distinguish drug-
induced parkinsonism from cases of nigrostratal degeneration (Lorberboym
et al. 2006).

A number of environmental factors can contribute to the development of
Parkinson's disease. This, in a large cohort study, $[^{123}I]$ioflupane uptake in the
striatum was more reduced in Parkinson's disease patients with a history of
occupational exposure to hydrocarbon vapors, than in unexposed patients,
suggesting that environmental factors exacerbate disease progression (Canesi
et al. 2007). Occupational exposure to manganese can evoke a rigid akinetic

disorder resembling Parkinson's disease, known as manganism. There was only a minor reduction in striatal [^{99m}Tc]TRODAT-1 binding in a group of manganism patients (Huang *et al.* 2003), which may account for the lack of efficacy of DOPA in treating that disorder. In monkeys intoxicated with manganese, there was a transient 50% increase in the striatal binding of [^{11}C]CFT; several weeks later the binding had returned to normal levels, suggesting an acute regulatory response, possibly related to recruitment of DAT to the cell surface (Chen *et al.* 2006).

Given the plethora of ligands available for DAT imaging, there have been lamentably few systematic comparisons of their utility. The uptake of [^{123}I]β-CIT and [^{123}I]FP-CIT was measured in the same groups of six Parkinson's patients and healthy control subjects (Seibyl *et al.* 1998). Binding ratios were measured at 20 h post injection for [^{123}I]FP-βCIT, and at 5 h post injection for [^{123}I]FP-β-CIT, reflecting the faster kinetics of the latter compound. Although the binding ratio for [^{123}I]β-CIT in healthy putamen (6.3) exceeded that of [^{123}I]FP-β-CIT (3.3), the latter compound was nonetheless slightly more sensitive at discriminating Parkinson's disease patients from controls. The sensitivity for detecting progression of nigrostriatal loss in Parkinson's disease has been compared for [^{123}I]FP-β-CIT and [^{99m}Tc]TRODAT-1 in a large cohort (Van Laere *et al.* 2004). Both tracers have relatively fast kinetics, obtaining their maximal binding in the striatum some 3 h after injection. However, [^{123}I]FP-β-CIT has superior binding ratio in the putamen relative to the occipital cortex, and could detect declining DAT as a function of disease duration, to which [^{99m}Tc]TRODAT-1 was relatively insensitive. In a more limited study, [^{123}I]altropane (Fischman *et al.* 1998) have compared favorably to FDOPA for the detection of nigrostriatal degeneration.

Declines in catecholamine innervation need not be restricted to the basal ganglia of patients with Parkinson's disease. Thus, in a PET study with [^{11}C]β-CFT, it was possible to detect reduced monoamine transporters not just in the striatum, but also in the orbitofrontal cortex and the amygdala of patients with early Parkinson's disease (Ouchi *et al.* 1999). Similarly, some reduction in [^{11}C] methylphenidate *p*B can be seen in the anterior cingulate cortex of the MPTP-treated monkeys, indicating loss of extrastriatal catecholamine fibers (Figure 11.2). This figure also shows that the MPTP model resembles idiopathic Parkinson's disease with respect to the relative preservation of the dopamine innervation to the nucleus accumbens.

11.4.3.   *Other neuropsychiatric disorders*

The influx of [^{11}C]β-CIT was reduced by 50% in the striatum of patients with Huntington's disease (Ginovart *et al.* 1997b). This is a somewhat perplexing finding, given that the degeneration of this disease is thought to be restricted to the medium spiny neurons of the striatum. Furthermore, the limited available data do not suggest any changes in the utilization of the presynaptic marker FDOPA in Huntington's disease (Otsuka *et al.* 1993). This discrepancy may be consistent with downregulation of DAT in otherwise intact nigorstriatal fibers of patients with Huntington's disease. Lesch–Nyhan syndrome, a devastating X-linked deficiency of hypoxanthine-guanine phosphoribosyltransferase, is associated with even more profound (70%) reductions in the binding of $[^{11}C]CFT$ in the striatum (Wong *et al.* 1996).

Machodo–Joseph disease, a hereditary spinocerebellar ataxia (SCA3) not always presenting with parkinsonian symptoms, was nonetheless associated with a substantial reduction in striatal $[^{99m}Tc]$-TRODAT-1 binding, which was also evident in asymptomatic carriers of the mutation (Yen *et al.* 2002). Parametric mapping with $[^{123}I]\beta$-CIT SPET in spinocerebellar ataxia (SCA2), a related condition, revealed loss of DAT in the putamen, and also in the caudate, midbrain, and pons (Scherfler *et al.* 2006a), as distinct from the more spatially restricted changes characteristic of Parkinson's disease. A similar pattern of widespread loss was evident in a $[^{123}I]\beta$-CIT study of multiple system atrophy (Berding *et al.* 2003). Symmetrical reductions of $[^{123}I]\beta$-CIT binding in striatum are more characteristic of multiple system atrophy than Parkinson's disease, which usually presents as an asymmetric condition (Knudsen *et al.* 2004). Thus, DAT imaging alone may not be adequate for the reliable differential diagnosis of Parkinson's disease and certain parkinsonian syndromes.

SPET with $[^{123}I]FP$-CIT reveals that DAT in caudate and putamen are intact in patients with Alzheimer's disease, as distinct from the condition of dementia with Lewy bodies, in which striatal DAT is substantially reduced (O'Brien *et al.* 2004). This tracer is less effective for the differential diagnosis of Parkinson's disease and dementia with Lewy bodies, although reduced DAT in the caudate nucleus, as opposed to the putamen, is more pronounced in the latter condition (Walker *et al.* 2004). The availability of $[^{11}C]$cocaine binding sites was 20% reduced in the striata of patients with HIV dementia, to an extent correlating with viral load (Wang *et al.* 2004).

Given the continuing currency of the dopamine hypothesis of schizophrenia, there have been relatively few investigations of DAT in that condition. In a $[^{18}F]$ CFT PET study, there was no difference in DAT availability between groups of untreated de novo schizophrenia patients and control subjects (Laakso *et al.* 2000a). In a $[^{123}I]\beta$-CIT SPET study, there was no evidence for abnormal levels of DAT in the striatum of a group of 24 patients with schizophrenia (Laruelle *et al.* 2000). These negative findings were replicated in a $[^{99m}Tc]$TRODAT-1 SPET study of an even larger cohort of patients (Schmitt *et al.* 2006). Among those patients with predominantly positive symptoms, DAT binding *declined* with increasing severity of these symptoms, which accounted for 50% of the variability in binding in a correlational analysis. In another [^{99m}Tc]TRODAT-1 study, overall striatal ligand binding was normal in patients with schizophrenia, but the asymmetric binding favoring the right side of healthy subjects was not evident in the schizophrenic subjects (Hsiao *et al.* 2003). This finding seems consistent with possible abnormalities in spontaneous turning bias reported among patients with schizophrenia. In a PET study of chronic, medicated patients, the striatal [^{18}F]CFT binding had declined by 15% (Laakso *et al.* 2001), which could be an effect of treatment or of disease progression.

The relationship between attention deficit hyperactiviy disorder (ADHD) and the density of DAT has been intensively studied using molecular imaging methods. A series of SPET studies in adolescents with ADHD have shown the presence of elevated levels of DAT in the basal ganglia (see for example Cheon *et al.* 2003; Dresel *et al.* 2000), and it has been claimed that [^{99m}Tc]TRODAT-1 binding in adult ADHD patients predicts good clinical reponse to treatment with methylphenidate (la Fougere *et al.* 2006). In a recent well-controlled [^{11}C]altropane PET study of 47 unmedicated ADHD patients, there was a significant increase in DAT specifically in the right caudate nucleus (Spencer *et al.* 2007). However, a [^{11}C]PE21 PET study showed no difference in the striatal DAT binding in a group of unmedicated ADHD patients (Jucaite *et al.* 2005), whereas others report a significant decrease in the striatal binding of [^{11}C]cocaine to DAT in unmedicated adults with ADHD (Volkow *et al.* 2007a). Thus, the initial consistent finding of increased striatal DAT of patients with ADHD is now called into question.

Striatal DAT measured with the SPET ligand [^{123}I]IPT was quite remarkably elevated (nearly doubled) in a group of never-medicated children with Tourette's disorder (Cheon *et al.* 2004), and somewhat elevated in adults with obsessive compulsive disorder, although the variability was quite high, suggesting a neurochemical heterogeneity within the affected population (Kim *et al.* 2003). Furthermore, a 37% increase in [^{123}I]β-CIT binding was seen in a completely independent study of Tourette's syndrome (Malison *et al.* 1995b). On the balance, results of these imaging studies link elevated striatal DAT with disorders of impulse control.

[^{99m}Tc]TRODAT-1 binding was slightly elevated in healthy subjects in proportion to signs of depressed affect (Newberg, Amsterdam, & Shults 2007), indicating the role of DAT in euthymia. The [^{11}C]RTI-32 *pB* for striatal DAT was significantly reduced in patients with major depression; an inverse correlation with neuropsychological test scores suggested that the greater reduction in DAT protected against symptoms (Meyer *et al.* 2001), perhaps in the manner of a compensatory change potentiating dopaminergic transmission. Others report [^{123}I]β-FP-CIT binding to be reduced specifically in depressed patients with anhedonia (Sarchiapone *et al.* 2006). There was a 10–20% increase in [^{123}I]β-CIT binding in the striatum of depressed patients following treatment with serotonin-selective reuptake blockers (Kugaya *et al.* 2003), an effect also seen following treatment of healthy subjects with the mixed noradrenaline/serotonin transporter ligand venlaflaxine (Shang *et al.* 2007). Nonetheless, the specific binding of [^{99m}Tc]TRODAT-1 was 20% elevated in the striata of a group of patients suffering from major depression prior to intitation of treatment (Brunswick *et al.* 2003), and was likewise elevated in a small group of patients with bipolar disorder (Amsterdam & Newberg 2007). Relative to age-matched controls, striatal [^{123}I]β-CIT binding was decreased in patients with social phobias (Tiihonen *et al.* 1997). The resolution of these disparate findings in mood disorder requires consideration of treatment effects, as well as specific symptomatology. Thus, for example, decreased DAT might manifest specifically in the dimension of anxiety, rather than depressed mood, per se.

11.4.4. *Drug abuse*

The specific binding of [^{99m}Tc]TRODAT-1 was reduced in the striata of patients suffering from alchoholism (Tiihonen *et al.* 1995), consistent with post mortem autoradiographic findings with [^{125}I]PE2I in patients dying with type I alcoholism (Tupala *et al.* 2001). In an [^{123}I]β-CIT SPET study of alcoholics, the decreased striatal binding normalized after 4 weeks abstinence (Laine *et al.* 1999). In contrast, the [^{11}C]methylphenidate *pB* was normal in another group of alcoholics (Volkow *et al.* 1996c). There was a slight increase in the striatal [^{123}I]β-CIT binding of smokers relative to non-smokers (Staley *et al.* 2001). However, others report decreased [^{99m}Tc]TRODAT-1 in the striata of a group of current smokers (Newberg *et al.* 2007). Given the comorbidity of smoking, alcohol abuse, and psychiatric disorders, particular emphasis must be placed on possible clinical heterogeneity within studies of smoking.

The concentration of binding sites for [^{3}H]CFT was increased by about 50% in membranes from the basal ganglia of cocaine users (Little *et al.* 1993). Likewise, the concentration of DAT was moderately increased in a [^{123}I]β-CIT SPET study of abstinent cocaine abusers (Malison *et al.* 1998a), in whom the elevated striatal DAT correlated with scores in the Hamilton Depression Rating Scale. Others, however, report that [^{11}C]cocaine uptake was globally reduced in the brain of cocaine users, without evidence for changes in specific binding within the basal ganglia (Volkow *et al.* 1996d). These disparate results do not entirely support the notion that increased expression of DAT could be a homeostatic response to chronic blockade of dopamine uptake by cocaine. Furthermore, prolonged medication with DOPA or the MAO inhibitor selegiline was without effect on [^{123}I]β-CIT binding in striatum of patients treated for Parkinson's disease (Innis *et al.* 1999). However, homeostatic regulation of DAT is likely impaired in subjects with a substantial degeneration of the nigrostriatal pathway.

A cumulative dose of 100 mg kg^{-1} amphetamine evoked a 20% reduction in [^{123}I]FP-CIT binding in rat striatum (Booij, de Bruin, & Gunning 2006), but similar results are not yet reported in human amphetamine users. The case for altered DAT is clearer in studies of methamphetamine toxicity. Thus, the [^{11}C]CFT *pB* was reduced by 20% in the caudate and putamen of abstinent methamphetamine users (McCann *et al.* 1998). While not crossing the threshold to frank parkinsonism, similar 20% reductions in [^{11}C]methylphenidate in striatum were associated with impaired performance in neuropsychological tests of cognitive and psychomotor function in former methamphetamine users (Volkow *et al.* 2001c). Although other studies showed eventual recovery of DAT following abstinence from methamphetamine (Volkow *et al.* 2001b), these findings raise the ominous prospect that the current generation of methamphetamine users may be at increased risk for acquiring parkinsonism. Injection of GDNF into the monkey striatum imparted some protection against methamphetamine-evoked declines in striatal [^{11}C]CFT binding (Melega *et al.* 2000). Additional loss of [^{11}C]CFT binding in the orbitofrontal cortex and amygdala of methamphetamine users suggested a basis for cognitive and behavioral difficulties (Sekine *et al.* 2003).

11.4.5.   *Psychostimulant action and euphoria*

The binding of cocaine and other psychostimulants to DAT can be assessed in human volunteers by measuring the dose-dependent displacement of [^{11}C]cocaine by a non-radioactive competitor. In this paradigm, the extent of euphoria experienced following administration of cocaine correlated positively with the occupancy of [^{11}C]cocaine-binding sites in the striatum, such that all subjects with greater than 60% occupancy of DAT experienced euphoria (Volkow *et al.* 1997a). The dose of cocaine producing a 50% displacement of [^{123}I]β-CIT sites (ED$_{50}$) was 2.8 mg kg^{-1} in cocaine-dependent subjects (Malison *et al.* 1995a) versus ED$_{50}$ of only 0.1 mg kg^{-1} when [^{11}C]cocaine itself was displaced by cocaine (Logan *et al.* 1997). This difference must surely be related to the very slow washout kinetics of [^{123}I]β-CIT binding, which thus disfavors its use in competition studies. This concept was further substantiated in baboon studies with cocaine against [^{11}C]methylphenidate, and methylphenidate against [^{11}C]cocaine, in which the ED$_{50}$s were in the order of 0.25 mg kg^{-1}, i.e. ten-fold lower than in similar competition studies against [^{123}I]β-CIT (Fowler *et al.* 1998a; Volkow *et al.* 1998b).

The action of cocaine at DAT has led to the search for longer-acting blockers which might be efficacious against cocaine addiction. Mazindol had an ED$_{50}$ of

30 mg kg^{-1} against [^{123}I]β-CIT sites, which was much too high for its safe use as a treatment for cocaine addiction (Malison *et al.* 1998b). Some monkeys self-administered the long-acting cocaine analog RTI-113, which might raise the specter of substituting one addictive drug for another, as first proposed by Sigmund Freud. However, response rates for a fixed schedule of cocaine were lowered by pretreatment with RTI-113, resulting in a 90% percent occupancy of DAT measured with [^{18}F]FECNT PET (Wilcox *et al.* 2002). In contrast, the same authors reported that RTI-112 did not itself evoke self-administration, but could nonetheless interfere with cocaine self-administration when high DAT occupancies were obtained (Lindsey *et al.* 2004).

In baboon striatum, [^{11}C]cocaine and [^{11}C]methylphenidate has similar rapid initial uptake, but the washout of the latter compound was considerably slower (Volkow *et al.* 1995a). In contrast to challenge with cocaine itself, a substantial displacement of [^{11}C]cocaine binding by methylphenidate did not invariably evoke experiences of euphoria in normal human volunteers (Volkow *et al.* 1999b). How to reconcile the difference in subjective experience evoked by two drugs binding to DAT? This discrepancy might be related to the lesser pharmacological specificity of cocaine, which also binds to serotonin uptake sites, but it may also be that the rapid pharmacokinetics of cocaine imparts a particular potential for abuse and self-administration. This claim was substantiated in a [^{11}C]altropane PET study, with scanning of healthy volunteers at intervals after oral methylphenidate (40 mg) administered as rapid- or slow-release tablets (Spencer *et al.* 2006). The slow-release tablets provoked a gradual decline in DAT availability lasting at least 7 h, but with little reporting of liking the drug effect. In contrast, the rapid-release drug evoked a rapid and more transient occupation of DAT, and consistent reports of drug-liking. Behavioral results in monkeys trained to self-administer tropane analogs revealed that the efficacy in promoting self-administration correlated with the association rate to DAT, measured in vitro (Wee, Carroll, & Woolverton 2006). Conceivably, euphoria imparted by the rapid kinetics of cocaine results in transient blockade of DAT, which is uncompensatable by homeostatic mechanisms of the dopamine fibers. Thus, PET informs us that a kick must be delivered swiftly if it is to be enjoyed.

12

Dopamine receptors

12.1. Pharmacology and biochemistry

The two classes of dopamine receptors, D_1 and D_2, were first distinguished on the basis of classical pharmacology (Kebabian & Calne 1979). In the late 1980s, the dopamine receptor genes were cloned from rodent brain expression libraries by hybridization with the genes for homologous GTP-binding protein-linked receptors (Neve & Neve 1997). These techniques subsequently revealed a further subdivision of the two classes of dopamine receptor. The D_1-like receptors consist of D_1 and D_5, while the D_2-like receptors consist of D_2, D_3, and D_4 receptors. In addition, alternate splicing of the D_2 gene product permits the expression of a short form of the D_2 receptor (D_2S), and a long form with an additional 29 amino acids (D_2L) at the third cytoplasmic loop (Giros *et al.* 1989).

Members of these two dopamine receptor classes have considerable sequence homology and broadly similar pharmacology. All of the dopamine receptors possess the 7-transmembrane domains which are characteristic of members of the large family of receptors that are coupled to GTP-binding proteins (G-proteins). Pharmacological specificity of dopamine receptors is imparted by the amino acid sequence of the agonist binding site, and transductional specificity is imparted by the nature of the intracellular G-protein binding domain. Thus, the dopamine D_1-like receptors are coupled to a G-protein activating cytosolic adenylate cyclase (G_s), whereas dopamine D_2-like receptors generally inhibit the activity of adenylate cyclase (G_i/G_o), although other signaling pathways have also been implicated.

The G-proteins afford the possibility of convergence and integration of the signal transduction pathways for multiple classes of neuroreceptors. For example, adenosine receptors (Mayfield *et al.* 1999) have independent effects on adenylate cyclase in some neurons also bearing dopamine receptors. The balance of all effects on the adenylate cyclase activity determines the rate of synthesis of the intracellular second messenger cAMP, which in turn regulates the activity of cAMP-dependent protein kinase enzymes. The phosphorylation of specific substrates by cAMP-dependent protein kinase has diverse consequences for the functional state of receptors, the activity of enzymes, and the conformation of structural proteins, and can ultimately alter the expression of genes.

The significance of the long and short isoforms of dopamine D_2 receptors is not fully understood. The ratio of the two isoforms is tissue-specific, but can be altered by treatment with sex steroids (Guivarc'h, Vernier, & Vincent 1995). Normally, the maturation of newly transcribed dopamine D_2 receptors proceeds by a series of steps involving glycosylation of the native protein and subsequent insertion into the plasma membrane. The post-transcriptional processing of the D_2L to the membrane-bound and fully glycosylated form is neither as complete nor as rapid as is the case for D_2S (Fishburn, Elazar, & Fuchs 1995). Thus, alternate transcription can influence the intracellular trafficking of dopamine D_2 receptors. The isoforms seem to be coupled to signal transduction pathways via distinct varieties of the G_i protein (Senogles 1994). The predominant isoform is D_2S in the soma and nigrostriatal projection fibers and D_2L in the medium spiny neurons of the striatum (Khan *et al.* 1998). The cellular localization of the short form suggests that it may be the presynaptic autoreceptor. This distinction may provide a partial explanation for the pharmacological specificity of dopamine autoreceptors, which are more sensitive to agonists than are the post-synaptic receptors. The G-protein binding is mediated by the variable sequence of the third cytoplasmic domain, predicting that ligands with specificity for D_2S or D_2L might conceivably be targeted against the third transmembrane sequence. However, current radioligands simply do not distinguish the isoforms of dopamine D_2 receptors.

12.2.   Neurochemical anatomy

D_1 and D_2 receptors make up the preponderance of dopamine receptors in the striatum. As noted in the introductory section on neurochemical anatomy, the dopamine receptors are partially segregated to specific cellular populations in the striatum, such that D_1 receptors are mainly located on striatal neurons projecting to the substantia nigra and external pallidum (the indirect pathway). The cloned D_5 receptor has similar pharmacology to the D_1 receptor, albeit with a considerably higher affinity for dopamine (Sunahara *et al.* 1991). Although radioligands distinguishing the dopamine D_1 and D_5 receptors have not yet been developed, the expression of D_5 receptors mapped with specific antibodies to dendrites of widely spread neurons of the cerebral cortex, diencephalon, and cerebellum (Ciliax *et al.* 2000), in spite of the sparse dopamine innervation of that tissue. In the striatum, D_5 receptors are associated mainly with interneurons, although some labeling of medium spiny projection neurons has also been observed (Rivera *et al.* 2002).

The relative segregation of dopamine D_1 and D_2 receptors to different populations of striatal neurons suggests that the full integration of dopamine signaling could be mediated by cross talk between dopamine-receptive neurons. Indeed, injections of fluorescent dye into single dopamine neurons (Grace & Bunney 1983) or dopamine-receptive neurons in the striatum (O'Donnell & Grace 1993) often result in the labeling of several neurons. Dyes, ions, and electrical currents can communicate freely between dye-coupled neurons via the gap junction, which serves to unite neurons into physiologically integrated units. Dopamine itself modulates the extent of dye coupling between striatal neurons. Whereas D_1 receptors have region-specific effects on dye coupling in the nucleus accumbens, D_3 receptor agonists increase the coupling between granule cells of the islands of Calleja of the ventral forebrain (Halliwell & Horne 1998).

Dopamine D_2 receptors have a particular association with striatal neurons projecting to the internal pallidum (the direct pathway) without an intervening synapse in the way-station of the subthalamic nucleus. The extent of co-expression of D_1 and D_2 receptors within individual striatal neurons has been a matter of debate, but in a study employing sensitive probes against mRNA, there was nearly complete segregation within the rat extended striatum (Le Moine & Bloch 1995). In contrast to this finding, co-expression of mRNA for D_1 and D_3 was present in approximately one quarter of neurons in the rat nucleus accumbens (Le Moine & Bloch 1996).

Whereas D_2 receptors are expressed throughout the forebrain, messages for the D_3 receptors one more restricted to forebrain structures innervated by the A10 dopamine neurons of the VTA. Additional sites for D_3 expression include limbic structures such as the hippocampus and also the substantia nigra (Bouthenet *et al.* 1991), where D_3 receptors may contribute to autoreceptor function. Binding studies with selective radioligands ($[^3H]$pramipexole for D_2 and $[^3H]$-(+)-7-OH-DPAT for D_3) revealed that D_3 receptors are preferentially expressed in the ventral striatum (Wallace, Owens, & Booze 1998). Likewise, autoradiographic studies with the dopamine D_3-selective antagonist $[^3H]$PD-128907 revealed most abundant binding in the nucleus accumbens and ventral forebrain of the rat (Bancroft *et al.* 1998). The proportion of D_3 to D_2 may be 25% in the nucleus accumbens, but only 4% in the dorsal caudate nucleus from human autopsy material (Piggott *et al.* 1999b).

The distribution of dopamine D_4 receptors can be assessed using the $D_{2/3/4}$ ligand [^{3}H]nemonapride in the presence of raclopride, to block the $D_{2/3}$ components; this procedure reveals most abundant D_4 binding in the hippocampus, limbic and frontal cortex, and relatively little binding in the basal ganglia (Tarazi, Kula, & Baldessarini 1997). However, [^{3}H]nemonapride proved to be a rather better ligand for the sigma receptors than for dopamine (Ujike, Akiyama, & Kuroda 1996). Using selective antibodies in conjunction with electron microscopy, D_4 receptors have been identified on axons of neurons of the rat nucleus accumbens, sometimes in direct apposition to TH-positive terminals (Svingos, Periasamy, & Pickel 2000). The dopamine D_4 receptor has attracted considerable attention, as the preferred site of action of the atypical antipsychotic medication clozapine (Wilson, Sanyal, & Van Tol 1998). However, progress in molecular imaging studies of D_4 receptors has been hampered by the lack of selective ligands.

12.3. Dopamine receptor signal transduction

Irrespective of their exact anatomical projections, all medium spiny neurons of the striatum possess a high expression of dopamine receptors and of a cAMP-regulated phosphoprotein (DARPP-32), which plays a key role in dopamine signal transduction. The state of phosphorylation of DARPP-32 is determined by the balance of activity of two enzymes, the cAMP-dependent protein kinase (PKA) and a calcium/calmodulin-dependent phosphatase known as calcineurin. Whereas activation of dopamine D_1 receptors directly stimulates cAMP production, which in turn stimulates phosphorylation of DARPP-32 in striatonigral neurons, dopamine D_2 agonists decrease DARPP-32 phosphorylation in striatopallidal neurons in a manner dependent upon membrane depolarization and calcium influx. This scenario is complicated by "cross talk" between populations of striatal projection neurons, such that D_2 receptors activation can override simultaneous D_1 activation (Lindskog *et al.* 1999). The anatomical basis of this intrastriatal connectivity could be mediated by striatal interneurons, by direct synaptic contact, or through heteroligomeric associations of the two receptor types, as discussed below.

The state of phopshorylation of DARPP-32 has consequences for the activity of signal transduction pathways in cells responsive to dopamine. Phosphorylation of DARPP-32 at one amino acid residue (Thr34) converts DARPP-32 into an inhibitor of protein phosphatase type 1, whereas phosphorylation at Thr74 is an inhibitor of PKA (Svenningsson *et al.* 2004). Striatal neurons respond to diverse signals by altered expression of c-*fos* and other so-called immediate-early genes.

The medium spiny neurons in DARPP-32 knockout mice had normal levels of dopamine receptors, but the *c-fos* expression in response to dopamine D_1 agonists was reduced, indicating attenuation of that pathway (Svenningsson *et al.* 2000). Among the many substrates of cAMP-dependent protein kinase is a transcription factor known as the cAMP-responsive element-binding protein (CREB); phosphorylated CREB binds to regulatory sites on nucleic acids regulating the expression of *c-fos* and other immediate-early genes. The extent of CREB phosphorylation reflects an integration of diverse inputs, and can also subserve a synergism between dopamine D_1 and D_2 receptors (Kashihara *et al.* 1999).

The extent of *c-fos* expression is the result of a multiplicity of factors converging to influence the medium spiny neurons. As such, *c-fos* and other immediate-early genes reveal the integrative function in the basal ganglia. In general, the expression of c-fos protein in rat striatal neurons is elevated by dopamine agonists. Blockade of D_2 receptors potentiates the increased *c-fos* expression in medium spiny neurons which is evoked by D_1 activation (Le Moine *et al.* 1997). Whereas directly acting dopamine agonists tend to produce patchy patterns of *c-fos* expression in rat striatum, cocaine and other dopamine re-uptake inhibitors produced a more even pattern of *c-fos* activation (Wirtshafter 2000). The basis of this discrepancy is an interesting matter for speculation. Whereas direct agonists may have their greatest effect on those dopamine receptors that are tonically the least activated, pure uptake blockers such as cocaine might activate a broader range of dopamine receptors.

Cortical and subcortical inputs are integrated in medium spiny neurons. The glutamatergic corticostriatal pathway is excitatory to medium spiny neurons, increasing the expression of *c-fos*. Thus, co-activation of dopamine D_1 receptors and NMDA-receptors is necessary for the full activation of *c-fos* expression in medium spiny neurons during the performance of a treadmill-running task (Liste *et al.* 1995). On the other hand, blockade of dopamine D_2 receptors decreased the threshold for activation of *c-fos* expression in medium spiny neurons by pharmacological stimulation of the cortex (Berretta, Sachs, & Graybiel 1999).

The phenomenon of priming is well established in the context of neurotoxic models of parkinsonism, and is thought to provide a model for levodopa-induced dyskinesias, which mar the clinical response to treatment in advanced cases of Parkinson's disease. In this condition, the formerly effective dose of DOPA evokes distressing movements of the limbs, indicative of sensitization to its agonist effects. In rats with unilateral 6-OHDA lesions, pre-exposure to a D_1 agonist results in large increases in the amount of cAMP formed upon subsequent activation of the same receptors (Pinna *et al.* 1997). This change occurs in the absence of large increases in the density of D_1 receptors. Increased cAMP levels in the striatum of dopamine-depleted rats result in turn in elevated phosphorylation of the CREB protein, which presumably changes the expression of diverse genes (Oh *et al.* 2003).

The control of cAMP synthesis by D_1 receptors in the striatum is mediated by the olfactory type G-protein α-subunit (Gαolf), concentrations of which are increased in the striatum of parkinsonian rats suffering from DOPA-induced dyskinesias (Corvol *et al.* 2004). The sensitivity of dopamine D_1 receptors can be assessed by measuring the agonist-evoked incorporation of GTPγS into brain cryostat sections. Using this technique, D_1 receptors were found to be supersensitive in parkinsonian monkeys with DOPA-induced dyskinesias. The absolute abundance of DARPP-32 was increased in the striata of the same animals (Guigoni *et al.* 2005). Thus, the integrity of signal transduction pathways emerges as more relevant to aspects of dopamine neurotransmission, than is the simple abundance of receptors.

As noted above, signaling via D_1 receptors has been assessed from the accumulation in the brain of cAMP, which is stimulated by agonists. The assay of D_2 signaling is more problematic, since it entails a reduction or no change in the intracellular concentration of cAMP. Classically, the state of activation of the D_2 pathway has been deduced from the inhibition of TH activity in dopamine neurons mediated by agonism at presynaptic autoreceptors. Alternately, the direct stimulation of adenylate cyclase by forskolin is opposed by treatment with dopamine D_2 agonists. Using this latter technique, the coupling of rat dopamine D_2 receptors expressed in clonal cells was shown to be mediated by inhibition of cAMP formation (Albert *et al.* 1990). Chronic activation of D_2 receptors can result in paradoxical stimulation of cAMP formation, which is not dependent upon expression of G_s protein, but rather upon a calcium-dependent mechanism (Vortherms *et al.* 2006). Recently, the efficacy of coupling of dopamine D_2 receptors to intracellular pathways in post-synaptic membranes has been measured autoradiographically or in membranes using the agonist-evoked association of radioactive GTPγS to G-proteins. In this paradigm, the increase in receptor numbers after haloperidol treatment was paralleled with an increase in agonist efficacy (Geurts, Hermans, & Maloteaux 1999).

12.4.   Agonist-induced internalization of dopamine receptors

The expression of dopamine D_1 receptors in transfected hamster ovary cells can be detected using fluorescent antibodies. Brief exposure of these cells to a dopamine D_1 agonist increased the intracellular cAMP concentration, followed by a rapid decline in the immunofluoresence, which returned to normal levels about 15 min after washing of the cells (Ariano *et al.* 1997). Furthermore, agonist treatment results in a rapid loss of mammalian D_1 binding sites expressed on the surface of ovary cells of the fall armyworm, an insect (Ng *et al.* 1995). Thus, agonists of D_1 receptors evoke a reversible translocation of the receptors from the plasma membrane site to an intracellular site, apparently mediated by an endocytotic mechanism. Agonists can also alter the subcellular distribution of dopamine D_1 receptors in living striatum. The D_1 receptors of rat medium spiny neurons are normally localized distal to the synapses, on the somatic plasma membranes and on dendritic spines. Treatment with a full dopamine D_1 agonist or with the indirect agonist amphetamine increased the immunoreactivity for D_1 receptors in the proximal dendrites; ultrastructural examination showed the receptors had been relocated from the plasma membrane to endocytotic vesicles (Dumartin *et al.* 1998).

The internalization of dopamine D_2 receptors was first demonstrated using the radioligand [^{3}H]spiperone. Accumulation of this ligand in living rat striatum was enhanced by electrical stimulation of dopamine release, and was attenuated by dopamine depletion with reserpine, suggesting an internalization process driven by binding of dopamine, the endogenous agonist. Treatment with chloroquine so as interfere with receptor recycling increased the [^{3}H]spiperone binding in microsomes, rather than the cell surface, revealing the occurrence of dynamic turnover of dopamine D_2 receptors (Chugani, Ackermann, & Phelps 1988). The pathway for agonist-induced internalization of dopamine D_2 receptors in COS-7 cells is mediated by phosphorylation of the receptors by specific protein kinases (Ito *et al.* 1999). Further use of subcellular fractionation methods showed that amphetamine treatment reduced cell-surface binding of the antagonists [^{3}H]raclopride and [^{3}H]spiperone, but enhanced accumulation only of the latter compound in intracellular compartments, suggesting that the agonist-induced internalization process disfavors the transfer of [^{3}H]raclopride into the cell (Sun *et al.* 2003). In that study, the [^{3}H]raclopride binding measured ex vivo continued to decrease for at least 6 h after amphetamine treatment, which is a matter of concern to the simple competition model, since amphetamine-evoked increases in interstitial dopamine tend to last only a few hours.

13

Imaging dopamine D_1 receptors

13.1. General aspects of D_1 receptors

In the presence of a D_2 antagonist, the binding of [^{3}H]dopamine to rat brain sections is very selective for dopamine D_1 sites, and is entirely displaced by low concentrations of the prototypic D_1 antagonist Sch 23390 (Herve *et al.* 1992). However, the D_1 receptors linked to adenylate cyclase may constitute a subset of the binding sites for [^{3}H]Sch 23390 (Andersen & Braestrup 1986). In the absence of sodium ion, two affinity states of dopamine D_1 receptors for dopamine can be distinguished. The high-affinity state of the receptor, which is sensitive to the presence of GTP, seems to constitute about one half of the total binding in membranes prepared from bovine caudate (Seeman *et al.* 1985). Likewise, increasing concentrations of a D_1 agonist displace [^{3}H]Sch 23390 from D_1 receptors in human caudate in a biphasic manner, revealing approximately equal proportions of $D_1{}^{Low}$ and $D_1{}^{High}$ states of the receptor. In contrast, others report the fraction of dopamine D_1 receptors in rat cryostat sections in a high-affinity state for dopamine to be only 20%, versus 77% for D_2 receptors (Richfield, Penney, & Young 1989).

The regulation of dopamine D_1 receptor expression in living brain is poorly understood. Steroid hormones play a role, since the striatal binding of [^{3}H]Sch 23390 in female rat decreased following ovariectomy, and varied across the estrus cycle (Levesque, Gagnon, & Di Paolo 1989). Prolonged treatment with a classical antipsychotic drug increased the concentration of D_2 receptors in rat striatum, but was without effect on the density of dopamine D_1 receptors (Huang *et al.* 1997). MPTP-lesions did not alter the density of D_1 binding sites in mouse striatum (Araki *et al.* 2000), and produced no changes (Graham *et al.* 1990), or only transiently increased D_1 binding in striatum of parkinsonian monkeys

(Decamp, Wade, & Schneider 1999). In an earlier MPTP study, the dopamine depletion tended to increase D_1 binding sites in monkey striatum to a greater extent in the caudal caudate-putamen than in the rostral regions (Graham, Sambrook, & Crossman 1993), but these effects were of marginal significance.

Changes in the population of dopamine D_1 receptors occurring in the functional agonist-binding state would be expected to modulate the sensitivity of dopaminergic signaling. Thus, partial inactivation of striatal dopamine D_1 receptors with the alkylating agent 1-ethoxycarbonyl-2-ethoxy-1,2-dihydroquinoline (EEDQ) resulted in relatively small declines in the dopamine-evoked stimulation of adenylate cyclase, which could suggest that the remaining receptors were more efficiently linked to signal transduction pathways (Trovero *et al.* 1992). Alternately, this observation may simply reveal the presence of a substantial reserve of receptors. Less consistent with the model of enhanced coupling, dopamine depletions did not change the abundance of D_1 antagonist binding sites in rat striatum, whereas the agonist-binding fraction had paradoxically declined to less than 25% of the total (Herve *et al.* 1992).

As suggested above, the D_1^{High} fraction may change in pathophysiological conditions. For example, in rats which had behavioral sensitization to the locomotor stimulant effect of cocaine, there was relatively reduced alkylation of the D_1 receptors by EEDQ, suggesting that the receptors were protected by increased occupation by dopamine in the sensitized condition (Burger & Martin-Iverson 1994). PET studies with the D_1 antagonist [^{11}C]Sch 23390 show that prolonged binge-like treatment with cocaine evokes a small but significant decline in the availability of D_1 receptors in rat striatum, although the effect on D_2 receptors was more pronounced (Tsukada *et al.* 1996). In brain samples from a small population of patients with schizophrenia, the affinity of the agonist-binding population of D_1 receptors was increased relative to normal control subjects (Mamelak, Chiu, & Mishra 1993).

13.2.   PET ligands for D_1 receptors

Several benzazepines possess 1000-fold preference of D_1 over D_2 receptors, with affinities in vitro close to 200 pM (Halldin *et al.* 1998). These compounds subsequently found use as ligands for autoradiographic studies of D_1 receptors in living brain; the most widely used tracer for PET studies of D_1 receptors are [^{11}C]NNC 112 and [^{11}C]Sch 23390. The distribution of binding sites for the D_1 antagonist [^{3}H]Sch 23390 in a sagital cryostat section of pig brain is illustrated in Figure 13.1. A dorsal–ventral gradient of specific binding can be discerned, with highest binding in the ventral striatum. A surface rendering of

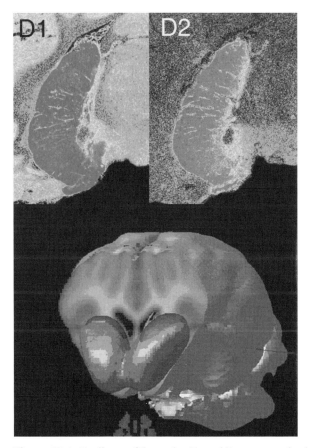

Figure 13.1 Gradients of dopamine D_1 and D_2 receptors in the brain of pig. The upper portion of the figure shows autoradiograms of the binding of (D_1) [^{3}H]Sch 23390 and (D_2) [^{3}H]raclopride in cryostat sections of pig brain, whereas the lower figures shows the surface renderings of the binding potential of (D_1, gold) [^{11}C]NNC 112 and (D_2, red) [^{11}C]raclopride in the striatum of living pig, projected onto the standard stereotaxic MR of pig brain. Images courtesy of Dr. Luciano Minuzzi, and Professor Pedro Rosa-Neto, Montreal Neurological Institute, McGill University. (For color version, see plate section.)

the specific binding of [^{11}C]NNC 112 in the brain of living pigs reveals the same trend towards peak binding in the ventral striatum (Rosa-Neto, Doudet, & Cumming 2004). Results of some quantitative studies of D_1 receptors are summarized in Table 13.1; while most abundant in the striatum, considerable amounts are also present throughout the cerebral cortex. However, displacement studies indicate that as much as 25% of the cortical binding of [^{11}C]NNC 112 and [^{11}C]Sch 23390 can be attributed to serotonin $5HT_2$ receptors (Ekelund *et al.* 2007).

Table 13.1. *Saturation binding parameters of ligands for dopamine D_1 receptors in brain*

	B_{max}, pmol g^{-1} (K_D, nM)	Reference
[^{3}H]Sch 23390 (2 nM), autoradiography, rat striatum ($n = 8$)	480 ± 50	Chen *et al.* 1997
Olfactory tubercle ($n = 8$)	480 ± 25	
[^{3}H]Sch 23390, autoradiography, rat striatum	280	Herve *et al.* 1992
Prefrontal cortex	37	
[^{3}H]dopamine, autoradiography, rat striatum (in presence of spiroperidol)	121	
[^{3}H]Sch 23390, autoradiography, adult human striatum	103 ± 17 (2 ± 1)	Montague *et al.* 1999
[^{3}H]Sch 23390, autoradiography*, rat striatum	480 ± 25 (2.1 ± 0.1)	Savasta, Dubois, & Scatton 1986
[^{3}H]Sch 23390, autoradiography, rat striatum	522 ± 38 (1.0 ± 0.2)	Carey *et al.* 1998
[^{3}H]Sch 23390, autoradiography, young rat striatum ($n = 8$)	232 ± 2 (1.9 ± 0.1)	Giardino 1996
Old rat striatum ($n = 8$)	111 ± 7 (1.5 ± 0.1)	
[^{3}H]Sch 23390, autoradiography, pig		Minuzzi *et al.* 2006
Caudate nucleus ($n = 4$)	227 ± 26 (1.5 ± 0.8)	
Nucleus accumbens ($n = 4$)	245 ± 32 (1.8 ± 1.0)	
Neocortex ($n = 4$)	59 ± 5 (2.9 ± 0.4)	
[^{125}I]Sch 23982, autoradiography*, rat striatum	9 ± 2 (0.09 ± 0.02)	Altar & Marien 1987
[^{125}I]Sch 23982, autoradiography*, rat striatum	17 ± 1 (0.09 ± 0.01)	Aiso *et al.* 1987
[^{3}H]Sch 23390, membranes, rat striatum	71 (0.45)	Hess *et al.* 1986
[^{3}H]Sch 23390, membranes, human striatum ($n = 121$)	16.5 ± 0.4	Seeman *et al.* 1987
[^{3}H]Sch 23390, membranes*, human caudate		Rinne, Lonnberg, & Marjamaki 1990
20 years old ($n = 10$)	22 ± 4	
60 years old ($n = 10$)	13 ± 4	
[^{3}H]Sch 23390, membranes*, human putamen		Rinne *et al.* 1991
Controls ($n = 33$)	13 ± 1	
Parkinson's disease ($n = 37$)	11 ± 1	
Parkinson's disease, with neuroleptics ($n = 12$)	13 ± 1	
[^{11}C]Sch 23390, PET, rat striatum at baseline	195 (50)	Tsukada *et al.* 1996
Binge cocaine treatment	195 (61)	
[^{11}C]NNC 112, PET, monkey ($n = 2$)		Chou *et al.* 1999
Striatum at baseline	78 (18)	
And 5 h after reserpine	78 (17)	
Neocortex at baseline	19 (13)	
And 5 h after reserpine	18 (14)	
[^{11}C]Sch 23390, PET, human		Karlsson *et al.* 2002
Caudate, healthy control ($n = 10$)	40 ± 11 (20 ± 6)	
Caudate, schizophreniform ($n = 10$)	36 ± 13 (17 ± 7)	

Note: Indicated are the maximal binding site density (B_{max}) and the apparent affinity (K_D). In some instances, number of subjects are not reported due to population-based estimation of kinetic parameters. *Results in vitro converted to pmol g^{-1} wet tissue, assuming 10% protein.

The association between dopamine D_1 ligands and receptors in living brain can be modulated by intracellular second messenger systems. Thus, intrastriatal infusions of cAMP analogs enhanced the binding of [^{3}H]Sch 23390 in rat striatum, an effect mediated by increased association rate (Abe *et al.* 2002). Co-injection of an inhibitor of PKA blocked the cAMP-mediated increase in ligand binding. Conversely, administration of the phosphodiesterase type IV inhibitor rolipram, which would be expected to increase cAMP levels, decreased the rate of association of [^{3}H]Sch 23390 (Hosoi *et al.* 2002). While these disparate results cannot be resolved, they reveal mechanisms by which affinity of D_1 receptors in living brain could be modulated.

13.3.   Imaging studies of D_1 receptors

13.3.1.   *Clinical studies*

Relative to rats aged 6 months, there was at 24 months a 25% reduction in dopamine D_1 receptors measured by [^{3}H]Sch 23390 autoradiography in vitro or by [^{11}C]Sch 23390 microPET (Suzuki *et al.* 2001). Likewise, the abundance of D_1 receptors in human striatum in a [^{3}H]Sch 23390 autoradiographic saturation binding study declined by 4% with each decade of healthy aging (Rinne, Lonnberg, & Marjamaki 1990), whereas the [^{11}C]Sch 23390 *pB* declined by 7% in caudate and 4% in putamen with each decade of healthy aging (Dagher *et al.* 2001). In the latter study, it was also shown that cigarette smoking did not acutely change the [^{11}C]Sch 23390 *pB* in the striatum. However, relative to non-smokers, there was a downward shift of about 10% in binding among smokers of all ages, a difference which was statistically significant in the ventral striatum. The binding of [^{11}C]Sch 23390 was 15% reduced in striatum of patients with major depression compounded by anger attacks (Dougherty *et al.* 2006) and of patients with autosomal-dominant frontal lobe epilepsy (Fedi *et al.* 2008). Given the anticonvulsant action of adenosine A_1 agonists, it may thus be relevant that such a drug reduced the binding of [^{11}C]Sch 23390 to D_1 receptors in striatum of anesthetized cats by 40% (Sakiyama *et al.* 2007).

The [^{11}C]Sch 23390 *pB* was reduced by 20% in the striatum of monkeys with MPTP-induced parkinsonism (Doudet *et al.* 2002). In contrast, there was a non-significant 10% reduction in D_1 binding in a PET study of Parkinson's disease patients (Turjanski, Lees, & Brooks 1997). Thus, the results of PET studies are consistent with the findings in experimental animals in vitro, which likewise failed to show consistent changes in the abundance of this receptor after dopamine depletion. The striatal binding of [^{11}C]NNC 756 to D_1 receptors (but not the D_2 binding) was slightly reduced in patients suffering from juvenile neuronal ceroid lipofuscinosis (Rinne *et al.* 2002), and in Alzheimer's disease patients (Kemppainen *et al.* 2000), in whom D$_2$ binding was likewise unaffected. The saturation binding parameters for [^{11}C]Sch 23990 were entirely normal in striatum of patients with schizophrenia (Karlsson *et al.* 2002). In contrast, the [^{11}C]Sch 23390 *pB* in the striatum was reduced by 40% in a PET study of patients with Huntington's disease (Ginovart *et al.* 1997b), in contrast to the 70% reduction seen in a post mortem autoradiographic study (Filloux *et al.* 1990), a discrepancy no doubt related to the greater disease progression in the patients dying with the disease. Indeed, results of a longitudinal PET study with [^{11}C]Sch 23390 indicate that D$_1$ receptors decline at a rate of 4.5% per year in symptomatic patients with actively progressing Huntington's disease, in comparison to 2% per year in asymptomatic carriers of the gene (Andrews *et al.* 1999). Thus, D$_1$ receptors may be especially vulnerable to certain neurodegenerative diseases of the striatum, but seem unaltered in Parkinson's disease.

D$_1$ receptor binding is not restricted to the basal ganglia, but can be readily detected by PET in the cerebral cortex (with the caveat of incomplete specificity). The cortical binding of [^{11}C]NNC112 was 20–50% higher in normal subjects with the more active Val/Val allele of COMT than in subjects with the Met/Met allele (Slifstein *et al.* 2008). The authors attributed this finding to relatively low cortical dopamine tonus, notwithstanding the paucity of evidence for upregulation of D$_1$ receptors in Parkinson's disease. The occurrence of reduced expression of DARPP-32 in post mortem frontal cortex suggests that D$_1$-mediated signaling may be impaired in patients with schizophrenia (Albert *et al.* 2002). The binding of [^{3}H]Sch 23390 was elevated in post mortem frontal cortex of patients with schizophrenia, an effect which was attributed to chronic antipsychotic treatment (Knable *et al.* 1996). In a study of patients with schizophrenia, increased binding of [^{11}C]NNC 112 in the dorsolateral prefrontal cortex correlated with the extent of impairment of working memory (Abi-Dargham *et al.* 2002). Elevated binding of [^{11}C]Sch 23390 to dopamine D$_1$ receptors in the frontal and temporal cortex was noted in healthy monozygotic twins of patients with schizophrenia, suggesting an endophenotype imparting increased genetic risk (Hirvonen *et al.* 2006). However, D$_1$ binding tended to be reduced in affected twins relative to healthy subjects. Nonetheless, in a saturation binding PET study with [^{11}C]Sch 23390, there was no evidence for any differences in the abundance or affinity of D$_1$ sites in the striatum or cortex of patients with schizopreniform disorder and healthy control subjects (Karlsson *et al.* 2002). Thus, the limited available evidence implicates an abnormality in D$_1$ signaling in the cortical regions rather than the striatum in the pathophysiology of schizophrenia.

13.3.2.   Competition at D_1 sites in living brain

Competition studies indicate that dopamine can displace some fraction of D_1 antagonists in vitro, predicting that competition from endogenous extra-cellular dopamine might be expected to reduce the apparent affinity of ligands in living brain. In slices of rat striatum maintained by superfusion, electrical stimulation at 2.5 Hz completely blocked the specific binding of [^{3}H]Sch 23390 (Gifford, Gatley, & Ashby 1996). However, the effect of endogenous dopamine on D_1 antagonist binding in living brain remains controversial. Paradoxically, acute treatment with reserpine reduces the in vivo binding of [^{3}H]Sch 23390 in rat striatum, by reducing the apparent affinity without changing the number of binding sites at saturation (Inoue *et al.* 1991). Other rat studies indicate that acute reserpine treatment reduced [^{3}H]Sch 23390 binding ex vivo, but was with-out effect on [^{11}C]NNC 112 binding measured in vivo by PET (Guo *et al.* 2003), again contrary to the expectation of a simple competition model. Acute depletion of dopamine with reserpine altered neither the apparent B_{max} nor the affinity of [^{11}C]NNC 112 in monkey brain, which seems to exclude an important competi-tion from tonic dopamine for D_1 radioligand binding sites (Chou *et al.* 1999). Likewise, depletion of catecholamine after oral administration of AMPT did not alter the binding of [^{11}C]Sch 23390 in human striatum (Verhoeff *et al.* 2002).

PET studies of D1 receptors after psychostimulant challenge have likewise failed to support simple competition from dopamine. Whereas [^{11}C]NNC 756 binding was readily displaced by excess non-radioactive Sch 23390, a challenge with amphetamine sufficient to produce a massive dopamine release in the striatum was without discernible effect on the radioligand binding (Halldin *et al.* 1998). Neither did an amphetamine challenge alter the striatal binding of [^{11}C]NNC 756 or [^{11}C]Sch 23390 in a PET study of baboons (Abi-Dargham *et al.* 1999). In this study, a continuous infusion design was used in order to impose an equilibrium condition, for the optimal detection of changes in receptor avail-ability. Together, the results of these studies preclude important competition between dopamine and D_1 ligands at binding sites in living brain.

14

Imaging dopamine D$_2$ receptors

14.1. General properties of D$_2$ ligands

14.1.1. Irreversible ligands

N-[^{3}H]methylspiperone ([^{3}H]NMSP) is a butyrophenone compound binding to at least two pharmacologically distinct sites in homogenates from the mammalian brain. Although the bindings had similar kinetics in the caudate and in the cortex, the preponderance of binding in the caudate could be displaced with dopamine D$_2$ antagonists, whereas most of the cortical binding was displaced with serotonin 5HT$_2$ antagonists (Lyon *et al.* 1986). The in vitro association kinetics for both sites was rapid, while dissociation kinetics was so slow as to be nearly irreversible in the time course of a PET study. Displacement studies in living mice likewise revealed that whereas 90% of the [^{3}H]spiperone binding in the frontal cortex was to serotonin receptors, 80% of the binding in the striatum was to dopamine D$_2$ receptors (Frost *et al.* 1987). With the caveat that functional selectivity is mainly imparted by the differing distributions of the two main binding sites, [^{11}C]NMSP and related compounds can potentially be used to measure dopamine and serotonin receptors in the same PET session (Borbely *et al.* 1999).

Displacement studies of [^{3}H]spiperone from rat brain membranes indicated the presence of considerable amounts of non-dopaminergic, non-serotonergic sites, although these were of ten-fold lower apparent affinity than were the identified components of the binding (List & Seeman 1981). Representative autoradiograms from rat striatum showing displacement of [^{3}H]spiperone with the D$_{2/3}$-selective antagonist butaclamol, and in the presence of ketanserin, reveal a complex pattern of residual binding, especially in the ventral striatum and in the superficial layer of the neocortex (Figure 13.1). The pharmacological identity of this binding remains uncertain, an unsatisfactory state of affairs which must be considered in the interpretation of PET studies with butyrophenone ligands.

The specific binding of [^{18}F]NMSP in monkey striatum continues to increase for at least 3 h after intravenous injection (Mach *et al.* 1995), and much of the specific binding of [^{3}H]spiperone was retained in the caudate of living mice for more than 24 h (Frost *et al.* 1987). Kinetic analysis of [^{11}C]NMSP uptake in living human striatum suggested that binding was essentially irreversible relative to the time course of a PET study, and that PET results were best quantified as k_3, defined as the product of the association constant (k_{on}) and the maximal number of receptors (B_{max}) (Wong, Gjedde, & Wagner 1986). Thus, the requirement for equilibrium binding is not obtained with [^{11}C]NMSP, as in the earlier case of [^{11}C]deprenyl. This state of affairs may not be true for all species; in living anesthetized pigs, the binding of [^{11}C]NMSP approaches an equilibrium V_d in the striatum, such that a *pB* can be calculated on the basis of 90 min long emission recordings (Rosa-Neto *et al.* 2004).

In addition to non-dopaminergic binding components, the binding properties of butyrophenones are further complicated by a lack of specificity between dopamine D$_2$-like receptor subtypes. Whereas the benzamide raclopride has similar high affinity for D$_2$ and D$_3$ receptors, spiperone binds equally to D$_2$, D$_3$, and D$_4$ receptors (Neve & Neve 1997), as noted above. Pretreatment with non-radioactive NMSP produced the expected complete inhibition of the specific binding of [^{3}H]raclopride or [^{3}H]NMSP in the striatum of freely moving mice (Inoue *et al.* 1999). In contrast, inhibition of [^{3}H]NMSP binding was incomplete at very high (3 mg kg^{-1}) doses of raclopride. This discrepancy could be due to the lesser pharmacological specificity of butyrophenone binding, or could reflect fundamental kinetic differences between the two radioligands.

14.1.2.   *Reversible binding of benzamides*

The substituted benzamide raclopride was first identified as a promising candidate for autoradiographic studies of dopamine D$_{2/3}$ receptors, based upon its reversible and displaceable binding in membranes from rat striatum, and in the striatum of living rats (Kohler *et al.* 1985). Shortly thereafter, the specific binding of [^{11}C]raclopride was measured by PET in human brain (Farde *et al.* 1986). The success of [^{11}C]raclopride has spawned a huge literature, and has given rise to the subsequent development of other benzamide ligands, including [^{18}F]desmethoxyfallypride and its high-affinity cogeners [^{18}F]fallypride and [^{11}C]FLB 457 for PET studies, and also [^{123}I]IBZM for SPECT studies of dopamine D$_{2/3}$ receptors.

While the ligands of moderate affinity such as [^{11}C]raclopride and [^{123}I]IBZM are admirably suited for quantifying dopamine receptors in the striatum, the

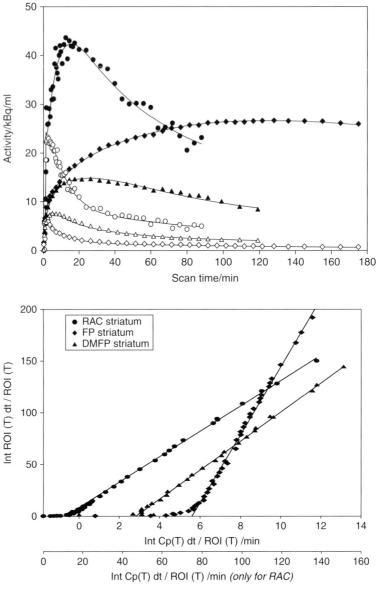

Figure 14.1 The kinetics of three different PET tracers for dopamine D$_{2/3}$ receptors in human brain. Representative time–activity curves in human striatum and cerebellum (upper figure) and the corresponding Logan plots (lower figure) for three benzamide ligands of differing affinity for dopamine D$_2$ receptors. Solid symbols represent the radioactivity concentrations in the striatum and open symbols show the cerebellum. Results are for the low-affinity ligands (•) [^{11}C]raclopride and (▴) [^{18}F]desmethoxyfallypride, and the high-affinity ligand (◊) [^{18}F]fallypride. Reproduced with permission from Siessmeier *et al.* (2005).

detection of these receptors has been problematic in extrastriatal regions, where the natural abundance of dopamine D$_2$ receptors is much lower. In Figure 14.1, time–radioactivity curves in human striatum are presented for ligands of high and low affinity, along with Logan plots of the corresponding binding. The more rapid state of equilibrium is evident in the plots for [^{11}C]raclopride and [^{18}F]desmethoxyfallypride, in contrast to the findings for [^{18}F]fallypride (Siessmeier *et al.* 2005). The figure also makes clear that the binding of [^{18}F]fallypride approaches equilibrium in human striatum only at 2 h after injection, which exceeds the practical time-limit of recordings with [^{11}C]-tracers.

As another instance of the new high-affinity ligands, the benzamide [^{11}C]FLB 457 binds with high specificity to dopamine D$_2$ receptors, with affinity in vitro (20 pM), some 50-fold higher than that of raclopride (Olsson *et al.* 1999). The *pB* of this ligand in human brain relative to an arterial or cerebellum input ranges from near unity in the cerebral cortex to 3 in the thalamus, and more than 20 in the striatum. In serial PET experiments using a range of specific activities, the saturation-binding parameters of [^{11}C]FLB 457 were estimated in extrastriatal structures, where the B_{max} was 5–10% of that found for [^{11}C]raclopride in the striatum (Olsson, Halldin, & Farde 2004). However, the quantitation of the *pB* for [^{11}C]FLB 457 and other high affinity [^{11}C]-labelled ligands in human striatum is problematic, because of the delay to obtain equilibrium. The situation could be compared to attempting to inflate a leaky zeppelin with a bicycle pump: equilibrium is not obtained before exhaustion sets in.

Reference tissue methods for the estimation of specific binding in the striatum generally assume absent specific binding in the cerebellum. While there was a small component of [^{11}C]FLB 457 specific binding in the cerebellum, its presence had little effect on the estimation of *pB* in the striatum (Asselin *et al.* 2007). Likewise, SPET studies of the high-affinity ligand [^{123}I]epidepride in patients treated for schizophrenia revealed the presence of a "non-negligible" specific binding component in the cerebellum (Pinborg *et al.* 2007). Although the use of the cerebellum as a non-binding reference region is likely to introduce bias everywhere, the relative magnitude of this bias will be greatest in cortical areas with the least specific binding.

As the available ligands for dopamine D$_2$-like receptors do not adequately distinguish subtypes, there is a pressing need to develop D$_3$-selective ligands for molecular imaging in vivo. D$_3$ sites are peculiar with respect to their apparent lack of coupling to intracellular G-proteins. Thus, the agonist ligand [^{125}I]-(+)-trans-7-OH-PIPAT could detect D$_3$ receptors in vitro, even when its binding was measured in the presence of a stable GTP analogue, which attenuated its binding to D$_2$ and serotonin sites (Kung *et al.* 1994). The D$_3$-selective antagonist [^{11}C]RGH-1756 had very low binding in the striatum of living monkeys, even following treatment with reserpine to abolish putative competition from endo-genous dopamine (Sovago *et al.* 2005), a failure that was attributed to the low abundance of the site and its restricted distribution in the ventral striatum and olfactory tubercle. Two benzamide ligands with considerable selectivity for D_4 receptors failed to reveal specific binding in living rat (Zhang *et al.* 2002), again apparently due to low abundance.

14.1.3. D_2 agonist binding sites in the brain

As is the case for D_1 receptors, D_2 receptors can also exist in high- and low-affinity states for agonists, as determined by their association with G-proteins. The displacement of [^{3}H]spiroperidol (in the presence of ketanserin to block serotonin receptors) from rat striatum membranes by increasing concentrations of dopamine or apomorphine is biphasic, with approximately equal components displaced at low and high concentrations of the agonists (Hamblin, Leff, & Creese 1984). Likewise, the displacement of [^{3}H]spiperone from receptors from bovine striatum by the agonist N-propylapomorphine (NPA) is biphasic; the two binding sites for NPA have calculated affinities of 100 pM (D_2^{High}) and 13 nM (D_2^{Low}) (Elazar & Fuchs 1991). These studies suggest that agonist ligands should likewise have very high affinity and selectivity for the subset of dopamine D_2 receptors in the high-affinity or agonist-binding state. It is presumably only this fraction of the total number of receptors that is coupled to intracellular second messenger systems. Thus, according to the affinity state model, agonist ligands should separate the wheat from the chaff by ignoring a non-functional population of receptors. Autoradiograms with [^{3}H]NPA and [^{3}H]raclopride nonetheless show roughly similar distribu-tions of the two ligands in rat brain cryostat sections (Figure 13.1).

In addition to G-protein coupling, several intrinsic factors can modulate the affinity of dopamine D_2 receptors for its agonists. For example, D_2 receptors purified from bovine striatum can be phosphorylated by cAMP-dependent protein kinase, which reduces the affinity for the agonist [^{3}H]NPA, without changing the total number of sites (Elazar & Fuchs 1991). Incubation of rat striatal membranes with the peptide neurotensin reduced the apparent affi-nity of [^{3}H]NPA for D_2 receptors (von Euler *et al.* 1991). Since this affinity change occurred in the presence of pertussis toxin, mediation by G-proteins can be excluded, suggesting instead an alosteric modulation of affinity by the peptide drug. However, the tripeptide L-propyl-L-leucyl-glycinamide and cer-tain peptidometic analogs increased the affinity of [^{3}H]NPA binding in vitro in a manner dependent upon coupling to G-proteins (Verma *et al.* 2005). In other studies, the proportion of [^{3}H]spiperone binding in rat striatum displaceable by low concentrations of apomorphine (i.e. D_2^{High}) increased within minutes

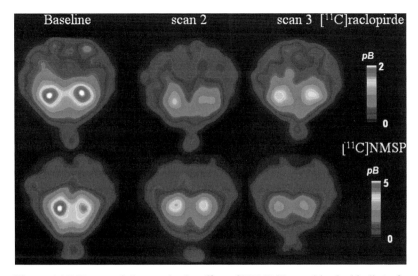

Figure 14.2 Temporal changes in the effect of MDMA (Ecstasy) in the binding of dopamine D$_2$ receptor ligands in pig brain. Groups of pigs were scanned at baseline with [^{11}C]raclopride (upper row) or [^{11}C]NMSP (lower row) and at 1 h (scan 2) or three hours (scan 3) after MDMA challenge. Modified with permission from Rosa-Neto *et al.* (2004). (For color version, see plate section.)

after estrogen treatment, indicating a rapid change in the coupling of receptors to intracellular G-proteins (Levesque & Di Paolo 1993). Thus, it should be considered that the affinity of dopamine D$_2$ sites for agonists is not static, but subject to modulation by diverse factors. Pharmacological modulation of affinity state would seem to be promising for medicinal chemistry, with potential benefits for the improved treatment of schizophrenia, for example.

The first ligand to be developed for PET studies of dopamine agonist binding sites was [^{11}C]NPA, which proved to have excellent binding properties in the brain of living monkey, and could be entirely displaced by haloperidol treatment, indicating selectivity for dopamine receptors (Hwang, Kegeles, & Laruelle 2000). The kinetics of [^{11}C]NPA was investigated in the brain of living pigs, in which it was noted that there was abundant binding in extrastriatal structures, including the midbrain and medial forebrain bundle (Cumming *et al.* 2003a). These results show a certain lack of identity of [^{11}C]NPA binding with that of [^{11}C]raclopride, which is almost entirely restricted to the striatum of pig brain (Figure 14.2).

The unusual pattern of dopamine D$_2$ agonist binding in the brain may be related to its selectivity for subtypes of dopamine D$_2$-like receptors. Indeed, the results of studies in vitro show that the agonist (+)-PHNO has markedly higher affinity for human dopamine D$_3$ receptors than for D$_2$ receptors expressed in cell lines (Freedman *et al.* 1994). This finding is consistent with the results of autoradiographic studies with [^{3}H]PHNO, which showed particularly dense binding in structures of the ventral forebrain, and relatively less binding in the dorsal striatum of rats (Nobrega & Seeman 1994). However, results of other studies in vitro, in which (+)-PHNO was used as a competitor against the binding of another agonist ([^{3}H]-domperidone), the former compound had similar affinities with respect to D_2 and D_3 receptors, specifically the high-affinity state of those receptor types (Seeman *et al.* 2005a).

PET studies with [^{11}C]-(+)-PHNO showed abundant reversible binding in the striatum, especially in the ventral striatum, and also considerable binding in the globus pallidus (Ginovart *et al.* 2007). It has been noted on the basis of the shape of dynamic time–activity curves in a human PET study with [^{11}C]-(+)-PHNO, that the tracer has distinct kinetics in the globus pallidus and in the striatum, suggesting the occurrence of multiple affinity states (Willeit *et al.* 2006). The preferential binding of [^{11}C]-(+)-PHNO in human globus pallidus, which was twice as high as that of [^{11}C]raclopride, may reflect preferential binding of the former compound to dopamine D_3 receptors (Graff-Guerrero *et al.* 2008), as has been demonstrated by displacement with selective antagonists in the brain of non-human primates (Narendran *et al.* 2006).

14.2.   Oligomeric associations of dopamine D_2 receptors

Immunoprecipitation of brain extracts or cells expressing dopamine D_2 receptors in conjunction with gel electrophoresis reveals that the receptors exist as monomers, which can be labeled with spiperone- and also nemonapride-like compounds, and dimers, which bind only benzamide ligands (Ng *et al.* 1996). The dimers could be dissociated into monomers by various chemical treatments, high temperature, or acidic conditions. In further studies, it was determined using specific antibodies that native D_2 receptors migrated in electrophoresis gels as monomers, dimers, trimers, tetramers, and even pentamers (Zawarynski *et al.* 1998). Hydrophobic interactions at transmembrane domain 4 of the receptors mediates homodimerization of D_2 receptors (Lee *et al.* 2003). Perplexing aspects of the responsiveness of different classes of different receptor ligands in response to psychostimulant challenge could be related to the state of equilibrium between monomers and aggregates of dopamine receptors, if this equilibrium is itself modulated by dopaminergic signaling (Logan *et al.* 2001).

In addition to homodimers, dopamine D_2 receptors can form associations with D_1 receptors. The D_1-D_2 heterodimer signal transduction pathway is mediated by a novel phospholipase C-dependent calcium signaling (So *et al.*

2005). Treatment with selective agonists and also blocking studies with specific antagonists revealed that activation of either receptor type was sufficient to evoked internalization of the entire hetero-oligomer complex expressed in kidney cells. In rat striatum, the detection of this signaling pathway was more evident in adult rats than in the (3-month-old) adolescent rats usually employed in neuropharmacology studies (Rashid *et al.* 2007). Doubtless, this interaction may account for some aspects of dopamine D_1–D_2 synergisms described above. However, still greater levels of complexity are present. Hetero-oligomers of adenosine A_2 and dopamine D_2 receptors are present in rat striatum (Fuxe *et al.* 2005), which may account for the modulation of the affinity state of dopamine D_2 receptors which is provoked by agonism of the adenosine receptors (Ferre *et al.* 1991). The observation of heteromeric association between dopamine receptors and diverse other classes of receptors indicates that cell membrane dopamine receptors may more properly be considered to exist as a mosaic rather than as singular entities of classical pharmacology (Agnati *et al.* 2005). This implies a level of complexity far surpassing the current state of development of molecular imaging studies.

14.3. Effects of denervation on D_2 receptors

Experimental parkinsonism has been used as a model for studying the modulation of dopamine D_2 receptor expression. After unilateral 6-OHDA lesions, the [^{3}H]spiroperidol B_{max} in rat brain autoradiograms increased by 25% relative to the binding in the intact side (Neve *et al.* 1984). Here, the specific binding was measured by displacement with butaclamol in order to isolate the $D_{2/3}$ component. The time course relationship between denervation and upregulation of dopamine receptors has been investigated using the rat 6-OHDA model (Chalon *et al.* 1999); 2 days after the lesion, striatal DAT binding with [^{125}I]PE21 in vitro has declined by one half, in association with a 30% increase in dopamine $D_{2/3}$ receptors measured with [^{125}I]IBZM. The peak upregulation occurred 5 days post lesion, when DAT binding was 99% depleted, and $D_{2/3}$ binding had increased by 53%. After prolonged MPTP-induced parkinsonism, the concentration of [^{3}H]sulpride specific binding was increased by 60% in parts of monkey putamen (Graham *et al.* 1990), but these increases were normalized in animals which had been treated with antiparkinsonian medication (Graham, Sambrook, & Crossman 1993). In another study, the specific binding of the D_2 receptor antagonist [^{125}I]IBF was elevated by 50% in the striatum of African green monkeys at 1 year after MPTP-intoxication (Elsworth *et al.* 1998). In these monkeys, an intrastriatal graft of fetal mesencephalic neurons essentially normalized the D_2 receptors, a response that occurred when the dopamine concentration at the site of the graft was restored to only 10% of normal.

In rat studies using [^{3}H]NPA over a range of specific activities, the B_{max} in normal striatum was close to 25 pmol g^{-1} (van der Werf, Sebens, & Korf 1984). Kainic acid lesions destroyed 80% of the striatal binding, indicating localization mainly to the medium spiny striatal neurons, rather than presynaptic auto-receptors. 6-OHDA lesions 1 week prior to the ex vivo study had no effect on the accumulation of [^{3}H]NPA in vivo, whereas the same authors report else-where that 6-OHDA lesions 3 weeks prior to the ex vivo study increased the striatal binding by 50% (van der Werf *et al.* 1983). Thus, quantitative studies with agonists concur with the antagonist studies, in also revealing a substantial upregulation of dopamine D_2 receptors in the dopamine-depleted condition. However, the bulk of evidence shows that receptor upregulation is a response to rather extreme and prolonged dopamine depletions.

14.4.   Competitive binding at D_2 receptors in living brain

14.4.1.   *Benzamide antagonists*

In unwashed slices from human or rat brain, the presence of endoge-nous dopamine can interfere with the binding of [^{3}H]raclopride to dopamine $D_{2/3}$ receptors (Seeman, Guan, & Niznik 1989). This observation led to the conjecture that a similar competition between endogenous dopamine and exogenous radi-oligand might occur during PET studies. In subsequent years, changes in the [^{11}C]raclopride *pB* has been used extensively for autoradiography studies puta-tively showing pharmacologically-evoked dopamine release in living striatum. The displacement can be quantified as a decline in *pB* calculated during a bolus infusion of radioligand. The amphetamine derivative methylenedioxymetham-phetamine (MDMA; "Ecstasy") evokes the simultaneous release of serotonin and dopamine, but only the dopamine competes at [^{11}C]raclopride binding sites. The time course of effects of MDMA challenge on [^{11}C]raclopride binding has been investigated in living pigs (Rosa-Neto *et al.* 2004). Relative to the baseline condition, there was a 30% reduction in striatal [^{11}C]raclopride *pB* at 1 h after MDMA, but the reduction was only 20% at 3 h after the challenge (Figure 14.2). This result reveals the transient nature of the competition, which is consistent with the time course of the amphetamine release reported in microdialysis studies. However, the interpretation of these findings must be moderated by the lack of appropriate control for possible effects of very prolonged anesthe-sia. The test–retest stability of [^{11}C]raclopride *pB* during prolonged anesthesia was first established by microPET study of rats (Figure 14.3, upper). There was

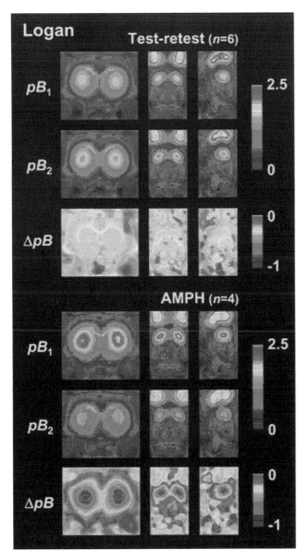

Figure 14.3 The effect of amphetamine challenge on [^{11}C]raclopride binding in rat brain. Mean parametric maps of [^{11}C]raclopride *pB* in rat brain, calculated by the reference tissue method of Logan of groups of living rats. Rows represent baseline results (*pB*$_1$), the second scan (*pB*$_2$) and the difference of the two binding maps (ΔpB) in a test–retest experiment (*n* = 6), and in a test of the effects of amphetamine challenge (*n* = 4). The parametric images are superposed on the rat brain histological atlas (gray scale), in identical coronal (*Z* = 19), horizontal (*Y* = 10) and sagittal (*X* = −11) planes. The ΔpB maps were blurred by 1 mm (FWHM). Reproduced with permission from Pedersen *et al.* (2007). (For color version, see plate section.)

no discernible change in binding between the first and the second scans, conducted 2 h apart (Pedersen *et al.* 2007). In another group of rats, amphetamine challenge was administered, and the pattern of altered *pB* was revealed by subtraction of the parametric maps from those in the baseline condition (Figure 14.3, lower).

In many molecular imaging studies of dopamine receptors, parametric maps of *pB* are calculated by the linearization of Logan, relative to time–radioactivity curve measured in the cerebellum, a non-binding reference region. However, this approach can lead to systematic bias in the voxel-wise estimation of *pB* (Cumming *et al.* 2003b). More robust estimates of specific binding can be obtained when the [^{11}C]raclopride is administered as an intravenous bolus followed by continuous infusion, so as to force the rapid approach to steady-state binding (Carson *et al.* 1997), thus in effect emulating the condition of DAT ligands at many hours after a bolus injection. The advantage of the bolus/infusion technique is that the simple binding ratio in the striatum approaches an equilibrium condition which is proportional to *pB*, thus obviating the need to carry out compartmental modeling of tracer uptake.

In monkey striatum, there was a good correlation between the amphetamine-evoked declines in [^{123}I]IBZM binding and the peak outflow of dopamine in striatal microdialysates (Laruelle *et al.* 1997b). Others show that it is the area under the curve of the increased interstitial dopamine that correlates best with [^{11}C]raclopride binding changes after acute amphetamine (Endres *et al.* 1997a). The displacement of [^{11}C]raclopride binding in living brain after challenge with amphetamine seems to be a general property of indirect agonists of dopamine transmission, as presented above for the case of challenge with MDMA. Both cocaine and methylphenidate evoked a 25% decline in [^{11}C]raclopride binding in living primate brain (Volkow *et al.* 1999a). Pretreatment with the DAT inhibitor GBR 12909 greatly attenuated the amphetamine-evoked reduction in [^{11}C]raclopride binding in the striatum of baboons (Villemagne *et al.* 1999), which seems somewhat paradoxical given that the pretreatment should have had the inherent effects of interstitial dopamine. However, this finding contrasts the direct release of dopamine with amphetamine, and the pharmacologically distinct mechanism of reuptake blockade by cocaine or methylphenidate, which potentiates the interstitial concentrations of spontaneously released dopamine. The two classes of psychostimulant may not have identical consequences in the competition binding paradigm. In normal humans, a single oral dose of amphetamine reduced striatal [^{11}C]raclopride binding by 13% at 2 h, and by 18% at 6 h after treatment, but had returned to normal at 24 h (Cardenas *et al.* 2004). The temporal changes in receptor availability were not completely explained by plasma amphetamine levels, which had only declined by one half between 2 and 24 h after dosing.

The amphetamine-challenge paradigm is based upon the release of intracellular pools of dopamine. Thus, the extent of the [^{11}C]raclopride binding reduction evoked by amphetamine was blunted in healthy human subjects after ingestion of a mixture of amino acids deficient in phenylalanine and tyrosine, the precursors for dopamine (Leyton *et al.* 2004). Conversely, it might be expected that a pharmacological treatment increasing the intracellular concentration of dopamine should potentiate the effect of amphetamine. Indeed, blockade of MAO-A with clorgyline increased the magnitude of the amphetamine-released dopamine in the interstitial fluid (Segal, Kuczenski, & Okuda 1992). However, pretreatment with pargyline at a dose sufficient to completely block the brain MAO was without significant effect, either on baseline [^{11}C]raclopride binding, or on the magnitude of the amphetamine-evoked binding changes in the striatum of living pigs (Jensen *et al.* 2006), and in rats (Pedersen *et al.* 2007). Perhaps rapid densitization of dopamine receptors following MAO inhibition masks the putative increases in the amphetamine-releasable dopamine pool.

The effects of tonic competition from endogenous dopamine on the availability of dopamine receptors can be tested in experimental animals treated with reserpine, alone, or in conjunction with AMPT in order to inhibit dopamine synthesis. Thus, the binding of [^{3}H]raclopride in rat striatum was substantially increased by pretreatment with reserpine (Young *et al.* 1991), as was the [^{11}C]raclopride *pB* in mouse (Cumming *et al.* 2002) and monkey striatum (Ginovart *et al.* 1997a) after reserpine treatment. The binding changes indicate that tonic extracellular dopamine normally is an effective competitor for dopamine D$_2$ binding sites, typically occupying some 40% of the binding sites. In the monkey study, the [^{11}C]raclopride *pB* was persistently elevated after reserpine treatment, consistent with the very long time required for recovery of brain dopamine following destruction of the synaptic vesicles. Saturation binding studies in vivo showed this increase was due to a decline in K_d^{app}, the apparent affinity, with no change in the B_{max}. This is to be expected, since K_d^{app} is defined as the intrinsic affinity reduced to some extent due to the competition from dopamine itself. However, it would be expected that B_{max} should eventually upregulate after prolonged dopamine depletion.

14.4.2.   *Butyrophenone antagonists*

The vulnerability of butyrophenone ligands to competition from endogenous dopamine has been a matter of some controversy. Stimulation of the nigrostriatal fibers in the medial forebrain bundle and amphetamine treatment both increased the accumulation of the D$_2$-like ligand [^{3}H]spiperone, whereas dopamine depletion with reserpine decreased the binding in vivo (Chugani, Ackermann, & Phelps 1988), neither of which results supports a model of competition from endogenous dopamine. However, these treatments did not alter the total number of binding sites measured in vitro, but instead changed the distribution of receptors between the plasma membrane and a microsomal compartment containing endocytotic vesicles. Apparently, the dissociation of agonists occurs upon internalization, but the internalized receptors remain available for binding with radiolabeled butyrophenones (Barbier *et al.* 1997), such that they can in some circumstances accumulate in response to dopamine release. The binding of an iodinated butyrophenone to dopamine D_2 receptors in living rat striatum could be blocked by pretreatment with haloperidol, but when tracer uptake had already occurred, its binding was insensitive to subsequent haloperidol treatment (Pellevoisin *et al.* 1993). These results show that, whereas butyrophenone ligands can be sequestered along with intracellular receptors (thus becoming less sensitive to displacement by other competitors), benzamides seem not to be internalized, but bind only to plasma membrane receptors.

In an early report, amphetamine treatment produced similar reductions (40%) in the specific binding of [^{11}C]raclopride and [^{3}H]NMSP in the striatum of living rats (Young *et al.* 1991). In contrast, amphetamine, methylphenidate, and other psychostimulants all paradoxically increased the binding of [^{3}H]spiperone in another study of living rat striatum (Vassout *et al.* 1993). In the first of these two studies, the effects of basal dopamine tonus were also investigated. Treatment of rats with reserpine increased [^{3}H]raclopride binding in rat striatum by 50% as expected, but was without effect on the binding in vivo of [^{3}H] NMSP. In yet another study, the [^{3}H]raclopride pB in mouse striatum nearly doubled after reserpine treatment, consistent with the effects of basal occupancy seen in other studies (Inoue *et al.* 1991). However, this study also reports that reserpine treatment decreased the rate of association of [^{3}H]NMSP to sites in mouse striatum by 50%, which is entirely unexpected on the basis of a simple competition model. This report should be interpreted with the caveat that the rate constants of association (k_3) and dissociation (k_4) of the butyrophenone were not obtained from time–activity curves from a population of mice, but were estimated from only a few time points.

In a monkey PET study, the rate of association (k_3) of the butyrophenone [^{18}F]N-methylspiroperidol to striatal dopamine receptors was in fact reduced following amphetamine treatment (Dewey *et al.* 1991). More recently, the psychostimulant MDMA was found to decrease the magnitude of k_3 (assuming irreversible binding), and also to reduce the equilibrium pB of [^{11}C]NMSP in the striatum of anesthetized pigs (Rosa-Neto *et al.* 2004). The magnitude of the effect increased with time, such that [^{11}C]NMSP binding had fallen by 50% at 4 h after the MDMA treatment. The same treatment evoked only a 20% decrease in the [^{11}C]raclopride *pB* at 1 h after MDMA treatment (Figure 14.2). However, 2 h later, when the [^{11}C]raclopride *pB* was returning toward baseline levels, the [^{11}C]NMSP *pB* had continued to decline relative to baseline levels, a finding that seems inconsistent with receptor internalization. Conceivably, some paradoxical effects of pharmacological on butyrophenone binding in rodent striatum may be unrelated to simple competition. For example, the hypothermia that typically follows reserpine treatment of rats, if the association kinetics of butyrophenones are temperature-dependent. However, this explanation seems to be unlikely, since the results of the pig study show that MDMA-evoked hyperthermia was associated with reductions in the striatal binding of [^{11}C]NMSP. In a microPET study of similar design, challenge with intravenous MDMA was without effect on striatal [^{11}C]NMSP binding (Figure 14.4), even while evoking substantially increased competition against the binding of [^{3}H]raclopride, which was measured ex vivo in the same animals. Thus, aspects of the pharmacological properties of dopamine receptors in pig brain may reflect idiosyncrasies of that experimental model.

A coherent explanation for all aspects of the inconsistent responsiveness of butyrophenone ligands to modulation of dopamine tonus remains to be proposed. Pharmacological treatments altering dopamine release can have no effect on butyrophenone binding in living brain, or can have the opposite effect to that expected on the basis of simple competition from the endogenous agonist. This discrepancy relative to the more orderly behavior of [^{11}C]raclopride has sometimes been attributed to the relatively higher affinity of butyrophenone ligands (Laruelle 2000). Indeed, the binding of butyrophenones to dopamine D_2 receptors is often considered to be nearly irreversible in the time course of a PET study, hence the prevalence of k_3 calculations noted above. However, the benzamide [^{18}F]fallypride, which has a similar high affinity to that of [^{11}C]NMSP, could be partially displaced from its receptors in anesthetized monkey striatum by amphetamine. Unexpectedly, this displacement was apparently due to an increase in k_{off}, the rate of dissociation from receptors (Mukherjee *et al.* 1997). However, the argument of high affinity fails to predict the vulnerability of the high-affinity ligand [^{18}F]fallypride to pharmacological challenges (Morris & Yoder 2007). In this latter study, it is shown that no single kinetic term is sufficient to predict the vulnerability of antagonists to competition from dopamine. Instead, the rank order of vulnerabilities of $D_{2/3}$ ligands can be predicted with a model incorporating the time–concentration curves for interstitial dopamine and for the radioligand, and also all the relevant rate constants for association and dissociation from the receptors. The model also predicts that the observed competition in vivo can depend sensitively on the time delay between pharmacological treatment and the tracer administration. Thus,

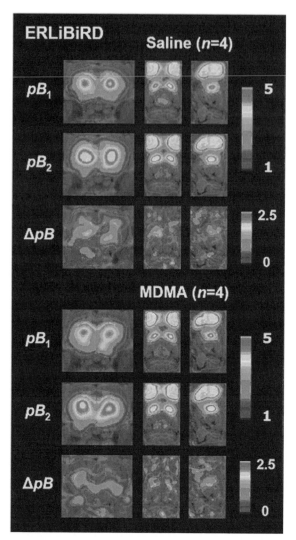

Figure 14.4 The effect of MDMA (Ecstasy) challenge on the binding of $[^{11}C]$NMSP in rat brain. Mean parametric images of $[^{11}C]$NMSP pB for groups of ($n=4$) rats, calculated by the ERLiBiRD reference tissue method. Rows represent baseline results (pB_1), the second scan (pB_2) and the difference of the two binding maps (ΔpB), in a test–retest experiment, and in a test of the effects of pharmacological challenge with MDMA (Ecstasy). The parametric images are superposed on the rat brain histological atlas (gray scale). The parametric images are co-registered to the rat brain cryo-atlas (gray scale), in identical coronal ($Z=18.5$), horizontal ($Y=10$) and sagittal ($X=-11$) planes. Images were blurred by 1.0 mm (FWHM). Figure courtesy of Dr. Søren Dinesen Østergaard, Aarhus University PET Centre. (For color version, see plate section.)

the simple relationship between the magnitude of the increased dopamine concentration observed in living striatum after amphetamine (the dopamine pulse) and [^{11}C]raclopride binding changes (Endres *et al.* 1997a) may reflect fortuitous kinetic circumstances peculiar to that particular competition paradigm.

Whereas saturation binding parameters can readily be measured in vitro using a whole range of radioligand concentrations, the B_{max} and apparent affinity of PET ligands are sometimes estimated using only two specific activities (Chou *et al.* 1999), in effect making a linear regression between two data points. Nonetheless, there is generally good agreement in the literature reports of the magnitude of the saturation binding parameters for [^{11}C]raclopride in the striatum of cat, monkey, and human (Table 14.1). In one such study of the amphetamine challenge paradigm, the treatment reduced B_{max} while also increasing the magnitude of K_d^{app} in the striatum of living cat (Ginovart *et al.* 2004), a finding that seems at odds with the conception of simple competition. Had the treatment only increased the competition from endogenous dopamine, the apparent affinity would indeed have decreased, but there should have been no reduction in the maximal number of binding sites. In other studies with three or four different specific activities, treatment with methamphetamine produced only the expected increase in [^{11}C]raclopride K_d^{app} in monkey striatum, without change in B_{max} (Doudet & Holden 2003). The saturation binding parameters were similar irrespective of whether the data were acquired sequentially in a single experimental day, or during three or four independent scanning days. In another monkey [^{11}C]raclopride study, the effects of the reuptake blockers methylphenidate or NS 2214 on saturation binding parameters depended upon the sequence of specific activities of tracers (Doudet, Ruth, & Holden 2006). These discrepancies may be related to violation of the assumption of steady-state changes in dopamine, which is likely to be less in the case of the relatively longer-acting methamphetamine challenge.

14.4.3. *Agonists*

The binding of [^{11}C]apomorphine to (presumably) dopamine D_2 agonist sites was elevated in the striatum of animals acutely pretreated with reserpine (Zijlstra *et al.* 1993), indicative of tonic competition from dopamine in living brain. Likewise, reserpine treatment doubled the [^{3}H]NPA binding in the striatum of living rats (van der Werf *et al.* 1983). Theory predicts that dopamine receptor agonists should have a greater vulnerability to competition from dopamine, than do antagonists. In particular, it can be assumed that dopamine is only able to interact in vivo with that fraction of dopamine D_2 receptors that are coupled to G-proteins. On the basis of displacement studies in vitro cited above, the magnitude of this fraction seems close to 50%. Consistent with this claim,

Table 14.1. *Saturation binding parameters for ligands of dopamine D_2 receptors in brain*

	B_{max}, pmol g^{-1} (K_D, nM)	Reference
[³H]spiroperidol, autoradiography*, rat striatum Intact (n=4)	121±9 (0.7±0.1)	Neve *et al.* 1984
6-OHDA lesioned (n=4)	150±13 (0.8±0.1)	
[¹²⁵I]iodosulpiride, autoradiography, rat striatum (n=4)	390±20 (8±1)	Ridd, Kitchen, & Fosbraey 1998
[³H]raclopride, autoradiography, rat striatum (n=8)	257±13 (2.9±0.4)	Minuzzi & Cumming,
[³H]spiperone, autoradiography, rat striatum (n=8)	277±13 (0.9±0.3)	unpublished observations
[³H]raclopride, autoradiography, pig caudate (n=4)	102±7 (1.9±0.4)	Minuzzi *et al.* 2006
[³H]raclopride, autoradiography, rat striatum (n=6)	267±15 (2.1±0.3)	Minuzzi and Cumming,
[³H]NPA, striatum (n=6)	286±36 (0.9±0.3)	unpublished
[³H]raclopride, olfactory tubercle (n=6)	137±7 (2.2±0.3)	observations
[³H]NPA, olfactory tubercle (n=6)	60±7 (0.5±0.2)	
[³H]PD 128907, autoradiography*, rat striatum	101±35 (144±100)	Hillefors *et al.* 1999
Island of Calleja (n=5)	45±21 (8±10)	
[³H]spiperone, membranes, rat striatum	31 (0.07)	Leslie & Bennett, Jr. 1987
[³H]spiperone, ex vivo, rat striatum	34 (14)	
[³H]spiroperidol, membranes*, human putamen		Rinne, Lonnberg, &
At 20 years (n=6)	23±4	Marjamaki 1990
At 60 years (n=8)	17±4	
[³H]spiroperidol, membranes*, human putamen		Rinne *et al.* 1991
Control (n=33)	17±1	
Parkinson's disease (n=37)	14±1	
Parkinson's disease, treated with neuroleptics (n=12)	25±2	
[³H]raclopride, membranes, rat striatum	20 (2)	Hall *et al.* 1990
Human putamen	10 (4)	
[³H]NMSP, membranes, rat striatum	20 (0.3)	
Human putamen	10 (0.2)	
[¹¹C]NMSP, membranes, rat striatum	33 (0.08)	Lyon *et al.* 1986
Human caudate nucleus	10 (0.11)	
[¹¹C]NMSP, PET, normal human striatum		Wong *et al.* 1997a
25 years old (n=12)	19±8	
50 years old (n=12)	13±7	
[¹¹C]raclopride, PET, normal human putamen (n=4)	14±2 (4±1)	Farde *et al.* 1986
[¹¹C]raclopride, PET, monkey striatum (n=2)		Ginovart *et al.* 1997a
Baseline	34 (8.6)	
Five hours post reserpine	33 (5.5)	
[¹¹C]raclopride, PET, normal cat striatum		Ginovart *et al.* 2004
Baseline (n=3)	23±3 (12±1)	
After amphetamine (n=3)	16±2 (16±2)	

Table 14.1. (*cont.*)

[^{11}C]raclopride, PET, normal monkey striatum		Doudet & Holden 2003
Baseline ($n=4$)	20±3 (11±2)	
After methamphetamine ($n=4$)	22±2 (20±4)	
[^{11}C]raclopride, PET, normal human striatum		Rinne *et al.* 1993
Third decade ($n=10$)	35±7 (11±3)	
Eighth decade ($n=4$)	26±2 (12±2)	
[^{11}C]raclopride, PET, normal human striatum ($n=20$)	28±7 (9±2)	Farde *et al.* 1995
[^{11}C]raclopride, PET, healthy human caudate ($n=14$)	27±8 (11±3)	Rinne *et al.* 1995
Parkinson's disease caudate ($n=10$)	29±8 (11±5)	
Healthy putamen ($n=14$)	30±7 (12±4)	
Parkinson's disease putamen ($n=10$)	43±9 (12±4)	
[^{11}C]NMSP, PET, human caudate		Wong *et al.* 1986
Healthy normal ($n=11$)	17±3	
Untreated schizophrenia ($n=10$)	42±4	
[^{11}C]raclopride, PET, human striatum		Hietala *et al.* 1994
Healthy normal ($n=8$)	29±5 (9±1)	
Alcoholics ($n=9$)	26±5 (10±2)	
[^{11}C]raclopride, PET, human striatum		Pohjalainen *et al.* 1998b
Male ($n=33$)	26±7 (10±3)	
Female ($n=21$)	27±7 (11±2)	
[^{3}H]NPA, ex vivo, rat striatum	27±2	van der Werf, Sebens, & Korf 1984
[^{3}H]NPA, ex vivo, rat striatum	26±2	van der Werf, Sebens, &
[^{3}H]spiperone ex vivo rat striatum	73±5	Korf 1986
[^{3}H]raclopride, ex vivo, mouse striatum ($n=18$)	41±3 (10±1)	Ross & Jackson 1989a
[^{3}H]NPA, ex vivo, mouse striatum ($n=4$)	47±4 (9±1)	Ross & Jackson 1989a
[^{11}C]raclopride, PET, monkey stiatum ($n=3$)	27±4 (1.6±0.3)	Narendran *et al.* 2005
[^{11}C]NPA, PET, monkey striatum ($n=3$)	22±3 (0.2±0.1)	
[^{3}H]-(+)-PHNO, membranes, rat striatum ($n=16$)	12±1 (1.0±0.1)	Seeman, McCormick, & Kapur 2007
[^{11}C]raclopride, PET, cat striatum ($n=2$)	31 (10)	Ginovart *et al.* 2006
[^{11}C]-(+)-PHNO	31 (10)	
[^{11}C]FLB 457, PET, normal human thalamus ($n=10$)	1.7±1.5 (0.4±0.4)	Olsson, Halldin, &
Temporal cortex ($n=10$)	0.6±0.2 (0.3±0.2)	Farde 2004
[^{18}F]fallypride, PET, normal monkey ($n=3$)		Slifstein *et al.*, 2004
Striatum	27±8 (0.2±0.1)	
Thalamus	2.5±1.0 (0.2±0.1)	
Hippocampus	2.4±0.8 (0.2±0.1)	

Note: Indicated are the maximal binding site density (B_{max}) and the apparent affinity (K_D). In some instances, number of subjects are not reported due to population-based estimation of kinetic parameters.

* Estimated in presence of ketanserin, and results converted from fmol mg protein^{-1} to pmol g^{-1} wet tissue, assuming 10% protein.

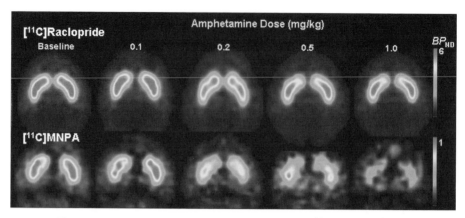

Figure 14.5 Differing vulnerability of an antagonist ([^{11}C]raclopride) and an agonist ([^{11}C]MNPA) to amphetamine challenge. Parametric maps show dose-dependent reductions in the availability of dopamine D$_{2/3}$ receptors in the striatum of monkeys, with consistently greater vulnerability of the agonist to amphetamine-evoked dopamine release. Modified from Seneca *et al.* (2006) and reproduced with permission of Dr. Sjoerd Finnema and Professor Christer Halldin, Karolinska Institute. (For color version, see plate section.)

experiment shows that the basal occupancy of dopamine D$_{2/3}$ receptors by dopamine in mouse striatum is greater with respect to the agonist [^{3}H]NPA than with respect to [^{11}C]raclopride (Cumming *et al.* 2002). Furthermore, the amphetamine challenge paradigm showed that the agonist was 1.7 times more sensitive to amphetamine-evoked dopamine release than was the antagonist ligand. Entirely similar findings were subsequently obtained in non-human primate brain using the PET tracer [^{11}C]NPA (Narendran *et al.* 2004), where it was furthermore calculated that 70% of dopamine D$_{2/3}$ receptors are in a high-affinity state for dopamine. The binding of the very similar agonist [^{11}C]MNPA in monkey striatum could be extensively blocked by pretreatment with non-radioactive raclopride, indicating specificity of the ligand (Finnema *et al.* 2005). The specific binding of [^{11}C]MNPA in living rat striatum was only slightly reduced by treatment with the D$_3$ antagonist BP897, suggesting selectivity for D$_2$ receptors (Seneca *et al.* 2008). In another monkey study, [^{11}C]MNPA proved to be twice as vulnerable as was [^{11}C]raclopride over a wide range of doses of amphetamine (Figure 14.5), yielding an estimated agonist-binding fraction of 60% (Seneca *et al.* 2006). PET studies in cat showed that the [^{11}C]-(+)-PHNO *pB* was two-fold greater than that of [^{11}C]NPA, and most importantly that the striatal [^{11}C]-(+)-PHNO binding was almost completely abolished (−83%) by treatment with amphetamine, in contrast to the more modest reductions observed for

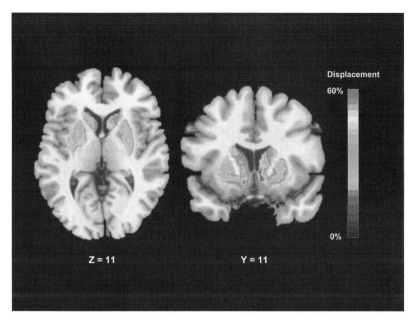

Figure 14.6 The effect of amphetamine challenge on [^{11}C]PHNO binding in human brain. The colour scale shows the percentage reduction in specific binding relative to the baseline condition, projected onto an anatomic atlas. The greatest relative declines are evident in the nucleus accumbens, and binding in the globus pallidus was nearly unaffected by the psychostimulant treatment. Figure reproduced with permission from Willeit *et al.* (2008). (For color version, see plate section.)

[^{11}C]raclopride after the same dose of amphetamine (Ginovart *et al.* 2006). In the first human study with [^{11}C]-(+)-PHNO and amphetamine challenge (Willeit *et al.* 2008), a dorsal–ventral gradient in the displaceability was clearly seen in the extended striatum, with 13% declines in the caudate, increasing to 25% in the ventral striatum (Figure 14.6). The rather extensive binding in the human globus pallidus seemed invulnerable to amphetamine challenge, although it could be displaced with a dopamine receptor antagonist (Willeit *et al.* 2006).

There emerges a broad consensus that agonist ligands are inherently fitter probes of competition in vivo. However, the original conjecture that agonists recognize a subpopulation of receptors (D_2^{High}) in vivo is being reassessed, as shall be discussed below (Chapter 16). The search for optimal agonist tracers continues. In spite of high affinity in vitro, [^{11}C]preclamol (Vasdev *et al.* 2006) and [^{18}F]fluoro-PHNO (Vasdev *et al.* 2007) failed to significanctly label dopamine receptors in living brain.

14.4.4.   Extrastriatal binding

The great preponderance of competition studies in vivo have consi-dered only the binding in living striatum. However, the advent of high-affinity ligands has made possible the assessment of competition at extrastriatal sites. In one study, treatment with methamphetamine was entirely without effect on the cortical binding of [^{11}C]FLB 457 in monkey brain, while decreasing striatal binding by 20% (Okauchi *et al.* 2001). In contrast, [^{18}F]fallypride binding could also be reduced in extrastriatal regions of human brain by an amphetamine challenge (Riccardi *et al.* 2006). Challenge with methylphenidate substantially decreased the [^{11}C]FLB 457 V_d in the thalamus and cerebral cortex of humans in a dose-dependent manner (Montgomery *et al.* 2007a).

14.5.   Clinical studies of dopamine D$_2$ receptors

14.5.1.   Aging and genetics

Across the rat lifespan, there was a 40% decline in the striatal abun-dance of dopamine D$_{2/3}$ receptors measured by [^{11}C]raclopride microPET and by [^{3}H]raclopride autoradiography in vitro (Suzuki *et al.* 2001). Food-restricted diet attenuated the decline in the striatal [^{11}C]raclopride binding with age in both normal rats and in obese Zucker rats (Thanos *et al.* 2007b). The density of [^{3}H]spiperone binding sites in samples from human post mortem brain declined by only 2% per decade (Seeman *et al.* 1987). In contrast, the simple binding ratio (striatum/cerebellum) of [^{76}Br]bromospiperone declined by 4% per decade of healthy human aging (Baron *et al.* 1986), as did the [^{11}C]raclopride pB in one PET study (Rinne *et al.* 1993). In other quantitative studies, the magnitude of k_3 for [^{11}C]NMSP in the striatum declined by 10% per decade (MacRae *et al.* 1987; Wong *et al.* 1997c), whereas the [^{11}C]raclopride pB in human striatum declined by 9% per decade of normal aging (Antonini *et al.* 1993; Volkow *et al.* 1996b). Together, these findings accentuate the need for rigorous age matching in PET studies of dopamine D$_2$ receptors.

Due to inherent limits of the spatial resolution of PET or SPECT, the specific signal measured in structures as small as the striatum can be substantially altered due to spillover of radioactivity, and intrusion of adjacent structures into the region of interest. As introduced in the chapter on FDOPA kinetics, the effects of partial volume generally lead to underestimation of the true magni-tude of dopamine binding parameters in the striatum, which is surrounded by "cool" regions lacking significant dopamine innervation. Thus, a study of partial volume effects in aged monkeys indicates that declining striatal volume results in over-estimation of the age-related loss of [^{11}C]raclopride binding (Morris *et al.*

1999). In a saturation binding study, the [^{11}C]raclopride B_{max} tended to decline more quickly in men than in women, and the magnitude of K_d^{app} was higher in women, implying greater basal occupancy by endogenous dopamine in the women (Pohjalainen *et al.* 1998b). These observations may likewise be related to gender differences in the rate of loss of striatal volume.

Age-related changes in dopamine D_2 receptor availability are not restricted to the extended striatum. The *pB* of the high-affinity ligand [^{11}C]FLB 457 in the frontal and temporal cortex declined by 10% per decade of normal aging, but thalamic binding did not decline with age (Talvik *et al.* 2003), perhaps because this central structure is relatively protected from partial volume effects. Similar rates of decline in extrastriatal binding of [^{11}C]FLB 457 were found in women as in men (Kaasinen *et al.* 2002a), although abundances were significantly higher in women than in an age-matched male group (Kaasinen *et al.* 2001a).

The abundance of striatal dopamine receptors within a population of rats can be quite variable. In a group of rats trained to press a lever to avoid an electric shock, the majority of the variance in response latency could be described by individual differences in the dopamine D_2 binding in vitro (Wilcox *et al.* 1988). Furthermore, an age-related decline in the abundance of dopamine D_2 receptors in rat striatum was linked to increases in behavioral response latency, i.e the time delay between stimulus and reaction (MacRae, Spirduso, & Wilcox 1988). Endurance training of aged rats significantly increased the B_{max} for [^{3}H]spiperone in rat striatal homogenates (MacRae *et al.* 1987). It can thus be predicted that age-related changes in motor function should likewise correlate with reduced dopamine receptor availability in human brain.

In a large group of subjects comprising an extended range of ages, there was a highly significant correlation between [^{11}C]raclopride *pB* in the caudate and putamen and the maximal rate of finger-tapping (Volkow *et al.* 1998a), as predicted on the basis of rat studies. The relationship persisted after correction for age-effects, and furthermore correlated with executive function, as measured by performance of the Stroop test and the Wisconsin Card Sorting Test. Perceptual speed can be measured by the trail-making task ("connect the dots"), and in a task in which subjects must identify certain configurations of dots. The speed of performance of both tasks declined with the age of healthy subjects, in a manner correlating with the declining [^{11}C]raclopride *pB* (Backman *et al.* 2000). There was a positive correlation between striatal [^{11}C]raclopride *pB* and spatial working memory, as measured by parts of the CANTAB test battery. In this study, effects of age were removed by "partialling," and the main correlation was with the most difficult cognitive tasks (Reeves *et al.* 2005). Finally, the availability of [^{11}C]raclopride binding sites in both limbic and sensorimotor divisions of striatum correlated with aspects of cognitive function in healthy middle-aged subjects (Cervenka *et al.* 2008). Thus, the performances of both motor and cognitive tasks covary with the availability of dopamine D$_2$ receptors in healthy human striatum. The binding of [^{11}C]FLB 457 to dopamine receptors in the hippocampus of healthy young men had a very high correlation with scores in neuropsychological tests, especially pertaining to memory function (Takahashi *et al.* 2007).

Dopamine receptors are not equally distributed between the two cerebral hemispheres; complex asymmetry in the binding of [^{11}C]raclopride could be seen in the striatum of normal female pigs (Cumming *et al.* 2003b), consistent with results in a meta-analysis of imaging studies in humans, showing a 5% predominance of dopamine D$_2$ receptor availability on the right side (Larisch *et al.* 1998). Since most subjects are right-handed, this PET result suggests a greater availability of dopamine receptors (i.e. lower occupancy) in the striatum regulating the control of the non-dominant side. More recently, asymmetry of [^{18}F]desmethoxyfallypride binding in the striatum of healthy subjects was shown to decline with age (Vernaleken *et al.* 2007b), consistent with results of an autoradiographic study in vitro of the aging rat (Giardino 1996). Contrary to the preceding literature in normal subjects, Tomer *et al.* (2008) found a preponderance of D$_2$ receptors on the left side of healthy subjects, the extent of which asymmetry correlated with the personality trait *incentive motivation*. Others found a left predominance of D$_2$ receptors in patients with schizophrenia but not in healthy control subjects (Schroder *et al.* 1997), which might subserve the reported abnormal bias in spontaneous turning reported elsewhere for these patients. Thus, changes in the symmetrical disposition of dopamine receptors should be interpreted in the context of contributions of age, pathophysiology, and possibly gender.

In the normal human population there are polymorphisms in the putative promoter region of the D$_2$ receptor gene, and in the gene itself. In a study of 56 healthy subjects, there was a significant association between the active promoter allele and [^{11}C]raclopride *pB*, and a negative association between the non-coding TaqA1 and TaqB1 alleles and [^{11}C]raclopride *pB* (Jonsson *et al.* 1999). Whereas another [^{11}C]raclopride study in 54 subjects reports a similar association between the TaqA1 allele and low availability of dopamine receptors (Pohjalainen *et al.* 1998a), an [^{123}I]IBZM study of 70 subjects failed to identify an association with TaqA1 (Laruelle, Gelernter, & Innis 1998). While these imaging studies represent commendable efforts to define the genetic basis for dopamine receptor expression, it seems likely that only multi-center studies with hundreds of subjects may be able to obtain definitive results. In a post mortem genetic study of 20 normal subjects and 20 alcoholics (a trait which is associated with the A1 allele), there was a highly significant association between the A1 allele and the age-corrected [^{3}H]raclopride B_{max} in membranes from the putamen (Ritchie & Noble 2003). Given the low abundance of some alleles in the general population, this result shows that pre-selecting subjects with genetic markers can enhance the statistical power of PET studies.

14.5.2.   Neurological disorders

The phenomenon of D_2 upregulation in dopamine-depleted striatum of experimental animals is documented in Section 14.3. Consistent with these findings in animal models of parkinsonism, the density of D_2 binding sites was nearly doubled in parts of the putamen of patients dying with Parkinson's disease (Piggott *et al.* 1999a). However, the binding of [^{11}C]NMSP in vivo was only slightly increased in the putamen of patients with Parkinson's disease, contralateral to the side of the main symptoms (Kaasinen *et al.* 2000). More consistent with the results in experimental animals, the availability of [^{11}C]raclopride binding sites was elevated in the putamen of untreated patients with Parkinson's disease (Antonini *et al.* 1997). Likewise, here was a 40% increase in B_{max} in the putamen of Parkinson's patients in a PET saturation binding study with [^{11}C]raclopride (Rinne *et al.* 1995). Prolonged treatment with DOPA resulted in a reduction in this binding, just as in experimental animals treated for acquired parkinsonism. Similar observations have been made in the course of DOPA treatment of patients with parkinsonism associated with mutations of the *parkin* gene (Scherfler *et al.* 2006b). It might be considered that competition from endogenous dopamine could interfere with the detection of upregulation of dopamine D_2 receptors in PET studies of living brain, assuming that some occupancy of receptors by dopamine occurs, even in an advanced stage of Parkinson's disease. However, altered competition was not evident in the measurements of $K_d{}^{app}$ in the saturation study cited above (Rinne *et al.* 1995).

The binding of [^{11}C]raclopride in the striatum of Parkinson's disease patients declined by 2–3% per year, i.e. several times faster than the declines seen with aging in healthy subjects (Antonini *et al.* 1997). Particularly severe loss of striatal D_2 binding has been linked to the emergence of DOPA-evoked motor fluctuations, a disabling aspect of advanced Parkinson's disease (Hwang *et al.* 2002). Likewise, the binding of the high-affinity ligand [^{11}C]FLB 457 in the cerebral cortex declined by 10% per year in patients with Parkinson's disease, also several times faster than in healthy subjects (Kaasinen *et al.* 2003).

In the striatum of non-genotyped patients with focal dystonia, there was a 30% decline in the [^{18}F]spiperone k_3 (Perlmutter *et al.* 1998) and a similar decrease in the binding ratio for [^{123}I]epidepride (Naumann *et al.* 1998), whereas there was a 12% reduction in [^{11}C]raclopride binding in essential blepharospasm patients (Suzuki *et al.* 2008) and a 19% decline in [^{11}C]raclopride binding in non-symptomatic carriers of the DYT1 dystonia mutation (Asanuma *et al.* 2005). Thus, decreased D$_2$ receptor availability throughout the striatum seems inadequate to account for the focal nature and incomplete penetrance of the dystonia phenotype. In striatum of patients with DOPA responsive dystonia and in non-symptomatic carriers of the disorder, there was a 15% increase in [^{11}C]raclopride binding, consistent with the functional dopamine denervation (Kishore *et al.* 1998). Striatal [^{11}C]raclopride binding was normal in patients with idiopathic restless legs syndrome (Tribl *et al.* 2004), although others report increased binding of [^{11}C]FLB 457 in the striatum and extrastriatal regions, a finding which was not subject to the diurnal changes characteristic of the clinical syndrome (Cervenka *et al.* 2006).

Profound changes in post-synaptic receptors are to be expected in Huntington's disease, in which the hallmark pathology is the loss of medium spiny neurons bearing dopamine D$_1$ and D$_2$ receptors. Thus, the *pB* of [^{11}C]raclopride in the striatum was reduced by 40% in a PET study of patients with Huntington's disease (Ginovart *et al.* 1997b). The binding of [^{11}C]raclopride in the striatum declined by 6.5% per year in patients with actively progressing Huntington's disease (Andrews *et al.* 1999), i.e. nearly ten times faster than in the course of normal aging. Furthermore, [^{11}C]raclopride *pB* was significantly reduced in asymptomatic carriers of Huntington's disease mutation, to an extent correlating significantly with product of the subject's age and the number of repeats of the CAG triplet coden in the mutant Huntington's gene (van Oostrom *et al.* 2005). The binding ratio of [^{123}I]IBZM was substantially decreased in striatum of de novo patients with Wilson's disease, but returned to the normal range after a period of chelation therapy (Schwarz *et al.* 1994).

[^{11}C]Raclopride binding is not notably reduced in the striatum of patients with Alzheimer's disease (Kemppainen *et al.* 2000), although, in another study, reduced [^{11}C]raclopride binding in the striatum was associated with severe behavioral pathology (Tanaka *et al.* 2003). [^{11}C]FLB 457 binding was reduced in the hippocampus of patients with Alzheimer's disease to an extent correlating with cognitive deficits (Kemppainen *et al.* 2003). This seems likely to be a non-specific indicator of neuronal loss in temporal structures.

14.5.3.   *Psychiatric disorders*

Controversy still surrounds the disparate findings of altered dopamine D$_2$ receptor binding of schizophrenia, which was an early clinical finding of molecular imaging. The rate of association of [^{11}C]NMSP (k_3) to dopamine D$_2$-like receptors in striatum was measured in healthy control subjects and in patients with schizophrenia, first in a baseline condition, and again after partial blockade of dopamine D$_2$ receptors with haloperidol (Wong *et al.* 1986). The individual estimates of k_3 were plotted as an inverse function of the plasma haloperidol concentrations in order to estimate the B_{max}. Using this method, the population-mean of B_{max} was considerably higher in the group of schizophrenics than in normal volunteers. Expansion of the earlier group to include 18 drug-naïve patients, and controlling for an apparent gender difference in the clinical group, showed similar results (Tune *et al.* 1993). Using a similar method, others failed to find a significant difference in [^{11}C]NMSP binding between control and schizophrenic patients, claiming that the specific signal measured in the presence of haloperidol was too low to permit adequate quantification of the binding site density (Nordstrom *et al.* 1995). Results of a further expansion of the original cohort suggested that the disagreement between laboratories could reflect greater dispersion of the B_{max} estimates among the schizophrenic group, and also the presence of greater age-related declines (Wong *et al.* 1997a).

In post mortem studies using the D_2 ligand [^{3}H]nemonapride, the $D_{2/3}$ binding component was only slightly increased in the brain of patients with schizophrenia, whereas the D_4 component of the binding was substantially increased (Seeman, Guan, & Van Tol 1993), possibly reflecting the premorbid treatment with neuroleptics in that subject group. However, this finding in vitro also suggests that the Baltimore PET result of increased [^{11}C]NMSP may be related specifically to D_4 receptors.

Given the problematic aspects of butyrophenone binding studies, the majority of investigations of schizophrenia have made use of benzamide radioligands. The concentration of [^{11}C]raclopride binding sites in the striatum was similar in a group of drug-free schizophrenics and healthy controls (Farde *et al.* 1990). No difference in striatal [^{11}C]raclopride binding was found in a more recent study of a large cohort of drug-naïve patients with schizophrenia (Talvik *et al.* 2006). Relatively increased [^{11}C]raclopride binding in the left caudate nucleus of homozygotic twins of patients with schizophrenia nonetheless suggests that genetic risk may be associated with increased binding (Hirvonen *et al.* 2005).

There have been relatively few investigations of extrastriatal dopamine D_2 receptors in patients with schizophrenia. The [^{11}C]FLB 457 pB was significantly reduced in parts of the right thalamus of drug-naïve patients with schizophrenia (Talvik *et al.* 2003), whereas others report an increase in [^{123}I]epidepride binding in the right thalamus of the patients (Glenthoj *et al.* 2006). [^{123}I]Epidepride binding was reduced in the insular cortex of unmedicated patients (Tuppurainen *et al.* 2003), in a manner correlating with the extent of general psychopathology. Binding of the same ligand was 15% reduced in the midbrain (Tuppurainen *et al.* 2006) in a small group of patients with schizophrenia; the latter finding could be consistent with downregulation of autoreceptors in the substantia nigra.

The [^{11}C]NMSP B_{max} was elevated in bipolar patients with psychosis, but not in non-psychotic patients (Wong *et al.* 1997a). As in the case of the schizophrenia group, this difference seemed to be occurring in association with a more rapid loss of receptors with age in the psychotic group. However, the striatal [^{11}C]raclopride pB was entirely normal in bipolar patients with non-psychotic mania, nor did treatment with the mood stabilizer divalproex sodium alter this binding (Yatham *et al.* 2002a). This disagreement could reflect the terms of definition of psychosis, or be another manifestation of the unresolved discrepancies between PET results with different ligands.

The abundance of [^{123}I]IBZM did not significantly differ in patients with major depression and healthy control subjects. However, after correction for age, the binding was found to be lower in those who subsequently responded to antidepressant treatment (Klimke *et al.* 1999). The lower binding tended to increase with treatment, while the converse was seen for non-responders, suggesting that the condition of depression is heterogenous with respect to baseline dopamine $D_{2/3}$ receptor availability, and with respect to receptor plasticity. [^{11}C]Raclopride binding was decreased in the dorsal striatum of a group of patients with depression, but results of this study are confounded by possible effects of antidepressant medication (Montgomery *et al.* 2007). Furthermore, increased [^{11}C]raclopride pB was detected bilaterally in the putamen of depressed patients with psychomotor retardation as measured by the performance of a finger-tapping test, suggesting that this symptom of depression reflects low basal occupancy by endogenous dopamine (Meyer *et al.* 2006b). Consistent with this notion, effective treatment with total sleep deprivation decreased striatal [^{123}I]IBZM binding in a small group of depressed patients (Ebert *et al.* 1994), perhaps revealing a normalization of the basal occupancy.

After controlling for age-related declines, the [^{11}C]NMSP B_{max} was within the normal range in the striatum of patients with Tourette's syndrome (Wong *et al.* 1997b). However, within the clinical group there were several outliers, with B_{max} values above the 95% confidence limits for the regression with age, suggesting the presence of clinical heterogeneity within the population. The availability of [^{11}C]raclopride binding sites in the anteroventral striatum increased in women during recovery from anorexia nervosa, suggesting that low basal occupancy might be a state marker of that disorder (Frank *et al.* 2005).

14.5.4.   Receptor occupancy during treatment with antipsychotic medication

PET has been used to assess the extent of occupancy of dopamine D_2 receptors during treatment with antipsychotic drugs. In patients with schizophrenia treated with haloperidol, [^{11}C]FLB 457 PET showed 60–80% occupancy of receptors in the thalamus and cortex, similar to the occupancies found for

[^{11}C]raclopride in the striatum (Farde *et al.* 1997). This occupancy has been used operationally to define the threshold between therapeutic efficacy and the syndrome of extrapyramidal side effects, which emerge when occupancy is greater than 80%. There is an important distinction to be made between typical antispsychotic drugs like haloperidol, which mainly interact with dopamine D$_2$ receptors, and the atypical antipsychotics like clozipine, which exert a greater antagonism against serotonin 5HT$_{2A}$ receptors, and which seem to preferentially bind to dopamine receptors in extrastriatal regions. Thus, a SPECT study with [^{123}I]epidepride in patients treated with the atypical neuroleptic amisulpride showed 80% occupancy of dopamine receptors in extrastriatal regions, versus only 50% occupancy in the striatum (Bressan *et al.* 2003). Another atypical antipsychotic, ziprasidone, evoked 76% occupancy of serotonin 5HT$_2$ receptors in the presence of only 56% occupancy at [^{11}C]raclopride binding sites (Mamo *et al.* 2004a). In a PET study with the high-affinity D$_{2/3}$ ligand [^{18}F]fallypride, therapeutic doses of clozapine occupied 55% of receptors in the cortex, versus only 40% in the striatum (Grunder *et al.* 2006). These results suggest that the antipsychotic benefits were obtained via more sensitive blockade of dopamine receptors outside the striatum, and without the extrapyramidal side effects resulting from substantial blockade of striatal receptors, in addition to effects mediated by serotonin receptor blockade. However, this interpretation should be made with caution, since (as noted above) the presence of specific binding in the cerebellum may result in relatively greater bias and relative error in regions of low receptor abundance.

Occupancy studies with the atypical antipsychotic quetiapine against [^{11}C]raclopride showed that peak occupancies at dopamine receptors of about 60% were obtained only transiently, declining to 14% in less than a day, even in patients obtaining a good and persistent clinical response (Tauscher-Wisniewski *et al.* 2002). In addition, atypical antipsychotic drugs seem to discriminate populations of dopamine receptors within the extended striatum. In a competition study against [^{123}I]epidepride, risperidone and amisulpride both showed a distinct preference for dopamine receptors in the caudate, i.e. limbic and associative regions, rather than the putamen (Stone *et al.* 2005). The atypical antipsychotic olanzipine has the same D$_2$ occupancy against [^{18}F]setoperone (70–80%) as did haloperidol throughout the extended striatum, but had distinctly lower occupancy (40%) in the substantia nigra, where presynaptic autoreceptors may predominate (Kessler *et al.* 2005). Antipsychostic doses of the dopamine receptor partial agonist aripiprazole obtained nearly complete occupancy for striatal [^{11}C]raclopride binding sites, without evoking extrapyramidal symptoms (Yokoi *et al.* 2002). Together, these results indicate that antipsychotic action is much more complex than simple blockade of dopamine receptors in the striatum, but can be mediated by serotonin receptors, cortical dopamine receptors, preferential blockade in different brain regions, or via partial activation of striatal dopamine receptors.

14.5.5.   Receptor occupancy by agonists

The effects of pharmacological challenge with the indirect agonist DOPA on D$_2$ receptor availability will be discussed Section 15.2.3. There have been few PET studies of dopamine receptor occupancy by direct agonists. Complete occupancy in human brain by the partial agonist aripiprazole was noted above (Yokoi *et al.* 2002). Very high doses of the D$_2$ agonist [+]-PD 128907 could substantially displace [^{11}C]raclopride binding in normal monkey striatum (Kortekaas *et al.* 2004), a finding to be discussed below in the context of the true population of agonist sites (Chapter 16). Prolonged treatment with the dopamine agonist lisuride at an effective antiparkinsonian dose (1 mg p.d.) reduced putamenal [^{11}C]raclopride binding by 19% relative to the baseline condition of de novo Parkinson's disease patients (Antonini *et al.* 1994). Prolonged treatment of patients with pergolide likewise reduced [^{11}C]raclopride binding by 14% (Linazasoro *et al.* 1999), whereas chronic lisuride or pramipexole decreased [^{123}I]IBZM binding by 5% (Schwarz *et al.* 1996); in these chronic studies, occupancy cannot be distinguished from downregulation of receptor expression. However, acute treatment with a low dose of the agonist apomorphine (0.03 mg kg^{-1}) decreased [^{11}C]raclopride binding by 9% in the more intact putamen of asymmetric Parkinson's disease patients and by 15% on the side contralateral to the main symptoms, whereas 0.06 mg kg^{-1} evoked 18 and 30% reductions (de la Fuente-Fernandez *et al.* 2001). This kind of asymmetric occupancy was also found in a study of rhesus monkey with unilateral MPTP lesions; the D2 agonist LY 1711555 (0.3 mg kg^{-1}) evoked 35% displacement of [^{123}I]IBZM in intact striatum and 45% displacement on the dopamine-depleted side (Vermeulen *et al.* 1994). In rats with hemi-parkinsonism, bromocriptine evoked a time- and dose-dependent displacement of striatal [^{3}H]raclopride binding measured ex vivo. This displacement was as high as 50%, in which circumstance the agonist-evoked rotational behavior reached its peak (Atsumi *et al.* 2003). In summary, the limited available results suggest that antiparkinsonian effects are obtained with only partial occupancy by agonists, perhaps consistent with the contrary finding that 80% blockade is required to evoke extrapyramidal symptoms.

15

Factors influencing D_2 binding in living brain

15.1. Pharmacological modulation

15.1.1. Dopamine antagonists

Just as the abundance of striatal dopamine D_2 receptors increases after prolonged dopamine depletion, chronic pharmacological blockade can also result in receptor upregulation. For example, chronic neuroleptic treatment increased dopamine $D_{2/3}$ receptor binding site density in rat striatum by 19%, whereas the specific binding to D_4 receptors increased two-fold (Schoots *et al.* 1995). In another study, chronic haloperidol treatment increased [^{3}H]spiperone binding (in the presence of a $5HT_2$ antagonist) in rat striatum membranes by 40%, but the antipsychotic treatment was without effect on the apparent fraction of those receptors which could be displaced by agonists, i.e. D_2^{High} (MacKenzie & Zigmond 1984). Similar increases in D_2 antagonist binding have also been seen in the striatum of monkeys after prolonged pharmacological blockade with receptor antagonists (Huang *et al.* 1997).

Pharmacologically evoked changes in dopamine receptor availability can be extremely long-lasting. In a primate PET study, daily treatment with raclopride ($10\,\mu g\,k\,g^{-1} \times 30$ days) increased the striatal binding of the D_2-selective antagonist [^{18}F]fluoroclebopride by 12–20%, an increase which persisted for 1 year in two of the three monkeys investigated (Czoty, Gage, & Nader 2005). In a case report of two patients with schizophrenia who had undergone treatment with haloperidol for many years, a non-smoker had a 98% increase in [^{11}C]raclopride *pB* and suffered from tardive dyskinesia, whereas a smoker, treated at a much higher haloperidol dose, had somewhat lower elevation in *pB*, and no tardive symptoms (Silvestri *et al.* 2004). Given the high prevalence of smoking among people with schizophrenia, it is tempting to speculate that nicotine may be serving to moderate pathological responses to chronic antipsychotic treatment.

15.1.2.   Anesthesia

The effects of anesthesia can be an important confounding factor in brain imaging studies of dopamine D_2 receptors. For example, [^{11}C]raclopride binding has been successfully measured in the striatum of awake cats trained to remain still during the scanning period. Relative to this condition, anesthesia with halothane increased the pB by one third (an effect which could be attributed to increased cerebral blood flow), whereas anesthesia with ketamine was without effect on the binding in vivo (Hassoun et al. 2003). In other PET studies, the binding kinetics of [^{11}C]NMSP are also sensitive to the type of anesthesia used during the emission recording. In particular, the [^{11}C]NMSP k_3 to receptors in monkey striatum was considerably lower with isofluorane than with ketamine anesthesia (Kobayashi et al. 1995). As with halothane, the [^{11}C]raclopride pB in monkey striatum increased with isofluorane anesthesia, an effect apparently due to decreased rate of dissociation of the radioligand.

15.1.3.   Drugs of abuse

In chronic cocaine users, the [^{11}C]raclopride pB was reduced by 15% throughout the extended striatum, in both limbic and sensorimotor divisions (Martinez et al. 2004). In a group of chronic cocaine users, the simple ratio of [^{11}C]NMSP uptake in the striatum to that in the cerebellum was substantially reduced, but returned to normal after prolonged abstinence (Volkow et al. 1990). Thus, it would seem that the post-synaptic effects of chronic cocaine-use can resolve with time. Similarly, in rats exposed to cocaine in a "binge pattern," there was a transient 20% decrease in striatal [^{11}C]NMSP binding, which normalized after several weeks' abstinence (Maggos et al. 1998). Among human methamphetamine users, there was a 10–15% reduction in striatal [^{11}C]raclopride binding, the extent of which correlated with reduced glucose consumption in the orbitofrontal cortex (Volkow et al. 2001a). Effects of abstinence from methamphetamine on D_2 binding seem not to have been documented, but the changes in DAT predict an eventual normalization of post-synaptic markers also.

The rate of decline in striatal [^{11}C]raclopride pB with age was 50% higher in a small group of chronic alcoholics than in healthy controls (Volkow et al. 1996c). Nonetheless, in abstinent alcoholics the [^{11}C]raclopride pB was only slightly reduced in the striatum, although the saturation binding parameters were not significantly altered (Hietala et al. 1994), whereas others report that reduced [^{11}C]raclopride pB persists after prolonged abstinence from alcohol (Volkow et al. 2002c). Furthermore, the [^{18}F]desmethoxyfallypride pB sites were reduced in the ventral striatum of alcoholics, the extent of which reduction correlating with the severity of craving evoked by visual cues (Heinz *et al.* 2005). Thus, imaging studies clearly link alcoholism with abnormality in dopamine receptor availability, with the usual caveat that these results may be confounded by changes in tonic occupancy. In a rodent model, precipitous withdrawal from alcohol evokes a long-lasting increase in the fraction of $[^3H]$raclopride in rat striatal membranes sensitive to GTPγS, and a similar increase in the fraction of $[^3H]$PHNO binding, both of which findings suggest a sensitization by enhanced coupling of the receptors to signal transduction pathways (Seeman, Tallerico, & Ko 2004). In the absence of other changes, alcohol-induced sensitization might be expected to increase the occupancy of receptors by tonic dopamine, resulting in some of the observed reductions in D_2 receptor availability in vivo.

15.2.   Clinical studies of psychostimulant-evoked dopamine release

15.2.1.   *Schizophrenia spectrum disorders*

The displacement of the SPET ligand $[^{123}I]$IBZM from dopamine D_2 receptors in the striatum has been used to assess the release of dopamine by amphetamine, assuming that its binding in vivo occurs in competition with the endogenous ligand. In a meta-analysis of earlier studies, acute amphetamine challenge reduced $[^{123}I]$IBZM binding by 7.5% in the striatum of normal control subjects and by 17% in a group of patients (*n*=34) with schizophrenia (Laruelle *et al.* 1999). The positive symptoms of the patients were acutely exacerbated by amphetamine challenge in proportion to the reduction in $[^{123}I]$IBZM binding. Similar findings have been observed in a study employing $[^{11}C]$raclopride and the bolus plus infusion method. Here, the binding ratio of $[^{11}C]$raclopride in the striatum declined by 16% after intravenous amphetamine in normal volunteers versus 22% in patients with schizophrenia (Breier *et al.* 1997). These findings have been widely interpreted to reveal the presence of a supernormal amphetamine-releasable dopamine pool in the cytosol of dopamine terminals of patients, although an alternate explanation will be presented below.

The amphetamine-evoked reductions in striatal $[^{123}I]$IBZM in a group of patients with schizotypal personality disorder (−12%) exceeded that in healthy control subjects (−7%), equaled that found in schizoprhrenia patients during remission (−10%), and was considerably elevated (−24%) in the personality disorder patients with psychotic exacerbations (Abi-Dargham *et al.* 2004). The authors of this study concluded that both psychotic traits and state could be separately manifest in hyper-reactivity to amphetamine challenge.

Furthermore, amphetamine-evoked [^{123}I]IBZM reductions were in the normal range in a group of euthymic bipolar patients (Anand *et al.* 2000), further implicating the potentiation of receptor occupancy by amphetamine challenge as a state marker for psychosis.

Just as benzamide binding can be displaced by psychostimulant challenge, the binding in living brain is tonically reduced by endogenous dopamine. The effects of acute reserpine-evoked dopamine depletion on benzamide binding in animal brain have been noted above. However, reserpine would be poorly tolerated by human subjects; the less toxic alkaloid tetrabenazine seems not to have been tested in dopamine depletion paradigms. Instead, partial and transient dopamine depletion can be obtained by treatment with AMPT, which is used clinically for the treatment of pheochromocytoma. A dose of 4.5 gr AMPT, evoking a substantial decline in plasma catecholamine metabolites, also evoked a 13% increase in [^{11}C]raclopride binding in the striatum of normal humans (Verhoeff *et al.* 2002). In an [^{123}I]IBZM SPET study, the extent of increased striatal binding after AMPT-induced dopamine depletion was highly variable, but correlated very well with the extent of dysphoria experienced by the subjects (Voruganti *et al.* 2001a). This suggests that consistent detection of disease-related changes in receptor availability may have been obscured by dispersion in the basal occupancy of dopamine receptors within populations of patients with schizophrenia. Indeed, [^{123}I]IBZM SPET results reveal a greater increase of dopamine receptor availability in response to dopamine depletion with AMPT in patients with schizophrenia (Abi-Dargham *et al.* 2000). Whereas the treatment increased striatal binding by only 9% in control subjects, there was a 17% increase in the group with schizophrenia. Dopamine depletion with AMPT has also revealed basal occupancy of cortical dopamine D$_{2/3}$ receptors in normal subjects through with [^{123}I]epidepride, which increased by 10% in the cerebral cortex (Fujita *et al.* 2000), whereas a similar AMPT treatment failed to evoke any measurable change in cortical [^{18}F]fallypride binding (Riccardi *et al.* 2007). It must be considered that these AMPT studies in humans cannot reveal the entire occupancy changes which might be evoked in experimental animals treated with reserpine; since the AMPT is a competitive TH inhibitor, even high plasma concentrations will result in incomplete inhibition of dopamine synthesis (Laruelle *et al.* 1997a).

A parsimonious explanation for increased vulnerability of [^{11}C]raclopride binding to an indirect agonist is that the amphetamine-sensitive dopamine pool in nigrostriatal dopamine fibers is elevated in patients with psychosis. This scenario seems consistent with the several reports of elevated AAADC activity in the striatum of patients, as cited in Chapter 5.5.6. However, the possible contribution of post-synaptic factors cannot be excluded, as argued above in the context of alcohol abuse. Thus, it seems remarkable that the massive dopamine release evoked by amphetamine (Endres *et al.* 1997a) can displace only 50% of [^{11}C]raclopride binding in vivo. Insofar as this ceiling effect may be established by the agonist-binding fraction, the amphetamine challenge paradigm in patients with schizophrenia may actually reveal sensitization of the dopamine receptors, rather than elevated dopamine release. In this scenario, the amphetamine-stimulated dopamine release is sufficient to displace a greater amount of the D$_2$ receptor ligand in the brain of patients.

The phenomenon of sensitization to the psychomotor stimulant effects of amphetamine is well established. Microdialysis studies show that prior exposure to psychostimulants potentiates the dopamine release in the rat nucleus accumbens, with somewhat disaparate results in the shell and cores divisions (Cadoni, Solinas, & Di 2000; Pierce & Kalivas 1995). Although such small structures may never be resolvable in PET studies of human brain, previous exposure to amphetamine sensitizes the vulnerability of [^{11}C]raclopride binding, especially in the ventral striatum of healthy volunteers (Boileau *et al.* 2006). Remarkably, this sensitization was apparent as much as 1 year after the priming doses (Figure 15.1). Furthermore, increased reactivity to amphetamine was associated with reduced baseline binding throughout the striatum, and sensitization of the subject rating of the "energetic" subscore in the Profile of Mood States (POMS) test. These findings may indicate that the amphetamine-releasable pool of dopamine is persistently enhanced by only a few previous exposures to amphetamine. However, experiments in rats also implicate postsynaptic factors in amphetamine sensitization. In striatal membranes from rats with behavioral sensitization to the effects of amphetamine, [^{3}H]-(+)-PHNO binding had increased, as had the displaceability of the agonist [^{3}H]domperidone by low concentrations of dopamine (Seeman, McCormick, & Kapur 2007). Together, these results indicate that sensitization is mediated by a shift in fraction or propensity of dopamine D$_2$ receptors to be coupled to intracellular G-proteins. In a comparison of diverse animal models of schizophrenia, including pharmacological treatments, gene knockouts, and cesarean delivery, the common element was found to be increased D$_2$^{High} levels, suggesting that the paths of schizophrenia converge on this common pathophysiological mechanism (Seeman *et al.* 2005b). This hypothesis is readily amenable to testing in PET studies with the new dopamine agonist ligands.

There is some evidence for lateralization of the amphetamine-evoked [^{11}C]raclopride binding changes. T-statistic maps show that the sensitization phenomenon was most evident in the right striatum of humans (Figure 15.1). This finding resonates with the somewhat asymmetric changes in [^{11}C]raclopride *pB* after methylphenidate (Figure 15.2), and of [^{11}C]PHNO *pB* after amphetamine (Figure 14.6). In contrast, no asymmetry was evident in the [^{11}C]raclopride

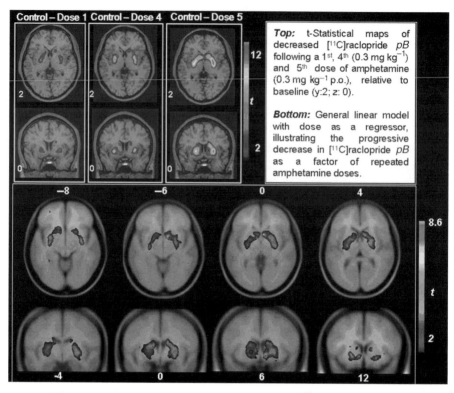

Figure 15.1 Sensitization of amphetamine-evoked [^{11}C]raclopride binding changes in human brain. A series of T-statistic maps show the progressive enhancement of the effect of amphetamine challenge on [^{11}C]raclopride binding in healthy volunteers receiving five doses of amphetamine over a period of one year. Figure reprinted with permission from Boileau *et al.* (2006). (For color version, see plate section.)

binding changes evoked by amphetamine in the rat (Figure 14.3), or by MDMA challenge in the pig (Figure 14.2), whereas the effects of nicotine challenge were greatest in the left striatum (Cumming *et al.* 2003b). Asymmetric reactivity of dopamine innervations may thus be a peculiarity of human brain.

15.2.2.   *Other psychiatric disorders and substance abuse*

In spite of some controversies surrounding its clinical use, oral methylphenidate remains the mainstay pharmacotherapy for attention-deficit hyperactivity disorder (ADHD). Its therapeutic action is presumably due to enhancement of interstitial dopamine levels following DAT blockade. In support of this claim, a single dose of methylphenidate (60 mg) to healthy adults resulted in 60% blockade of DAT labeled with [^{11}C]cocaine, and an 18% reduction in [^{11}C]raclopride binding to post-synaptic receptors (Volkow *et al.* 2002a). In adolescent patients with ADHD, oral methylphenidate at the therapeutic dose

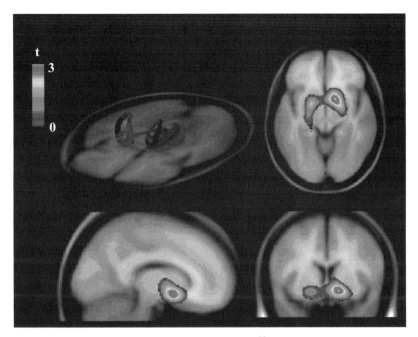

Figure 15.2 The effect of oral methylphenidate on [^{11}C]raclopride binding in human brain. T-statistic map of voxels in which oral administration of methylphenidate reduced the availability of binding sites for [^{11}C]raclopride in the brain of a group of adolescent patients with diagnosis of attention deficit hyperactivity disorder. Figure reproduced with permission from Rosa-Neto *et al.* (2005). (For color version, see plate section.)

decreased [^{11}C]raclopride binding especially in the right striatum (Figure 15.2) (Rosa-Neto *et al.* 2005). This t-statistic map shows the spatial extent of brain regions in which there was a significant difference between the mean para-metric *pB* map at the baseline and that after the pharmacological challenge. The clusters are distinctly positioned toward the ventral portion of the extended striatum, consistent with the large body of literature indicating a greater sensi-tivity of the ventral striatum to psychostimulant-evoked dopamine release. The figure also indicates substantial lateralization of the effect to the right hemisphere.

The methylphenidate challenge reduced [^{11}C]raclopride binding to a highly variable extent in the ADHD patients, perhaps reflecting individual differences in the absorption of the drug after oral administration. However, the binding decrease in the striatum correlated with individual scores for impulsivity and inattention (Rosa-Neto *et al.* 2005b), which seems consistent with findings cited above of increased DAT in patients with impulse control disorders. Others report the precise opposite in young adults with ADHD, in whom the severity of symptoms assessed with the Connors Adult Rating Scale correlated inversely with the magnitude of reduction of striatal [^{11}C]raclopride binding after a challenge with intravenous methylphenidate (Volkow *et al.* 2007b), a reduction which was also noted in the extra-striatal regions not normally assessed using [^{11}C]raclopride. Among the factors possibly accounting for these contradictory results are differences in patient demographics and psychological testing instruments, or the use of intravenous rather than oral methylphenidate in the latter study, which might have resulted in rapid adaptive changes in the vulnerability of dopamine receptors to increased competition from endogenous dopamine, i.e desensitization.

Chronic treatment of rats with oral methylphenidate evoked an initial decrease in [^{11}C]raclopride binding measured by microPET, but a 20% increase was evident after 8 months of treatment (Thanos *et al.* 2007a). This increase was associated with a decreased rate of lever responses in order to self-administer cocaine, consistent with the notion that high receptor availability is protective against psychostimulant use. The relationship between cocaine and methylphenidate use and dopamine receptor availability changes is reciprocal. Thus, detoxified patients with a history of cocaine dependency were insensitive to the acute effects of methylphenidate on [^{11}C]raclopride binding (Volkow *et al.* 1997b). This loss of sensitivity could be attributed to the decline in the density of DAT known to occur following chronic cocaine use. Interestingly, the effect of cocaine on [^{11}C]raclopride binding was briefer than that of methylphenidate, perhaps due to more rapid elimination of cocaine from the brain.

In cocaine-dependent subjects, the baseline [^{11}C]raclopride *pB* was reduced by 10% throughout the extended striatum, but the amphetamine-evoked reductions were nearly absent, in contrast to the usual 10–15% reductions seen in healthy subjects (Martinez *et al.* 2007). In patients with alcohol dependence, there was a similar blunting of the [^{11}C]raclopride binding changes evoked by amphetamine to that seen in cocaine users. (Martinez *et al.* 2005a), a finding that was replicated with a methylphenidate challenge and linked to abnormal uptake of FDG in orbitofrontal cortex of the alcoholics (Volkow *et al.* 2007c). However, the amphetamine-induced [^{11}C]raclopride binding changes in first-degree relatives of alcoholics was entirely normal (Martinez *et al.* 2005b), suggesting that the blunted response to amphetamine seen in alcoholics is an acquired trait, rather than an endophenotype.

Dopamine transmission has also been implicated in the pathophysiology of depression. To test the hypothesis that the responsiveness of dopamine release should be blunted in depressed individuals, [^{123}I]IBZM uptake was measured in patients before and after amphetamine challenge. After age-correction, there was no significant difference in the observed binding changes compared to that in a group of healthy control subjects (Klimke *et al.* 1999). Nonetheless, baseline binding was lower and amphetamine-evoked changes were higher in those patients who responded well to treatment with antidepressants, consistent with dopaminergic mediation in at least a subset of depressed patients. In another [^{123}I]IBZM study, there was no difference in the amphetamine-evoked binding changes between a group of unmedicated patients with depression and healthy age-matched controls (Parsey *et al.* 2001).

15.2.3. Parkinson's disease

DOPA is, like amphetamine, an indirect agonist, but differs from amphetamine in that its action is mediated by serving as the precursor for dopamine synthesis. Having no inherent effect on dopamine release, DOPA should therefore have less effect in the competition paradigm. Indeed, in healthy elderly subjects, DOPA did not alter [^{11}C]raclopride binding at rest, presumably because autoregulation of dopamine release was still intact (Floel *et al.* 2008). However, the DOPA treatment slightly enhanced the effect of training in a cognitive task on the apparent release of dopamine in caudate nucleus. In contrast, treatment of Parkinson's disease patients with DOPA evoked an acute decline in striatal [^{11}C]raclopride binding (Tedroff *et al.* 1996), thus firmly linking the therapeutic action of DOPA to enhanced dopamine release from the remaining dopamine innervation. It is known that the treatment of advanced Parkinson's disease is marred by the emergence of motor complications, especially the DOPA dyskinesias, which may be a consequence of impaired dopamine storage. Thus, DOPA challenge evoked a two-fold higher [^{11}C]raclopride displacement in striatum of patients with DOPA dyskinesia than in patients with stable Parkinson's disease (de la Fuente-Fernandez *et al.* 2004). Furthermore, the magnitude of DOPA-evoked reductions in [^{11}C]raclopride *pB* in the putamen of patients with advanced Parkinson's disease did not correlate with improved clinical symptoms such as rigidity and bradykinesia, but rather with dyskinesias scores (Pavese *et al.* 2006). Finally, a group of Parkinson's disease patients who abused dopaminergic drugs had a substantially greater DOPA-induced [^{11}C]raclopride binding change than was typical of the condition (Evans *et al.* 2006). These observations seem akin to the earlier discussion about amphetamine-sensitization. New agonist PET ligands may help elucidate the contribution of post-synaptic sensitization mechanism to DOPA dyskinesias.

Oral methylphenidate, which blocks the reuptake of dopamine, but has no intrinsic capacity to release dopamine, did not evoke changes in [^{11}C]raclopride binding in patients with Parkinson's disease (Koochesfahani *et al.* 2006). However, this study was carried out during pause of medication, so it might be speculated that methylphenidate would have retained its indirect action at post-synaptic receptors had the subjects been on DOPA.

15.3. Other pharmacological challenges altering dopamine receptor binding

15.3.1. Nicotine, smoking, and caffeine

Subcutaneous nicotine (20 μg kg^{-1}) decreased the specific binding of [^{11}C]raclopride in the striatum of anesthetized monkeys by 12%, an effect which was blocked by treatment with the GABA-transaminase inhibitor γ-vinyl GABA (Vigabatrin), a drug potentiating inhibitory neurotransmission (Dewey *et al.* 1999). In anesthetized pigs, an intravenous high dose of nicotine (500 μg kg^{-1}) bilaterally reduced [^{11}C]raclopride binding by 10% in the ventral striatum of anesthetized pigs. Similar effects of a low dose (40 μg kg^{-1}) were of marginal significance, but were most distinct in the ventral striatum (Cumming *et al.* 2003b). Infusion of nicotine via microdialysis paradoxically increased [^{11}C]raclopride in rat striatum (Tajima *et al.* 2007), but this may be a consequence of the very high drug concentration applied (100 mM), which may have had local toxic effects. Nicotine-induced 5–10% declines in [^{11}C]raclopride binding were seen in the striatum of isoflurane-anesthetized monkeys, but were absent in awake monkeys, drawing into question the pertinence of studies in anesthetized animals (Tsukada *et al.* 2002). Nonetheless, smoking after a period of withdrawal was initially reported to evoke very substantial declines (−30%) in [^{11}C]raclopride *pB* in the ventral striatum of habitual smokers (Brody *et al.* 2004), a finding that was considerably less pronounced (−10%) in a later study (Scott *et al.* 2007). A number of genetic factors, including DAT alleles and dopamine D$_4$ (but not D$_2$) receptor alleles, substantially contributed to the individual effects of smoking on [^{11}C]raclopride binding. However, the major genetic factor was the allele of COMT, discussed above in the context of vulnerability to schizophrenia (Brody *et al.* 2006). These genetic factors may in turn relate to the relationship between smoking-induced [^{11}C]raclopride binding changes and hedonic response (Barrett *et al.* 2004; Brody *et al.* 2008) discussed below.

Chronic nicotine treatment reduced the density of [^{3}H]NPA binding sites in rat striatum and nucleus accumbens without altering the density of antagonist binding sites (Janson *et al.* 1992). Thus, long-term exposure to nicotine in tobacco smoke may result in a shift in the population distribution of dopamine D$_2$ receptors towards a desensitized state. Conceivably, this phenomenon may underlie the syndrome of nicotine dependency, suggesting another potential application of new agonist PET ligands.

In a group of healthy, habitual coffee drinkers, 200 mg caffeine significantly decreased the [^{11}C]raclopride *pB* in the thalamus, and tended to decrease binding in the ventral striatum, where the [^{11}C]raclopride binding correlated with the extent of arousal by caffeine (Kaasinen *et al.* 2004a). Given the considerable comorbidity of smoking and drinking coffee, it would be interesting to test for synergistic effects of nicotine and caffeine on dopamine receptor availability.

15.3.2.   Inhibitory substances

The anticonvulsant γ-vinyl-GABA has long been used for the treatment of seizure disorders, and has also been promoted for the treatment of diverse addictions. Treatment of rats with γ-vinyl-GABA substantially blocks the ability of heroin or ethanol to increase the dopamine concentration measured in microdialysates from rat nucleus accumbens; the dopamine releasing effect of methamphetamine was also partially blocked by γ-vinyl-GABA (Gerasimov et al. 1999). Consistent with this finding, γ-vinyl-GABA, and also the GABA-A agonist lorazepam decreased the binding of [^{11}C]raclopride in the striatum of anesthetized baboons (Dewey et al. 1992). Ethanol is also thought to act by potentiation of GABA-ergic inhibitory transmission. An intoxicating dose of ethanol (1 mg kg^{-1}) reduced [^{11}C]raclopride binding specifically in the ventral striatum of healthy humans (Boileau et al. 2003), consistent with the purported common mechanism of action of abused substances via mesolimbic dopamine systems. Baseline [^{11}C] raclopride binding correlated with the extent of "high" experienced during controlled intoxication (Yoder et al. 2005). However, the effect of ethanol on [^{11}C] raclopride binding were highly heterogeneous within a group of healthy subjects, with some subjects showing increases in receptor availability (Yoder et al. 2007).

15.3.3.   Others

Pharmacological agonism of dopamine D$_2$ receptors in the rat nucleus accumbens prevents the somatic symptoms of naloxone-induced withdrawal from opiates (Harris & Aston-Jones 1994). Furthermore, microdialysis studies indicate an important modulation of dopamine release in the ventral striatum by opiate agonists. Nonetheless, there have been few PET investigations of opiate/dopamine interactions. The opiate analgesic alfentanil reduced [^{11}C]raclopride binding in the human putamen by 6%, a result which must be interpreted with some caution, since the treatment was found to slightly increase end-tidal pCO$_2$, which might well have altered cerebral perfusion (Hagelberg et al. 2002). The baseline [^{11}C]raclopride pB was significantly lower (15%) than normal in the putamen of a group of opiate-dependent subjects, but precipitation of naloxone withdrawal did not alter the binding, suggesting that opioid effects, at least in addicts, do not tonically modulate dopamine receptor occupancy (Wang et al. 1997). Alfentanyl treatment increased binding of the high-affinity ligand [^{11}C]FLB 457 in parts of the frontal and cingulate cortices, to an extent correlating with the change in euphoria (but not analgesia) between the two scans (Hagelberg et al. 2004).

In addition to nicotinic modulation cited above, additional cholinergic interactions with dopamine transmission can be mediated by the muscarinic receptors. In a PET study of conscious monkeys, treatment with the muscarinic cholinergic antagonist scopolamine did not alter the B_{max} of [^{11}C]raclopride, but increased the magnitude of K_d^{app} (Tsukada *et al.* 2000a), implying that competition from endogenous dopamine was increased in the drugged condition. However, there were no concomitant changes in the interstitial dopamine concentration measured by microdialysis in the same animals. In the same report, other PET studies of scopolamine challenge revealed an increase in β-[^{11}C]DOPA utilization, and an increase in DAT availability measured with β-[^{11}C]CFT. Together, these results suggest that [^{11}C]raclopride can decline when the flux of dopamine across the plasma membrane is increased, irrespective of changes in the interstitial concentration.

NMDA blockade with ketamine has served as a model for behavioral and cognitive changes resembling schizophrenia. In healthy humans, the amphetamine-induced reductions in striatal [^{123}I]IBZM binding doubled after treatment with a psychoactive dose of ketamine (Kegeles *et al.* 2000), supporting the notion that schizophrenia may be related to a dysregulation of dopamine transmission by excitatory inputs. Ketamine alone at a dose evoking a dissociation state in healthy humans was without discernible effect on [^{11}C]raclopride *pB* (Kegeles *et al.* 2002), while others reported a 15% decline in [^{11}C]raclopride *pB* (Vollenweider *et al.* 2000). This difference might reflect the constant infusion method used in the former report versus bolus injection in the latter study. In a monkey study, ketamine infusion decreased [^{11}C]raclopride *pB* in the absence of concomitant increases in interstitial dopamine concentrations measured by microdialysis (Tsukada *et al.* 2000b). As in the case of the scopolamine study, the ketamine treatment also increased β-[^{11}C]DOPA and β-[^{11}C]CFT uptake in monkey striatum. In contrast, administration of phencyclidine, another NMDA antagonist, decreased the availability of [^{11}C]raclopride sites and the availability of DATs labeled with [^{11}C]cocaine, an effect possibly mediated by competition at DAT (Schiffer, Logan, & Dewey 2003). These disparate findings accentuate the problematic nature of PET studies conducted in anesthetized animals, and the imperfect relationship between interstitial dopamine levels and [^{11}C]raclopride binding changes. As noted above, ketamine reduced the binding of [^{11}C]raclopride especially in the ventral striatum of awake humans (Vollenweider *et al.* 2000), but had no effect on [^{11}C]raclopride binding in another study, in which the ketamine also transiently evoked psychotic symptoms (Aalto *et al.* 2002).

The release of serotonin in the brain is potently stimulated by fenfluramine by an amphetamine-like mechanism. Thus, the [^{11}C]raclopride V_d in human striatum was decreased by 20% a few hours after treatment with fenfluramine (Smith *et al.* 1997). Blockade of serotonin uptake with the antidepressant citalopram likewise reduced [^{11}C]raclopride binding in human striatum, although to a lesser extent than did the direct serotonin releaser (Tiihonen *et al.* 1996). Psilocybin is a hallucinogen acting mainly as an agonist at serotonin 5HT$_{2A}$ receptors. A psychotomimetic dose of psilocybin reduced the [^{11}C]raclopride *pB* in human caudate nucleus by 20% (Vollenweider *et al.* 1999), similar in magnitude to the decreases reported after amphetamine challenge. These observations suggest that direct or indirect serotonin agonists potentiate the release of dopamine in the basal ganglia, and may also be relevant to the mechanism of antipsychotic action of the atypical neuroleptic clozapine, which has occupied serotonin receptors. An action via serotonin 5HT$_{1A}$ receptors can be excluded since the selective agonist flesinoxan was without effect on [^{11}C]raclopride binding in healthy human subjects (Bantick *et al.* 2005). Nonetheless, a psychoactive dose of the serotonin agonist LSD evoked a 15% reduction of [^{11}C]raclopride *pB* in the striatum of living pig. This interaction peaked at 3 h after drug administration, suggesting that effects mediated by dopamine receptors could account specifically for a late component of the psychopharmacology of LSD (Minuzzi *et al.* 2005).

The scenario of simple competition from dopamine mediated indirectly by serotonin release is however not entirely consistent with the results of a PET study in awake primates. Here, administration of the 5HT$_2$ antagonist ketanserin decreased striatal [^{11}C]raclopride binding, while also increasing (slightly) the interstitial dopamine concentration measured simultaneously in microdialysates (Tsukada *et al.* 1999). In this study, a number of other stimulant agents were also tested, including methamphetamine. All of these drugs reduced [^{11}C]raclopride *pB* in a dose-dependent manner, and to a similar maximal extent (−25%). However, there was no simple relationship between these binding changes, and the increased interstitial dopamine, which had a ten-fold range between the strongest and the weakest dopamine release.

In a single case study, smoking cannabis decreased the binding of [^{123}I]IBZM by 20% in the striatum of a patient with schizophrenia (Voruganti *et al.* 2001b). This isolated finding surely merits further investigation, given the identification of early cannabis as a risk factor for development of psychosis (Semple, McIntosh, & Lawrie 2005).

15.4. Transcranial magnetic stimulation, deep brain stimulation, and sensory stimulation

The advent of transcranial magnetic stimulation (TMS) had opened new channels for investigations of brain function in living subjects. In this procedure, a probe is placed on the scalp, and an oscillating electromagnetic field is directed at the underlying cerebral cortex, which can evoke sensory or motor effects, depending on the cortical target. Stimulation of the motor cortex of anesthetized monkeys reduced [^{11}C]raclopride binding in the putamen and ventral striatum, suggesting an unexpected modulation by the motor cortex of mesolimbic dopamine release (Ohnishi *et al.* 2004), somewhat in contrast to findings in healthy humans, in whom the motor cortex stimulation mainly resulted in reduced binding in the ipsilateral putamen (Strafella *et al.* 2003). In contrast, TMS of the prefrontal cortex of healthy humans evoked [^{11}C]raclopride binding reductions mainly in the ipsilateral caudate nucleus (Strafella *et al.* 2001), even though anatomical connectivity might have predicted changes also in the ventral striatum.

In patients with Parkinson's disease, TMS of the sensorimotor cortex evoked a substantial decline in [^{11}C]raclopride *pB* in the ipsilateral putamen. The magnitude of this effect was smaller when the stimulation was applied to the side opposite to the major motor symptoms, consistent with an action mediated by the stimulated release of dopamine. However, the spatial extent of the [^{11}C]raclopride binding reductions was greater on the more affected side, which led the authors to speculate that the spatial domain of action of dopamine is increased during the early stages of nigrostriatal degeneration (Strafella *et al.* 2005). An extensive regimen of TMS to the dorsolateral prefrontal cortex reduced [^{123}I]IBZM binding in the ipsilateral striatum by 10% in patients with depression (Pogarell *et al.* 2006), even though clinically effective TMS for the treatment of depression failed to evoke measurable [^{11}C]raclopride binding changes in another study (Kuroda *et al.* 2006).

Stimulation of the subthalamic nucleus for the treatment of Parkinson's disease is without any effect on striatal [^{11}C]raclopride binding (Hilker *et al.* 2003; Strafella, Sadikot, & Dagher 2003; Thobois *et al.* 2003). Nonetheless, clinically effective stimulation of the subthalamic nucleus attenuated the DOPA-evoked reductions in striatal [^{11}C]raclopride binding, suggesting that fluctuations in dopamine release had been stabilized (Nimura *et al.* 2005).

Electrical stimulation of the paw of anesthetized cats evoked a substantial decline in [^{11}C]raclopride *pB* in the striatum contralateral to the side of sensory stimulation (Inoue *et al.* 2004). However, in another study, electrical stimulation of the paw or median nerve was entirely without effect on striatal [^{11}C]raclopride binding in anesthetized cats or awake humans (Thobois *et al.* 2004). The effect of exercise on [^{11}C]raclopride binding has also been a matter of some controversy. In one study of human subjects, aerobic exercise on a treadmill for one half hour was without effect on striatal [^{11}C]raclopride binding in a scan initiated a few minutes after completion of the running (Wang *et al.* 2000).

However, when scanning was undertaken during performance of a laborious foot extension task, there was a reduction in [^{11}C]raclopride binding in the putamen contralateral to the exercise in healthy subjects, in contrast to a resting scan (Ouchi *et al.* 2002). Perplexingly, a reduction was also seen during exercise in Parkinson's patients, but it was in the ipsilateral putamen.

15.5. Personality

In spite of inbreeding and shared environmental factors, individual rats can have distinct patterns of behavior. The occurrence of this variability has been exploited to investigate the relationship between dopamine and response to novelty. When placed in an unfamiliar cage, those rats spending a long time in exploration of the novel environment can be identified as "high responders." Microdialysis studies of these rats showed that the exploration was associated with a greater elevation in interstitial dopamine than that seen in the low responders (Saigusa *et al.* 1999). While behavioral response to a novel environment did not in a simple manner predict the rate of amphetamine self-administration of individual rats (Klebaur *et al.* 2001), the locomotor response to a novel environment did predict the rate of acquisition of nicotine self-administration (Suto, Austin, & Vezina 2001).

Pigs, like rats and people, are curious animals; they will naturally investigate an unfamiliar object with their snout, and the duration of this probing can be used as an index of novelty seeking. In a group of pigs, the duration of this exploratory behavior correlated with the individual response in the [^{11}C]raclopride/amphetamine challenge paradigm (Lind *et al.* 2005), suggesting that common mechanisms may subserve psychostimulant action and exploratory behavior. In a microPET study, the availability of binding sites for [^{18}F]fallypride was reduced in rats expressing trait impulsivity; this biomarker further predicted a high rate of self-administration of cocaine (Dalley *et al.* 2007), a finding which resonates with the well-established link between impulsivity, drug-seeking, and dopamine.

Based upon the results of animal studies, the index of novelty seeking has obvious implications for the phenomenon of psychostimulant drug use by humans. Not all healthy subjects respond identically to the same challenge with amphetamine; in a group of healthy males, the magnitude of the [^{11}C]raclopride binding change correlated positively with scores in the novelty-seeking trait (Leyton *et al.* 2002). In another group of normal subjects, high novelty-seeking scores predicted higher sensitization to the effects of repeated amphetamine challenge on [^{11}C]raclopride binding (Boileau *et al.* 2006). The [^{11}C]raclopride *p*B was lower in those normal subjects who reported enjoying the effects of methylphenidate, than in those who found it aversive (Volkow *et al.* 1999d). In the context of the competition paradigm, this kind of result is formally ambiguous, since lower availability in vivo could mean fewer receptors, or greater basal occupancy. However, the bulk of evidence supports the notion that personality, especially on the scale of novelty seeking, is a predisposing factor for psychostimulant abuse.

As noted above, of the various human personality traits linked to dopamine transmission, the strongest association has been with novelty or sensation seeking. The Zimmerman Sensation-seeking Scale has been used to assess measured sensation seeking in a group of 18 male subjects also investigated with [^{11}C]raclopride-PET. There was a negative correlation between sensation seeking and the baseline [^{11}C]raclopride *pB* in the striatum (Möller & Kumakura, unpublished observations). As usual, it is uncertain if the high sensation seekers have higher basal occupancy, or lower absolute abundance of receptors. There was a significant negative correlation between [^{11}C]FLB 457 binding in the right insular cortex and the novelty-seeking trait in a group of 24 healthy young men (Suhara *et al.* 2001). This correlation was also found bilaterally in the insular cortex of a large series of patients with Parkinson's disease, indicating that this relationship between novelty seeking and cortical dopamine receptors is independent of the integrity of the dopamine innervation (Kaasinen *et al.* 2004c).

Results of studies linking baseline [^{11}C]raclopride *pB* to personality can be very sensitive to the particular psychological test-battery employed. Thus, [^{11}C]raclopride binding correlated with ratings of personal detachment scores as defined by the Karolinska Scales of Personality, but no such correlation could be found using the NEO Personality Inventory (revised), which did however reveal a correlation with depression (Kestler *et al.* 2000). Furthermore, striatal [^{11}C]raclopride binding correlated with the index of personal detachment from the Karolinska test, but did not correlate with the detachment score of Cloninger (Breier *et al.* 1998). In a group of post-menopausal women, socially desirable responding – the telling of "whites lies" – had a very significant (*p*=0.002) inverse correlation with [^{11}C]raclopride binding in the putamen (Reeves *et al.* 2007). In women who had recovered from anorexia nervosa, the [^{11}C]raclopride *pB* in the dorsal caudate correlated with harm-avoidance scores, which the authors note is a personality trait which may persist after recovery (Frank *et al.* 2005).

15.6.   Pain and stress

Dopaminergic systems are implicated in the central processing of pain. In a study of healthy males, the threshold for pain evoked by the cutaneous application of heat had an inverse correlation with baseline [^{11}C]raclopride pB in the right putamen, but there was no such association with simple tactile sensation (Martikainen *et al.* 2005). A similar study with the high-affinity ligand [^{11}C]FLB 457 did not reveal any correlations with pain threshold or "response bias or attitude" and baseline binding in extrastriatal regions (Pertovaara *et al.* 2004). When using pain as an activation condition, efforts must be made to design a painful stimulus remaining constant during the recording session. This condition can be met using a continuous infusion of hypertonic saline in the jaw muscle, with feedback control of the rate of infusion so as to clamp the subjective pain rating, and with isotonic saline infusions as a "placebo" substitute for painful stimulus. Use of this careful design revealed pain-evoked reduction in [^{11}C]raclopride pB in the caudate and putamen (Scott *et al.* 2006). These reductions correlated with the sensory experience of pain, but only in the ventral striatum, where the correlations were with the negative affective and fearful components of the pain rather than with the sensory aspects. A single intramuscular injection of hypotonic saline caused pain, the extent of which correlated with [^{11}C]raclopride binding decreases in normal subjects. The same stimulus evoked greater pain in patients with fibromyalgia, but there was no correlation between pain scores and the binding changes (Wood *et al.* 2007), indicating abnormal central processing of pain in this syndrome.

Psychosocial stress can be inflicted by instructing subjects to perform a mathematical task, while providing feedback implying to the subject that their performance is inadequate. Using this paradigm, [^{11}C]raclopride pB changes were measured in subjects with personal histories of high and low parental bonding. Relative to the resting baseline condition, the task evoked a significant pB reduction in the ventral striatum and putamen of the group with low parental bonding. These changes furthermore correlated with salivary cortisol levels, an independent marker of stress (Pruessner *et al.* 2004). In another use of a mental arithmetic stressor task, there were no [^{11}C]raclopride pB changes (Montgomery, Mehta, & Grasby 2007), but this group was not stratified by parental bonding, which must have isolated a stress-vulnerable subgroup in the other study. Performance of the Montreal Card Task for cognitive set shifting, a test of frontal executive function, was associated with a reduction of [^{11}C]raclopride pB in the striatum (Monchi, Ko, & Strafella 2006). While this was intended to link cognitive functions mediated by the frontal cortex to increased dopamine release in subcortical structures, it seems equally possible that the interpretation may be confounded by the effects of stress. Psychological stress evoked a reduction in striatal [^{11}C]raclopride binding in a subset of schizotypal subjects which was not evident in healthy control subjects (Soliman *et al.* 2008). This finding was co-expressed with defects in a visual task subserved by the frontal cortex, suggesting that cortical and subcortical abnormalities can be risk factors for psychosis.

A social stress paradigm involving a sham job application and mathematical task evoked an increase in serum cortisol levels, the extent of which correlated with the magnitude of the amphetamine-evoked [¹¹C]raclopride pB reductions in the ventral striatum of a large group of subjects (Wand *et al.* 2007). High cortisol response furthermore correlated with the subjective positive aspects of the amphetamine treatment. In the absence of stress, cortisol levels correlated with placebo-evoked reductions in [¹¹C]raclopride pB in the right dorsal putamen, and with amphetamine-evoked reductions in the left ventral striatum and left dorsal putamen (Oswald *et al.* 2005). While these studies no doubt link responsiveness of the dopamine system to stress, cortisol levels need not be causal, but rather an indicator of the vulnerability of the nervous system to stress or pharmacological challenge. Subsequent studies revealed a powerful interaction between the trait of impulsivity and amphetamine-evoked [¹¹C] raclopride pB changes (Oswald *et al.* 2007); whereas high impulsivity trait in the group as a whole was associated with relatively blunted binding reductions in the right ventral striatum, stratification of the subjects by their life-history of stressful events showed that the effect of impulsivity on amphetamine response was much greater in the subgroup which had not experienced stress.

15.7.   Motivation, craving, and placebo

The motivational and rewarding properties of psychostimulants have a close relationship with dopamine release. Thus, amphetamine reduces [¹¹C]raclopride binding in all divisions on the human striatum, but the extent of euphoria correlates specifically with reduced binding in the ventral striatum, and to a much lesser extent in the dorsal associative striatum (Drevets *et al.* 2001; Martinez *et al.* 2003). Likewise, the intensity of the "high" experienced after administration of intravenous methylphenidate correlated precisely with the reductions in [¹¹C]raclopride pB in the striatum (Volkow *et al.* 1999c). The design of this latter study made exemplary use of placebo, so that effects of anticipation can be excluded. In a similar study using the bolus plus infusion paradigm, the reduction in [¹¹C]raclopride pB evoked by methylphenidate correlated with the reported euphoria, and also with the baseline anxiety (Udo de Haes *et al.* 2005), suggesting that stress and the propensity to experience reinforcement are indeed inextricably bound.

Dopaminergic systems serve a role in motivational aspects of appetite and feeding. For example, the amount of sucrose consumed by individual rats correlates with the dopamine-evoked increase in GTPγS binding in cryostat section, indicating an association between sensitivity of dopamine D_2 receptors and the salience of sucrose (Tonissaar *et al.* 2006). In human PET studies, contrasting the condition of eating to satiety with the fasting condition did not reveal any feeding-evoked changes in [^{11}C]raclopride *pB* in human striatum. However, pretreatment with methylphenidate resulted in feeding-related changes in the dorsal, but not ventral, striatum of healthy humans (Volkow *et al.* 2002b). The implication is that small increases in dopamine release induced by feeding alone were potentiated or unmasked by blockade of DAT. Paradoxically, this finding might imply that psychostimulants, which are generally anorexigenic, should *increase* the salience of food.

Consumption of palatable foods in contrast to a fasting condition was itself sufficient to reveal decreased [^{11}C]raclopride *pB* in the dorsal caudate and putamen of lean subjects, such that individual changes correlated with the subjects' own assessment of the pleasantness of their particular meal (Small, Jones-Gotman, & Dagher 2003). This study is notable for revealing the neurochemical basis of a fondness for Sushi. Although the lack of feeding-related effects in the ventral striatum seems somewhat at odds with results in the animal literature, these studies might predict greater responsiveness of dopamine release in obese subjects. This seems not to have been explicitly tested, although the body mass index (BMI) of a group of obese subjects correlated inversely with the baseline striatal [^{11}C]raclopride *pB* (Wang *et al.* 2001).

Tobacco smoking reduced craving in withdrawn smokers, but only reduced striatal [^{11}C]raclopride binding in proportion to the extent of euphoria experienced after smoking (Barrett *et al.* 2004), which is evidently quite variable, even among smokers. In that study, the dopamine D_2 receptor availability actually increased after smoking in those few subjects reporting dysphoria. Similarly, nasal administration of nicotine did not alter the mean [^{11}C]raclopride *pB* in a group of smokers, but regression analysis showed that subjective rating of increased happiness correlated with individual reductions in dopamine receptor availability (Montgomery *et al.* 2007b). In healthy subjects, controlled ethanol infusions evoked subjective sensations of "intoxication" which correlated with the baseline [^{11}C]raclopride *pB* in the left nucleus accumbens (Yoder *et al.* 2005). As a general rule, drugs or behaviors with a relatively weak propensity to increase dopamine release may alter [^{11}C]raclopride binding in a manner depending on the individuals' "set point" of receptor occupancy at the time of baseline scanning.

Effects of amphetamine can be quite variable in the [^{11}C]raclopride competition paradigm. Although there was no gender difference in the baseline [^{11}C]raclopride *pB*, the amphetamine-evoked [^{11}C]raclopride *pB* reductions were greater in men than in women, as were the subjective ratings of euphoria evoked by the drug

(Munro *et al.* 2006). Furthermore, the amphetamine-evoked [^{11}C]raclopride binding changes in the left striatum correlated with the positive rating of the drug effect (Oswald *et al.* 2005). In the context of the occupancy model, higher baseline [^{11}C]raclopride binding and greater psychostimulant-evoked changes may together reveal a predisposition to experience greater reward. However, inconsistent with this model, higher [^{11}C]raclopride *pB* was noted in healthy subjects with a family history of alcoholism (Volkow *et al.* 2006), a finding which was interpreted to indicate a protection, i.e. the opposite of vulnerability.

In a landmark PET study, playing a video game for monetary reward elicited reduction in striatal [^{11}C]raclopride binding (Koepp *et al.* 1998). Interpretation of this study is, however, complicated by the element of motor skill learning, which may have confounded the effects of reward *per se*. Indeed, performing a difficult finger apposition task without reward was sufficient to reduce [^{11}C]raclopride binding in the striatum (Badgaiyan, Fischman, & Alpert 2003). The same authors subsequently found evidence for dopamine release in the bilateral caudate and left putamen during implicit learning of a right-handed complex motor task (Badgaiyan, Fischman, & Alpert 2007), with additional activation in the right putamen during explicit learning of the same task, when the subjects could give an accurate account of the learned motor sequence (Badgaiyan, Fischman, & Alpert 2008). However, performance of a mathematical task for monetary reward resulted in decreased striatal [^{11}C]raclopride binding relative to the condition of a neutral visual task (Volkow *et al.* 2004). This finding would seem to isolate reward from pure motor effects, although these binding changes, as in the case of a feeding study, were only apparent in subjects pretreated with methylphenidate. In another cognition study, subjects engaged in a task with monetary reward at either a fixed or a variable reward schedule, contrasted with a sensorimotor control condition, without any reward (Zald *et al.* 2004). Here, specifically, the variable response task evoked a pattern of reduced and increased [^{11}C]raclopride binding, with the predominant effects suggesting decreased dopamine transmission in the striatum. The authors interpreted their results in the context of the work of Schultz showing that activity of dopamine neurons depends on prediction error. In a follow-up study with a different kind of unpredictable monetary reward, the same group replicated the finding of a paradoxical suppression of striatal dopamine release (Hakyemez *et al.* 2008).

As noted above, there has been some tendency to confuse the release of dopamine in the brain with the reward itself, rather than as the herald that an unexpected reward (or punishment) has taken place. Neither should treatment for a medical condition be confused with reward, especially given that some aspects of therapeutic effects of a drug might be conditioned based upon past experience. In a [^{11}C]raclopride-PET study, the anticipation of treatment with apomorphine evoked a 20% decline in *pB* in the striatum of Parkinson's disease patients, which was attributed to the effect of placebo (de la Fuente-Fernaudez *et al.* 2001). In another study of patients with Parkinson's disease, "placebo" transcranial stimulation evoked reductions in [^{11}C]raclopride binding, most notably on the side contralateral to the main symptoms (Strafella, Ko, & Monchi 2006).

Strictly speaking, a true placebo effect was not demonstrated in either of the above studies, since clinical improvements were not documented during the PET scanning sessions. However, others showed that the expectation of receiving caffeine by habitual coffee drinkers reduced [^{11}C]raclopride *pB* in the thalamus (Kaasinen *et al.* 2004b). While quantitation of [^{11}C]raclopride binding in that structure is problematic, this study also linked putamenal [^{11}C]raclopride *pB* in the putamen to the extent of arousal after receiving placebo caffeine. In another [^{11}C]raclopride study of craving, habitual cocaine users were scanned in a baseline condition, and again while listening to an audiotape alluding to cocaine use, which evoked varying degrees of craving in the subjects. Individual reductions in [^{11}C]raclopride binding in the second scan, which ranged from 0 to 10%, correlated with the intensity of craving experienced by the subjects (Wong *et al.* 2006).

Conditioning based upon previous experience can acutely modulate [^{11}C]raclopride binding. Thus, a group of healthy young subjects were administered amphetamine on three occasions in the environment of the PET suite (Boileau *et al.* 2007). A few weeks later, they were scanned with [^{11}C]raclopride after administration of nothing, or a placebo tablet identified as amphetamine. In this contrast, the placebo evoked a 22% decline in *pB* in the ventral striatum (as much as did amphetamine itself), and a lesser reduction in the dorsal striatum, which the authors interpreted in the context of the reward prediction error signaled by dopamine release in the ventral striatum. In general, there is a need for a clearer physiological distinction between the binding changes evoked by placebo or by conditioning and the unconditioned changes evoked by the drug itself. The PET studies in awake monkeys showing partial dissociation between [^{11}C]raclopride binding changes and interstitial dopamine concentrations seem relevant in this context; the same PET end point might well be obtained by diverse distinct mechanisms, only some of which are indicative of altered dopamine release.

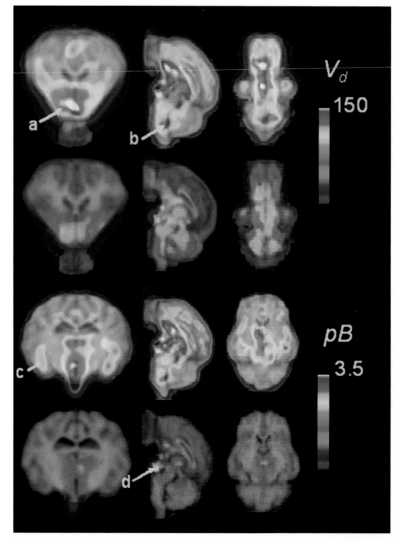

Figure 8.2 Parametric maps of the distribution volume (here, V_d, $ml\,g^{-1}$) and binding potential (pB) for $[^{11}C]$harmine in the brain of Göttingen minipigs. Each image is the mean of five separate determinations in the untreated condition and after acute pargyline treatment, co-registered to the common stereotaxic MR coordinates (grey scale). Relative to the V_d maps [X=0, Y=−15, Z=20], the pB maps [X=0, Y=−5, Z=7] are shown in planes 13 mm posterior and 10 mm ventral. Zones of particular interest are indicated as follows: (a) the ventral forebrain, (b) vicinity of the locus coeruleus, (c) the amygdala and hippocampal formation, and (d) the pituitary gland. Reproduced with permission from Jensen *et al.* (2006).

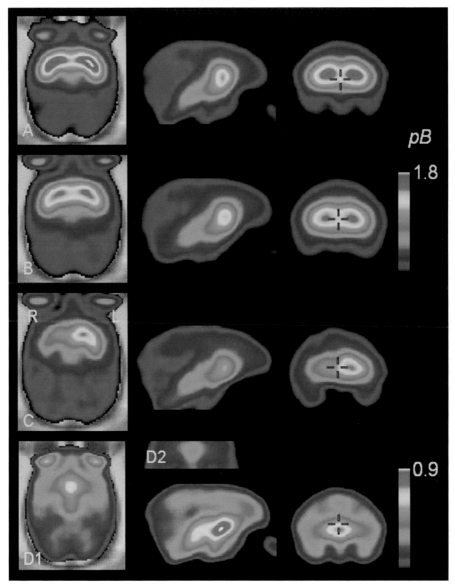

Figure 9.1 The binding potential (pB) of (+)[^{11}C]dihydrotetrabenazine (+[^{11}C]DTBZ)
for monoamine vesicles in the brain of monkeys. Mean parametric maps were
calculated in (A) normal young ($n = 7$), (B) normal aged ($n = 4$) rhesus monkeys, (C) aged
monkeys with unilateral intracarotid infusion of MPTP ($n = 3$), and (D) monkeys of
intermediate age with systemic MPTP administration (N = 6). Mean parametric maps
are co-registered to the MR template, shown as gray-scale in the horizontal plane
images. A sector containing the striatum in the horizontal plane from the MPTP
group (D2) is presented with identical intensity scaling as in the intact animals. The
cursor in the coronal plane images indicates the position (0,10,10) in the MR
coordinate system. Reproduced with permission from Doudet *et al.* (2006).

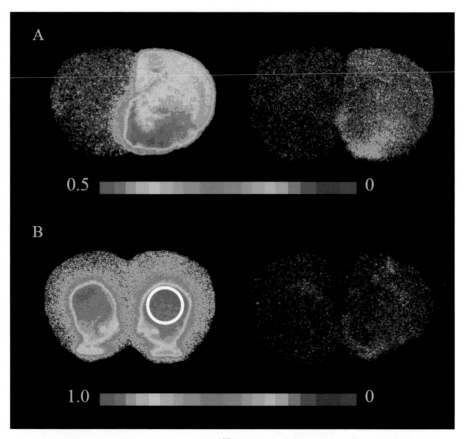

Figure 11.1 The ambivalence of [^{125}I]RTI-55 for transporters of dopamine and serotonin. Autoradiograms with [^{125}I]RTI-55 in coronal cryostat sections from a rat with unilateral destruction of the serotonin innervation. [^{125}I]RTI-55 (10 pM) was employed under conditions specific for SERT (A) and DAT (B). Total binding is shown to the left and non-specific binding to the right. The scale is in units of fmol mg^{-1} tissue. Figure courtesy of Dr. Søren Dinesen Østergaard, Aarhus University PET Centre.

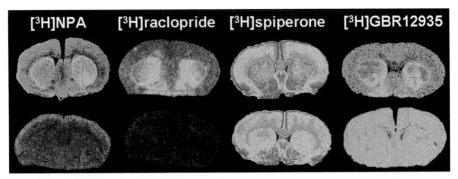

Figure 11.2 Autoradiograms of dopamine D_2 and DAT ligands in rat brain cryostat sections. Dopamine binding sites are labeled with the agonist [^{3}H]NPA, the benzamide antagonist [^{3}H]raclopride, and the butyrophenone antagonist [^{3}H] spiperone, in the presence of ketanserin. Also illustrated is the distribution of dopamine transporters labeled with [^{3}H]GBR 12935. All autoradiograms were obtained with ligand concentrations close to the affinities in vitro. The lower row shows the non-specific binding in the presence of butaclamol, in the case of receptor ligands. Figure courtesy of Dr. Luciano Minuzzi, Montreal Neurological Institute, McGill University.

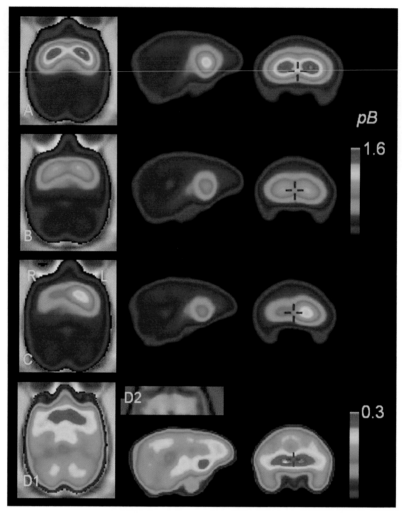

Figure 11.3 The binding potential (*pB*) of [^{11}C]methylphenidate for catecholamine uptake sites in the brain of monkeys. Images show the mean parametric maps in (A) normal young (*n* = 6), (B) normal aged (*n* = 4) rhesus monkeys, (C) aged monkeys with unilateral intracarotid infusion of MPTP (*n* = 3), and (D) monkeys of intermediate age with systemic MPTP administration (*n* = 6). Mean parametric maps are co-registered to the MR template, shown as gray-scale in the horizontal plane images. A sector containing the striatum in the horizontal plane from the MPTP group (D2) is presented with identical intensity scaling as in the intact animals. The cursor in the coronal plane images indicates the position (0,10,10) in the MR coordinate system. Reproduced with permission from Doudet *et al.* (2006).

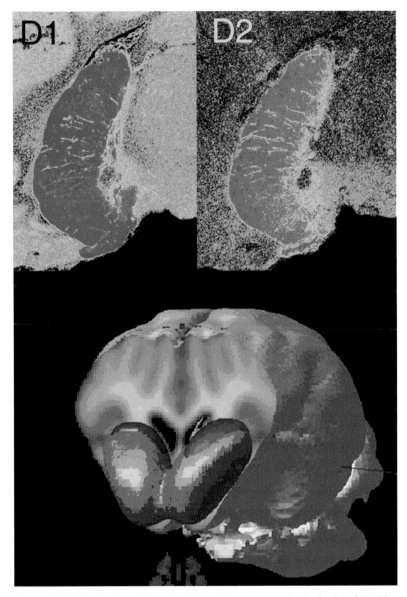

Figure 13.1 Gradients of dopamine D_1 and D_2 receptors in the brain of pig. The upper portion of the figure shows autoradiograms of the binding of (D_1) [^{3}H]Sch 23390 and (D_2) [^{3}H]raclopride in cryostat sections of pig brain, whereas the lower figures shows the surface renderings of the binding potential of $(D_1$, gold) [^{11}C]NNC 112 and $(D_2$, red) [^{11}C]raclopride in the striatum of living pig, projected onto the standard stereotaxic MR of pig brain. Images courtesy of Dr. Luciano Minuzzi, and Professor Pedro Rosa-Neto, Montreal Neurological Institute, McGill University.

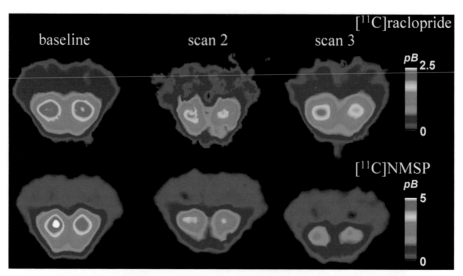

Figure 14.2 Temporal changes in the effect of MDMA (Ecstasy) in the binding of dopamine D_2 receptor ligands in pig brain. Groups of pigs were scanned at baseline with $[^{11}C]$raclopride (upper row) or $[^{11}C]$NMSP (lower row) and at 1 h (scan 2) or three hours (scan 3) after MDMA challenge. Modified with permission from Rosa-Neto *et al.* (2004).

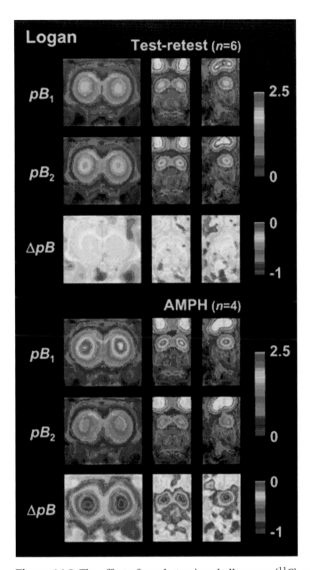

Figure 14.3 The effect of amphetamine challenge on [^{11}C]raclopride binding in rat brain. Mean parametric maps of [^{11}C]raclopride pB in rat brain, calculated by the reference tissue method of Logan of groups of living rats. Rows represent baseline results (pB_1), the second scan (pB_2) and the difference of the two binding maps (ΔpB) in a test–retest experiment ($n=6$), and in a test of the effects of amphetamine challenge ($n=4$). The parametric images are superposed on the rat brain histological atlas (gray scale), in identical coronal ($Z=19$), horizontal ($Y=10$) and sagittal ($X=-11$) planes. The ΔpB maps were blurred by 1 mm (FWHM). Reproduced with permission from Pedersen *et al.* (2007).

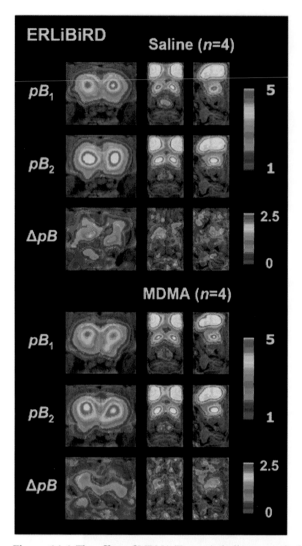

Figure 14.4 The effect of MDMA (Ecstasy) challenge on the binding of [^{11}C]NMSP in rat brain. Mean parametric images of [^{11}C]NMSP pB for groups of ($n = 4$) rats, calculated by the ERLiBiRD reference tissue method. Rows represent baseline results (pB_1), the second scan (pB_2) and the difference of the two binding maps (ΔpB), in a test–retest experiment, and in a test of the effects of pharmacological challenge with MDMA (Ecstasy). The parametric images are superposed on the rat brain histological atlas (gray scale). The parametric images are co-registered to the rat brain cryo-atlas (gray scale), in identical coronal ($Z = 18.5$), horizontal ($Y = 10$) and sagittal ($X = -11$) planes. Images were blurred by 1.0 mm (FWHM). Figure courtesy of Dr. Søren Dinesen Østergaard, Aarhus University PET Centre.

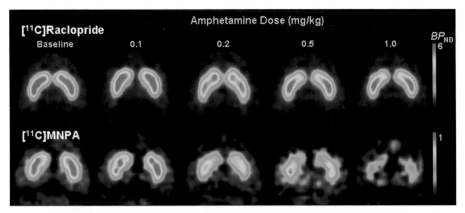

Figure 14.5 Differing vulnerability of an antagonist ([^{11}C]raclopride) and an agonist ([^{11}C]MNPA) to amphetamine challenge. Parametric maps show dose-dependent reductions in the availability of dopamine D$_{2/3}$ receptors in the striatum of monkeys, with consistently greater vulnerability of the agonist to amphetamine-evoked dopamine release. Modified from Seneca *et al.* (2006) and reproduced with permission of Dr. Sjoerd Finnema and Christer Halldin, Karolinska Institute.

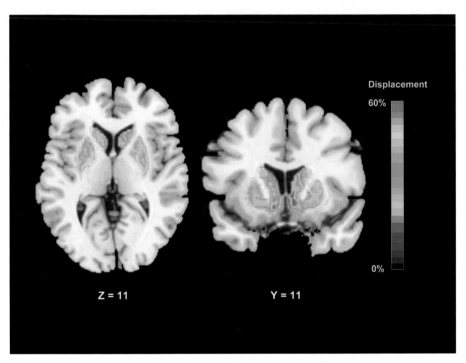

Figure 14.6 The effect of amphetamine challenge on [^{11}C]PHNO binding in human brain. The colour scale shows the percentage reduction in specific binding relative to the baseline condition, projected onto an anatomic atlas. The greatest relative declines are evident in the nucleus accumbens, and binding in the globus pallidus was nearly unaffected by the psychostimulant treatment. Figure reproduced with permission from Willeit *et al.* (2008).

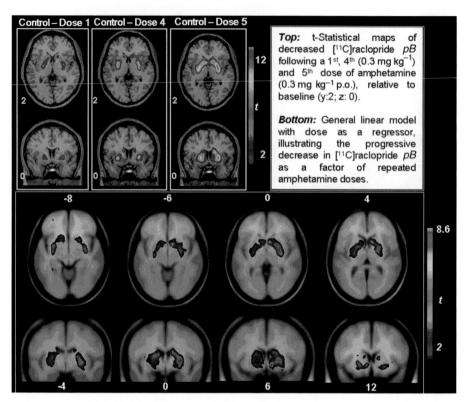

Figure 15.1 Sensitization of amphetamine-evoked [^{11}C]raclopride binding changes in human brain. A series of T-statistic maps show the progressive enhancement of the effect of amphetamine challenge on [^{11}C]raclopride binding in healthy volunteers receiving five doses of amphetamine over a period of one year. Figure reprinted with permission from Boileau *et al.* (2006).

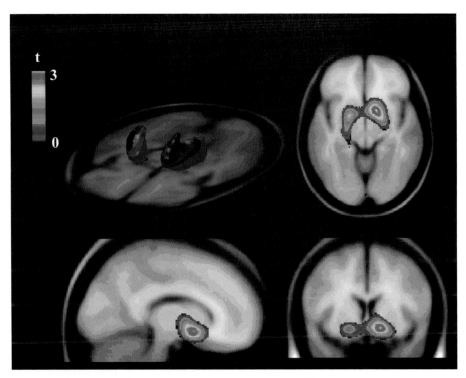

Figure 15.2 The effect of oral methylphenidate on [¹¹C]raclopride binding in human brain. T-statistic map of voxels in which oral administration of methylphenidate reduced the availability of binding sites for [¹¹C]raclopride in the brain of a group of adolescent patients with diagnosis of attention deficit hyperactivity disorder. Figure reproduced with permission from Rosa-Neto *et al.* (2005).

16

The absolute abundance of dopamine receptors in the brain

Most molecular imaging studies make use of a single injection of the radioligand at very high specific activity, such that the mass of substance is negligible. Consequently, the index of receptor availability (pB) is formally ambiguous, being a function of the number of receptors (B_{max}), divided by the apparent affinity of the ligand in vivo (K_d^{app}). Separate determination of the saturation binding parameters requires multiple tracer injections, such that a range of receptor occupancies are obtained. This chapter summarizes the relationship between PET estimates of dopamine receptor abundance, and estimates obtained using preparations in vitro. The various findings in the cases of dopamine D_1 receptors (Table 13.1) and D_2 receptors (Table 14.1) reveal the extent of agreement between the several quantitative methods.

The absolute density of dopamine receptors in the brain can be quantified using a variety of methods in vitro (Seeman 1987). The saturation binding parameters for a radioligand are measured under controlled conditions, using either washed membranes or brain cryostat sections. The experimentalist exposes the tissue samples to a range of radioliogand concentrations, ideally extending at least one order of magnitude to each side of the half-saturation concentration, K_d. The ionic composition of the incubation buffer, the incubation temperature, and the duration of incubation are determined entirely by laboratory procedures; the specific binding is measured relative to the binding in the presence of a non-radioactive competitor for the same site. After equilibrium is obtained, the samples are washed to remove excess unbound radioligand, and the radioactivity concentrations are measured. Then, the specifically bound radioactivity is plotted over the broad range of ligand concentrations, such that the magnitudes of B_{max} and K_d can be calculated separately. The Scatchard analysis, in which the ratio of Bound/Free is plotted as a function of the Free ligand concentration in the incubation medium remains widely used, in spite of the problem that the two axes are covariant. It is mathematically more appropriate to use non-linear methods for calculating the binding parameters from the equation,

$$\text{Bound} = B_{\text{max}}[\text{Free}]/(K_d + [\text{Free}]),$$

which arises from the definition of specific binding in the case of a saturable one-site model.

Ex vivo methods for the assay of saturation binding parameters likewise make use of radiopharmaceuticals at a range of concentrations. Living brain cannot be washed to remove endogenous competitors; in the case of some dopamine receptor ligands, the magnitude of K_d^{app} is altered by the extent of competition from endogenous dopamine in vivo, where

$$K_d^{\text{app}} = K_d(1 + C_{\text{DA}}/K_d^{\text{DA}}).$$

C_{DA} is the concentration of dopamine in the compartment containing the receptors (assumed to be constant during the experiment) and K_d^{DA} is the affinity of dopamine with respect to its own receptors. The extent of this competition with respect to [^{3}H]NPA has been estimated in mouse striatum by pharmacological blockade of dopamine release with γ-butyrolactone, from which it was calculated that the normally prevailing extracellular dopamine concentration is close to 50 nM (Ross 1991). This seems a rather high concentration, relative to estimates from zero net flux microdialysis studies, perhaps reflecting invalid assumptions about the magnitude of K_d^{DA} in living brain. Another complication is presented by the use of the cerebellum concentration for the measurement of [Free], the unbound radioligand concentration. Treatment with reserpine enhanced the uptake of [^{3}H]NPA in mouse cerebellum, thus substantially reducing the magnitude of K_d^{app}, without changing the B_{max} estimates (Ross & Jackson 1989b).

The design of PET studies for the assay of saturation binding parameters emulates the design of studies in vitro or ex vivo. In the first applications, [^{11}C] NMSP binding was measured in the striatum at baseline (high specific activity), and after administration of another competitor, haloperidol. Using the two measurements of k_3, the magnitude of B_{max} was then calculated relative to the plasma concentration of the antagonist (Wong et al. 1986). Alternately, saturation binding parameters have been estimated from the [^{11}C]raclopride pB measured in the striatum at two or more different specific activities (Farde et al. 1995). Using the high-affinity ligand [^{11}C]FLB 457, saturation binding parameters can likewise be estimated in extrastriatal regions of humans (Olsson, Halldin, & Farde 2004); B_{max} values in cortex were 5–10% of those in the striatum (Table 14.1).

Molecular imaging studies of B_{max} and K_d are technically difficult because of the requirement of several PET studies in each subject. Furthermore, subjects must be able to tolerate non-tracer doses of competitors for binding. How well do these estimates in vivo agree with those obtained in the biochemistry laboratory? Estimates of K_d in membranes and in cryostat sections are quite similar, but at least ten times higher than most of the corresponding estimates in living brain for the cases of dopamine D_1 ligands (Table 13.1) and D_2 ligands (Table 14.1). Part of this discrepancy, at least in the case of D_2 ligands, can be readily attributed to competition from endogenous dopamine, such that K_d^{app} always exceeds K_d measured in the absence of dopamine. However, this explanation is not sufficient for the case of D_1 ligands, which seem largely invulnerable to competition from dopamine in living brain. Additional factors such as the association of receptors with other membrane proteins or allosteric regulation may influence K_d^{app} in living brain, relative to observations in membranes or in cryostat sections.

Estimates of the magnitude of B_{max} of dopamine D_1 (Table 13.1) and D_2 ligands (Table 14.1) also reveal an interesting discrepancy based on methodology. While there is good agreement between B_{max} measurements made in membrane preparations and by PET (Seeman 1987), B_{max} estimates based upon quantitative autoradiography of cryostat sections are generally five-fold higher. This difference is best documented in the case of D_2 ligands, but two of the three PET studies of D_1 receptors also show considerably lower B_{max} than are seen in autoradiograms. Indeed, quantitative autoradiographic estimates of B_{max} with [^{3}H]Sch 23390 in vitro are ten-fold higher than SPET estimates obtained with its analog [^{123}I]Sch 23982 (Aiso et al. 1987; Altar & Marien 1987). Quantitation of autoradiograms with tritiated ligands is frequently made using plastic standard strips, designed to emulate the attentuation of signal from the brain tissue, whereas the binding of radioactivity in membranes is measured by scintillation spectroscopy, which is likely more accurate. However, it is difficult to contend that a calibration error could result in ten-fold disagreements in B_{max}.

The available results in vitro also address the question of the identity of the binding sites labeled with various classes of tritiated dopamine D_2 antagonists. For example, the B_{max} of the benzamide [^{3}H]domperidone in rat striatal membranes was identical to that of the [^{3}H]spiperone binding which could be displaced by butaclamol (Lazareno & Nahorski 1982), as were the abundances of the benzamide [^{3}H]sulpiride and [^{3}H]spiperone in membranes from intact rats, and also in rats with previous 6-OHDA lesions, which had increased B_{max} by 50% for both ligands (Urwyler & Coward 1987). Thus, if one properly considers the need to block the serotonin 5HT$_2$ component of butyrophenone binding, there emerges little evidence that the B_{max} for butyrophenone and benzamide ligands for D_2 receptors actually differ in striatum. This is especially hard to reconcile with the notion that [^{3}H]spiperone binds only with the monomeric form of dopamine D_2-like receptors, cited above. The B_{max} of spiperone for D_2 receptors *should* be less than that of raclopride, but it is not.

The relative abundance of agonist and antagonist binding sites has been another matter of controversy. The biphasic displacement of dopamine D_2 antagonists by increasing concentrations of agonists, cited above, and the GTP-evoked changes in ligand binding in vitro, have been interpreted to reveal that only some fraction of dopamine receptors are available for interaction with agonists (D_2^{High}). This fraction is generally found to be less than 50% in vitro. In this scenario, the fractional abundance of D_2^{High} sets the upper limit of how much displacement can be evoked by amphetamine challenge in molecular imaging studies in vivo, which also seems to be close to 50%.

The ex vivo B_{max} of [^{3}H]NPA binding sites in rodent striatum was approximately one half that of [^{3}H]spiperone (van der Werf, Sebens, & Korf 1986), perhaps consistent also with the results of PET studies showing that only one half of [^{11}C]raclopride binding is vulnerable to competition from dopamine in living brain. However, saturation binding studies in vitro do not reveal consistent differences in B_{max} for [^{3}H]NPA, [^{3}H]raclopride, or [^{3}H]spiperone in the striatum of cryostat sections, or in membranes (Table 14.1). In a PET study with high and low specific activities of the tracers, the [^{11}C]raclopride B_{max} in baboon striatum exceeded that of [^{11}C]NPA by 15% (Narendran *et al.* 2005), but this difference seems unlikely to have been significant, given that the standard deviation was less than the expected biological variability. Furthermore, with the single exception cited above, the available in vivo data do not consistently suggest important differences in the maximal binding of agonists and antagonists in living brain. In addition, the binding of [^{11}C]raclopride in living monkey striatum could be entirely displaced in a simple dose-dependent manner with the $D_{2/3}$ agonist (+)-PD-128907 (Kortekaas *et al.* 2004). This latter result suggests that agonist and antagonist sites are a single population in living brain. Similarly, ex vivo studies showed that the binding of [^{11}C](+)-PHNO and [^{3}H]raclopride in rat striatum were both displaced by NPA with Hill slopes close to unity, consistent with the presence of a single site (McCormick *et al.* 2008).

This scenario is difficult to reconcile with the results of receptor occlusion studies: [^{3}H]NPA binding in rat striatal membranes had returned to normal within hours after treatment with the alkylating agent phenoxybenzamine, whereas the return of [^{3}H]spiperone binding was delayed by 1 day (Hall, Jenner, & Marsden 1983). How then can the two ligands be labeling the same receptors? While a multiplicity of factors may contribute to this issue, the discrepant estimates of B_{max} may give an indication. Let us assume that there exists in living brain a large reservoir of dopamine receptors in an inactive form, not expressed on the cell membrane. These might be invisible to radioligands in vivo, and might be washed away in the course of membrane preparation, thus accounting for the similar B_{max} values by PET and in membranes. This hypothetical superabundance of receptors might be preserved within cryostat sections, but altered in such a way as to interact with radioligands, thus accounting for the five-fold greater abundance of D_2 receptors measured by this technique. This hypothesis might also account for discrepancies in the proportion of dopamine receptors in an agonist-binding state, which is approximately 50% on the basis of displacement studies in vitro. Nonetheless, the displacement of [^{3}H]raclopride binding by increasing concentrations of dopamine reveals only small amounts of $D_2{}^{High}$ in pig brain cryostat sections (Minuzzi et al. 2005). This conundrum might be resolved if G-proteins were abundantly present in vivo and in brain cryostat sections, but that a substantial fraction were lost during the preparation and washing of brain membranes; Gα is, after all, a soluble protein, at least in the presence of GTP. The dopamine receptors in membranes might then be resolved into high- and low-affinity states, in proportion to the remaining availability of G-protein.

17

Conclusions and perspectives

Presenting the life history of dopamine has been a matter of assigning quantities to the arrows depicted in the schematic diagram of Carlsson, introduced over 40 years ago (Figure 1.2). This endeavor has made use of a range of methods, extending from classical enzymology and receptor pharmacology, to modern molecular imaging techniques. All of these methods have been brought to bear on the implicit task of breathing life into a model, with the expectation that garnering enough specific information would allow the construction of an explicit model of dopamine neurotransmission. Needless to say, completion of this task remains to be fulfilled. But after 50 years of dopamine research, enough information has been gathered such that a biological model of considerable complexity can now be defined and constrained, encompassing the main elements of metabolic regulation, compartmentation, and anatomical connectivity of dopamine in the basal ganglia.

The neurochemical anatomy of the basal ganglia has a fine structure; many of its components in human brain are simply too small to be seen with PET. The spatial resolution of PET has dramatically increased in the past quarter century. Thus, it was nearly impossible to resolve the human caudate and putamen in the earliest PET images, which had a spatial resolution of 6–8 mm. Newer tomographs with a resolution of 4 mm allowed the defining of a region of interest encompassing the ventral striatum, which has attracted much attention due to its key importance in the rewarding properties of psychostimulants. The latest generation of tomographs has a spatial resolution of 2 mm, which should finally be sufficient for the task of anatomically resolving the nucleus accumbens, but will not resolve important functional divisions of that structure, i.e. the core and shell. It cannot be forseen that technical improvements in PET will ever allow the spatial resolution of the patch-matrix design of the extended striatum, which is at a scale of considerably less than 1 mm. Thus, it may be an axiom that molecular imaging researchers will always attempt to study anatomical structures a bit smaller than the useful limit imposed by the performance of their instruments.

The earliest phase of the life of dopamine is mediated by the activity of TH in the brain. A detailed account of the biochemical complexity of the modulation of this enzyme serves to provide the background of the main themes, which are compartmental modeling, and steady-state kinetics of elements in the dopamine life history. Thus, the activity of TH in living brain is assessed by measuring the accumulation of DOPA in the brain following pharmacological blockade of AAADC. However, the validity of this method can be called into question because of its violation of several steady-state assumptions, particularly the assumption that all DOPA formed in the brain is retained in the brain. The facilitated diffusion of DOPA from the brain highlights a key difference between conducting a reaction in a glass vessel, where reagents, substrates, and products are retained, and a similar reaction conducted in the crucible of the human brain.

The concept of compartmental modeling is introduced in the context of efforts to measure the activity of TH in living brain. Based upon experiment with [^{11}C]tyrosine, it is shown that the specific signal related to dopamine synthesis is overshadowed by the very extensive trapping of this tracer in brain protein. As such, it remains impossible to measure the actual rate of dopamine synthesis in living brain, even when TH is pharmacologically stimulated. The recycling of tyrosine from brain protein may be another factor limiting the utility of tracer methods for the assay of TH in vivo. Whereas FDOPA and other substrates of AAADC in part circumvent this limitation, it must always be recalled that the concentration of endogenous DOPA in the brain is unknown. Consequently, FDOPA-PET results are indicative of the *capacity* of the brain to make dopamine from exogenous DOPA, but do not reveal the actual rate of its synthesis. Furthermore, there remains a considerable discrepancy in the magnitude of the estimates of AAADC activity in vivo (0.1 min^{-1}) and in vitro (1 min^{-1}), which cannot be attributed solely to methodological factors. Nonetheless, FDOPA has proven very useful for clinical studies, especially of Parkinson's disease, and has been used as an end point in a large multi-Center study of the effect of treatment on disease progression.

For pragmatic reasons, the formation from FDOPA of the product [^{18}F]fluorodopamine has generally been assumed to be irreversible in living brain, at least on the timescale of the PET recording. However, new methods of kinetic analysis indicate that the loss of deaminated metabolites can never be neglected without some penalty for the accuracy of the model. A new steady-state model shows that the transient storage of [^{18}F]fluorodopamine is the most salient feature of FDOPA-PET studies in normal aging, Parkinson's disease, and schizophrenia. These results are consistent with the uncommitted nature of DOPA metabolism in living brain, from which it follows that modulation of AAADC activity can contribute to the net rate of dopamine synthesis. Thus, compartmental modeling unseats TH as the sole regulatory step in the dopamine pathway.

The reversibility of dopamine trapping emerges again in the context of MAO, which can be assayed using a number of PET ligands. The binding of irreversible MAO ligands indicates catalytic activity of the enzyme (V_{max}), whereas the reversible ligands associate with a binding site on the enzyme, which is proportional to B_{max} (studies of homospecific TH indicate that enzyme abundance and activity need not be synonymous). MAO inhibition is a useful pharmacological tool for studying the dynamics of dopamine catabolism in experimental animals. Nonetheless, there have been few clinical PET studies of MAO in living brain, greater emphasis having been placed on VMAT2 and other elements of the dopamine neuron. Results of the FDOPA steady-state model reveal that MAO and VMAT2 are inextricably linked, since whatever dopamine is not stored in vesicles must run the gauntlet of cytoplasmic MAO.

[^{11}C]DTBZ-PET is a very sensitive tracer for measuring the abundance of VMAT2 in monoamine terminals. Dopamine signaling following vesicular release is terminated by DAT, which transfers interstitial dopamine back to the presynaptic terminal. The prototypic DAT inhibtor is cocaine, which served as the point of departure for developing a range of tropane derivatives used in PET and SPET studies. Such agents are widely used for the diagnosis of nigrostriatal degeneration, but mostly suffer from a certain lack of pharmacological selectivity between DAT and serotonin transporters. In addition, the diagnostic value of DAT changes is complicated by the apparent modulation of DAT expression. In contrast, VMAT2 may be a more apt indicator of the density of dopamine innervations, with the caveat that VMAT2 ligands bind in several classes of monoamine neurons.

PET results obtained with dopamine D_1 receptors are discussed in a lamentably brief chapter. Although several specific ligands are available for PET studies, D_1 sites seem to be a "receptor without a disease," in that no specific ailment has been linked firmly to them. This seems a conceptual failing, in that we have failed to understand the functional significance of D_1 signaling. In contrast, D_2 receptors are discussed at great length, especially in the context of neurological and psychiatric disorders, and in the context of personality. Available tracers for dopamine receptors are rather lacking in specificity. Thus, serotonin receptors contribute to the specific binding of most D_1 receptor PET ligands. No truly selective ligands are available for the three main subtypes of the D_2-like receptors, nor can pre- and post-synaptic D_2 receptors (presumably

D_2-short and D_2-long) be distinguished with the available probes for molecular imaging. The natural abundance of dopamine receptors remains a perplexing issue. Although there is considerable agreement between B_{max} values obtained in membrane preparations and the results of quantitative PET studies, considerably higher estimates of B_{max} are obtained by quantitative autoradiography in cryostat sections. Also unresolved is the relative abundance of antagonist and agonist binding sites; displacement studies in membranes indicate roughly equal proportions of D_2^{High} and D_2^{Low} receptors, although saturation binding studies with agonist ligands, as well as recent displacement studies, simply do not support the claim that agonist sites comprise a subset of the total number of receptors in living brain.

Notwithstanding these reservations, there has emerged a large body of clinical research reporting subtle changes in D_2 receptor availability in diverse neurological conditions. Given the normal pattern of age-related changes, these changes are seldom pathognomonic of specific disease (the frank degeneration in Huntington's disease is an exception to this rule). The recent PET literature supports a notion of neurochemical typology, in which specific aspects of personality are manifest through the integrity of dopamine innervations and especially by transmission via dopamine D_2 receptors. It is here assumed that the availability of D_2 receptors in normal brain can be parsed into components defining aspects of personality and behavior, which constitutes an implicit bottom-up theory of the brain function. However, it is equally possible that aspects of personality and vulnerabilities manifest themselves through the dopamine system at hand, as was seen to be the case for the alcoholics, in whom striatal D_2 receptor availability and FDOPA uptake were normal, but nonetheless correlating with a behavioral measure of craving. All of these results must be interpreted with the caveat of spurious causality. For example, the association of declining motor reaction rates and dopamine receptor levels with age does not prove that one is the consequence of the other, since reaction rates might be controlled by a multitude of factors, all declining in parallel with D_2 receptor levels.

A great deal of attention has been placed on the competition occurring between dopamine and certain ligands for dopamine D_2 receptors, since this interaction seems to reveal information about the concentration of invisible dopamine in the interstitial fluid. Certainly, psychostimulants reduce the availability of benzamide binding sites in living brain, consistent with a simple competition model. However, the relationship is less clear in other contexts, in which altered receptor binding availability can be dissociated from dopamine release. The task is to determine when altered [^{11}C]raclopride binding reveals altered competition, and when it does not. This formal ambiguity can sometimes be resolved by using PET to measure the saturation binding para-meters, B_{max} and K_d^{app} at dopamine receptors. In general, a change in apparent affinity is attributed to altered competition from endogenous dopamine. Because of the formal ambiguity of changes in the magnitude of pB, it may be necessary to take the extreme position that only saturation binding studies are valid indicators of altered dopamine transmission.

In spite of persistent reservations about the absolute abundance of agonist binding sites, dopamine D_2 agonists have emerged as an important tool in the investigation of dopamine transmission by PET. The binding of agonists in living brain seems generally more fit than antagonists for detecting changes in the competition from endogenous dopamine. However, this may be due to factors other than agonism per se; it remains to be demonstrated that agonist PET ligands impart unique information about the coupling of receptors to intracel-lular second messenger systems in living brain: D_2^{High} and D_2^{Low} seem most clearly evident in membrane preparations.

Direct assay of signal transduction pathways has scarcely been attempted, but may prove more relevent to an understanding of the brain function than is the simple abundance of plasma membrane receptors. One of the very few available PET ligands for a signal transduction enzyme is [^{11}C]rolipram, an antagonist of phosphodiesterase type IV. Its uptake in the brain of awake monkeys is attenuated by antagonism of dopamine D_1 receptors; this effect was more pronounced in young than in aged rats (Harada et al. 2002). Furthermore, methamphetamine treatment increased [^{11}C]rolipram binding in the brain of living monkeys, without altering the availability of [^{11}C]Sch 23390 binding sites (Tsukada et al. 2001). These observations may set the stage for a systematic study of signal transduction in living brain, but contingent upon a more full development of medicinal chemistry and radiochemistry. The current poverty of PET ligands for signal transduction resembles the state of affairs 20 years ago, when only a very few ligands were available for the study of dopamine transmission.

References

Aalto, S., Hirvonen, J., Kajander, J., Scheinin, H., Nagren, K., Vilkman, H., Gustafsson, L., Syvalahti, E., & Hietala, J. 2002, "Ketamine does not decrease striatal dopamine D2 receptor binding in man", *Psychopharmacology (Berl)*, vol. **164**, no. 4, pp. 401–406.

Abdolmaleky, H. M., Cheng, K. H., Faraone, S. V., Wilcox, M., Glatt, S. J., Gao, F., Smith, C. L., Shafa, R., Aeali, B., Carnevale, J., Pan, H., Papageorgis, P., Ponte, J. F., Sivaraman, V., Tsuang, M. T., & Thiagalingam, S. 2006, "Hypomethylation of MB-COMT promoter is a major risk factor for schizophrenia and bipolar disorder", *Hum. Mol. Genet.*, vol. **15**, no. 21, pp. 3132–3145.

Abe, K., Hosoi, R., Momosaki, S., Kobayashi, K., Ibii, N., & Inoue, O. 2002, "Increment of in vivo binding of [3H]SCH 23390, a dopamine D1 receptor ligand, induced by cyclic AMP-dependent protein kinase in rat brain", *Brain Res.*, vol. **952**, no. 2, pp. 211–217.

Abi-Dargham, A., Gandelman, M. S., DeErausquin, G. A., Zea-Ponce, Y., Zoghbi, S. S., Baldwin, R. M., Laruelle, M., Charney, D. S., Hoffer, P. B., Neumeyer, J. L., & Innis, R. B. 1996, "SPECT imaging of dopamine transporters in human brain with iodine-123-fluoroalkyl analogs of beta-CIT", *J. Nucl. Med.*, vol. **37**, no. 7, pp. 1129–1133.

Abi-Dargham, A., Kegeles, L. S., Zea-Ponce, Y., Mawlawi, O., Martinez, D., Mitropoulou, V., O'Flynn, K., Koenigsberg, H. W., Van Heertum, R., Cooper, T., Laruelle, M., & Siever, L. J. 2004, "Striatal amphetamine-induced dopamine release in patients with schizotypal personality disorder studied with single photon emission computed tomography and [123I]iodobenzamide", *Biol.Psychiatry*, vol. **55**, no. 10, pp. 1001–1006.

Abi-Dargham, A., Mawlawi, O., Lombardo, I., Gil, R., Martinez, D., Huang, Y., Hwang, D. R., Keilp, J., Kochan, L., Van Heertum, R., Gorman, J. M., & Laruelle, M. 2002, "Prefrontal dopamine D1 receptors and working memory in schizophrenia", *J. Neurosci.*, vol. **22**, no. 9, pp. 3708–3719.

Abi-Dargham, A., Rodenhiser, J., Printz, D., Zea-Ponce, Y., Gil, R., Kegeles, L. S., Weiss, R., Cooper, T. B., Mann, J. J., Van Heertum, R. L., Gorman, J. M., & Laruelle, M. 2000, "Increased baseline occupancy of D2 receptors by dopamine in schizophrenia", *Proc. Natl. Acad. Sci. USA*, vol. **97**, no. 14, pp. 8104–8109.

234

Abi-Dargham, A., Simpson, N., Kegeles, L., Parsey, R., Hwang, D. R., Anjilvel, S., Zea-Ponce, Y., Lombardo, I., Van Heertum, R., Mann, J. J., Foged, C., Halldin, C., & Laruelle, M. 1999, "PET studies of binding competition between endogenous dopamine and the D1 radiotracer [11C]NNC 756", *Synapse*, vol. **32**, no. 2, pp. 93–109.

Adams, F., Schwarting, R. K., Boix, F., & Huston, J. P. 1991, "Lateralized changes in behavior and striatal dopamine release following unilateral tactile stimulation of the perioral region: a microdialysis study", *Brain Res.*, vol. **553**, no. 2, pp. 318–322.

Adams, J. R., van Netten, N. H., Schulzer, M., Mak, E., Mckenzie, J., Strongosky, A., Sossi, V., Ruth, T. J., Lee, C. S., Farrer, M., Gasser, T., Uitti, R. J., Calne, D. B., Wszolek, Z. K., & Stoessl, A. J. 2005, "PET in LRRK2 mutations: comparison to sporadic Parkinson's disease and evidence for presymptomatic compensation", *Brain*, vol. **128** (Pt 12), pp. 2777–2785.

Adell, A. & Myers, R. D. 1995, "Synthesis of dopamine and 5-HT in anatomical regions of the rat's brain is unaffected by sustained infusion of amperozide", *Pharmacol. Toxicol.*, vol. **77**, no. 5, pp. 341–345.

Agnati, L. F., Ferre, S., Burioni, R., Woods, A., Genedani, S., Franco, R., & Fuxe, K. 2005, "Existence and theoretical aspects of homomeric and heteromeric dopamine receptor complexes and their relevance for neurological diseases", *Neuromolecular. Med.*, vol. **7**, no. 1–2, pp. 61–78.

Ahlenius, S., Ericson, E., & Wijkstrom, A. 1993, "Stimulation of brain dopamine autoreceptors by remoxipride administration in reserpine-treated male rats", *J. Pharm. Pharmacol.*, vol. **45**, no. 3, pp. 237–239.

Ahlenius, S. & Salmi, P. 1994, "Behavioral and biochemical effects of the dopamine D3 receptor-selective ligand, 7-OH-DPAT, in the normal and the reserpine-treated rat", *Eur. J. Pharmacol.*, vol. **260**, no. 2–3, pp. 177–181.

Ahnert-Hilger, G., Nurnberg, B., Exner, T., Schafer, T., & Jahn, R. 1998, "The heterotrimeric G protein Go2 regulates catecholamine uptake by secretory vesicles", *EMBO J.*, vol. **17**, no. 2, pp. 406–413.

Aiso, M., Shigematsu, K., Kebabian, J. W., Potter, W. Z., Cruciani, R. A., & Saavedra, J. M. 1987, "Dopamine D1 receptor in rat brain: a quantitative autoradiographic study with 125I-SCH 23982", *Brain Res.*, vol. **408**, no. 1–2, pp. 281–285.

Albert, K. A., Helmer-Matyjek, E., Nairn, A. C., Muller, T. H., Haycock, J. W., Greene, L. A., Goldstein, M., & Greengard, P. 1984, "Calcium/phospholipid-dependent protein kinase (protein kinase C) phosphorylates and activates tyrosine hydroxylase", *Proc. Natl. Acad. Sci. USA*, vol. **81**, no. 24, pp. 7713–7717.

Albert, K. A., Hemmings, H. C., Jr., Adamo, A. I., Potkin, S. G., Akbarian, S., Sandman, C. A., Cotman, C. W., Bunney, W. E., Jr., & Greengard, P. 2002, "Evidence for decreased DARPP-32 in the prefrontal cortex of patients with schizophrenia", *Arch. Gen. Psychiatry*, vol. **59**, no. 8, pp. 705–712.

Albert, P. R., Neve, K. A., Bunzow, J. R., & Civelli, O. 1990, "Coupling of a cloned rat dopamine-D2 receptor to inhibition of adenylyl cyclase and prolactin secretion", *J. Biol. Chem.*, vol. **265**, no. 4, pp. 2098–2104.

Albert, V. R., Allen, J. M., & Joh, T. H. 1987, "A single gene codes for aromatic L-amino acid decarboxylase in both neuronal and non-neuronal tissues", *J. Biol. Chem.*, vol. **262**, no. 19, pp. 9404–9411.

Albert, V. R., Lee, M. R., Bolden, A. H., Wurzburger, R. J., & Aguanno, A. 1992, "Distinct promoters direct neuronal and nonneuronal expression of rat aromatic L-amino acid decarboxylase", *Proc. Natl. Acad. Sci. USA*, vol. **89**, no. 24, pp. 12053–12057.

Albin, R. L., Koeppe, R. A., Bohnen, N. I., Nichols, T. E., Meyer, P., Wernette, K., Minoshima, S., Kilbourn, M. R., & Frey, K. A. 2003, "Increased ventral striatal monoaminergic innervation in Tourette syndrome", *Neurology*, vol. **61**, no. 3, pp. 310–315.

Alexander, G. E. & Crutcher, M. D. 1990, "Functional architecture of basal ganglia circuits: neural substrates of parallel processing", *Trends Neurosci.*, vol. **13**, no. 7, pp. 266–271.

Alia-Klein, N., Goldstein, R. Z., Kriplani, A., Logan, J., Tomasi, D., Williams, B., Telang, F., Shumay, E., Biegon, A., Craig, I. W., Henn, F., Wang, G. J., Volkow, N. D., & Fowler, J. S. 2008, "Brain monoamine oxidase A activity predicts trait aggression", *J. Neurosci.*, vol. **28**, no. 19, pp. 5099–5104.

Almas, B., Le Bourdelles, B., Flatmark, T., Mallet, J., & Haavik, J. 1992, "Regulation of recombinant human tyrosine hydroxylase isozymes by catecholamine binding and phosphorylation. Structure/activity studies and mechanistic implications", *Eur. J. Biochem.*, vol. **209**, no. 1, pp. 249–255.

Altar, C. A. & Marien, M. R. 1987, "Picomolar affinity of 125I-SCH 23982 for D1 receptors in brain demonstrated with digital subtraction autoradiography", *J. Neurosci.*, vol. **7**, no. 1, pp. 213–222.

Amsterdam, J. D. & Newberg, A. B. 2007, "A preliminary study of dopamine transporter binding in bipolar and unipolar depressed patients and healthy controls", *Neuropsychobiology*, vol. **55**, no. 3–4, pp. 167–170.

Anand, A., Verhoeff, P., Seneca, N., Zoghbi, S. S., Seibyl, J. P., Charney, D. S., & Innis, R. B. 2000, "Brain SPECT imaging of amphetamine-induced dopamine release in euthymic bipolar disorder patients", *Am. J. Psychiatry*, vol. **157**, no. 7, pp. 1108–1114.

Anastasiadis, P. Z., Kuhn, D. M., & Levine, R. A. 1994, "Tetrahydrobiopterin uptake into rat brain synaptosomes, cultured PC12 cells, and rat striatum", *Brain Res.*, vol. **665**, no. 1, pp. 77–84.

Anden, N. E., Rubenson, A., Fuxe, K., & Hokfelt, T. 1967, "Evidence for dopamine receptor stimulation by apomorphine", *J. Pharm. Pharmacol.*, vol. **19**, no. 9, pp. 627–629.

Andersen, P. H. & Braestrup, C. 1986, "Evidence for different states of the dopamine D1 receptor: clozapine and fluperlapine may preferentially label an adenylate cyclase-coupled state of the D1 receptor", *J. Neurochem.*, vol. **47**, no. 6, pp. 1822–1831.

Andrews, T. C., Weeks, R. A., Turjanski, N., Gunn, R. N., Watkins, L. H., Sahakian, B., Hodges, J. R., Rosser, A. E., Wood, N. W., & Brooks, D. J. 1999, "Huntington's disease progression. PET and clinical observations", *Brain*, vol. **122** (Pt 12), pp. 2353–2363.

Anstrom, K. K. & Woodward, D. J. 2005, "Restraint increases dopaminergic burst firing in awake rats", *Neuropsychopharmacology*, vol. **30**, no. 10, pp. 1832–1840.

Antonini, A., Leenders, K. L., Reist, H., Thomann, R., Beer, H. F., & Locher, J. 1993, "Effect of age on D2 dopamine receptors in normal human brain measured by positron emission tomography and 11C-raclopride", *Arch. Neurol.*, vol. **50**, no. 5, pp. 474–480.

Antonini, A., Schwarz, J., Oertel, W. H., Beer, H. F., Madeja, U. D., & Leenders, K. L. 1994, "[11C]raclopride and positron emission tomography in previously untreated patients with Parkinson's disease: influence of L-dopa and lisuride therapy on striatal dopamine D2-receptors", *Neurology*, vol. **44**, no. 7, pp. 1325–1329.

Antonini, A., Schwarz, J., Oertel, W. H., Pogarell, O., & Leenders, K. L. 1997, "Long-term changes of striatal dopamine D2 receptors in patients with Parkinson's disease: a study with positron emission tomography and [11C]raclopride", *Mov. Disord.*, vol. **12**, no. 1, pp. 33–38.

Apud, J. A. & Weinberger, D. R. 2007, "Treatment of cognitive deficits associated with schizophrenia: potential role of catechol-O-methyltransferase inhibitors", *CNS Drugs*, vol. **21**, no. 7, pp. 535–557.

Arai, R., Karasawa, N., Geffard, M., Nagatsu, T., & Nagatsu, I. 1994, "Immunohistochemical evidence that central serotonin neurons produce dopamine from exogenous L-DOPA in the rat, with reference to the involvement of aromatic L-amino acid decarboxylase", *Brain Res.*, vol. **667**, no. 2, pp. 295–299.

Arai, R., Kimura, H., & Maeda, T. 1986, "Topographic atlas of monoamine oxidase-containing neurons in the rat brain studied by an improved histochemical method", *Neuroscience*, vol. **19**, no. 3, pp. 905–925.

Araki, T., Tanji, H., Kato, H., Imai, Y., Mizugaki, M., & Itoyama, Y. 2000, "Temporal changes of dopaminergic and glutamatergic receptors in 6-hydroxydopamine-treated rat brain", *Eur. Neuropsychopharmacol.*, vol. **10**, no. 5, pp. 365–375.

Ariano, M. A., Sortwell, C. E., Ray, M., Altemus, K. L., Sibley, D. R., & Levine, M. S. 1997, "Agonist-induced morphologic decrease in cellular D1A dopamine receptor staining", *Synapse*, vol. **27**, no. 4, pp. 313–321.

Arias-Montano, J. A., Martinez-Fong, D., & Aceves, J. 1991, "Gamma-aminobutyric acid (GABAB) receptor-mediated inhibition of tyrosine hydroxylase activity in the striatum of rat", *Neuropharmacology*, vol. **30**, no. 10, pp. 1047–1051.

Arias-Montano, J. A., Martinez-Fong, D., & Aceves, J. 1992, "GABAB receptor activation partially inhibits N-methyl-D-aspartate-mediated tyrosine hydroxylase stimulation in rat striatal slices", *Eur. J. Pharmacol.*, vol. **218**, no. 2–3, pp. 335–338.

Arnett, C. D., Fowler, J. S., MacGregor, R. R., Schlyer, D. J., Wolf, A. P., Langstrom, B., & Halldin, C. 1987, "Turnover of brain monoamine oxidase measured in vivo by positron emission tomography using L-[11C]deprenyl", *J. Neurochem.*, vol. **49**, no. 2, pp. 522–527.

Asanuma, K., Ma, Y., Okulski, J., Dhawan, V., Chaly, T., Carbon, M., Bressman, S. B., & Eidelberg, D. 2005, "Decreased striatal D2 receptor binding in non-manifesting carriers of the DYT1 dystonia mutation", *Neurology*, vol. **64**, no. 2, pp. 347–349.

Asselin, M. C., Montgomery, A. J., Grasby, P. M., & Hume, S. P. 2007, "Quantification of PET studies with the very high-affinity dopamine D2/D3 receptor ligand [11C]FLB 457: re-evaluation of the validity of using a cerebellar reference region", *J. Cereb. Blood Flow Metab.*, vol. **27**, no. 2, pp. 378–392.

Atkinson, J., Richtand, N., Schworer, C., Kuczenski, R., & Soderling, T. 1987, "Phosphorylation of purified rat striatal tyrosine hydroxylase by Ca2+/calmodulin-dependent protein kinase II: effect of an activator protein", *J. Neurochem.*, vol. **49**, no. 4, pp. 1241–1249.

Atsumi, M., Kawakami, J., Sugiyama, E., Kotaki, H., Sawada, Y., Sato, H., Yamada, Y., & Iga, T. 2003, "Pharmacokinetic and pharmacodynamic analyses, based on dopamine D2-receptor occupancy of bromocriptine, of bromocriptine-induced contralateral rotations in unilaterally 6-OHDA-lesioned rats", *Synapse*, vol. **50**, no. 2, pp. 110–116.

Aubert, I., Ghorayeb, I., Normand, E., & Bloch, B. 2000, "Phenotypical characterization of the neurons expressing the D1 and D2 dopamine receptors in the monkey striatum", *J. Comp. Neurol.*, vol. **418**, no. 1, pp. 22–32.

Axelrod, J. & Tomchick, R. 1958, "Enzymatic O-methylation of epinephrine and other catechols", *J. Biol. Chem.*, vol. **233**, no. 3, pp. 702–705.

Azzaro, A. J., King, J., Kotzuk, J., Schoepp, D. D., Frost, J., & Schochet, S. 1985, "Guinea pig striatum as a model of human dopamine deamination: the role of monoamine oxidase isozyme ratio, localization, and affinity for substrate in synaptic dopamine metabolism", *J. Neurochem.*, vol. **45**, no. 3, pp. 949–956.

Bach, A. W., Lan, N. C., Johnson, D. L., Abell, C. W., Bembenek, M. E., Kwan, S. W., Seeburg, P. H., & Shih, J. C. 1988, "cDNA cloning of human liver monoamine oxidase A and B: molecular basis of differences in enzymatic properties", *Proc. Natl. Acad. Sci. USA*, vol. **85**, no. 13, pp. 4934–4938.

Backman, L., Ginovart, N., Dixon, R. A., Wahlin, T. B., Wahlin, A., Halldin, C., & Farde, L. 2000, "Age-related cognitive deficits mediated by changes in the striatal dopamine system", *Am. J. Psychiatry*, vol. **157**, no. 4, pp. 635–637.

Badgaiyan, R. D., Fischman, A. J., & Alpert, N. M. 2003, "Striatal dopamine release during unrewarded motor task in human volunteers", *Neuroreport*, vol. **14**, no. 11, pp. 1421–1424.

Badgaiyan, R. D., Fischman, A. J., & Alpert, N. M. 2007, "Striatal dopamine release in sequential learning", *Neuroimage*, vol. **38**, no. 3, pp. 549–556.

Badgaiyan, R. D., Fischman, A. J., & Alpert, N. M. 2008, "Explicit motor memory activates the striatal dopamine system", *Neuroreport*, vol. **19**, no. 4, pp. 409–412.

Ballesteros, J., Maeztu, A. I., Callado, L. F., Meana, J. J., & Gutiérrez, M. 2008, "Specific binding of [3H]Ro 19-6327 (lazabemide) to monoamine oxidase B is increased in frontal cortex of suicide victims after controlling for age at death", *Eur. Neuropsychopharmacol.*, vol. **18**, no. 1, pp. 55–61.

Bancroft, G. N., Morgan, K. A., Flietstra, R. J., & Levant, B. 1998, "Binding of [3H]PD 128907, a putatively selective ligand for the D3 dopamine receptor, in rat brain: a receptor binding and quantitative autoradiographic study", *Neuropsychopharmacology*, vol. **18**, no. 4, pp. 305–316.

Bannon, M. J. & Roth, R. H. 1983, "Pharmacology of mesocortical dopamine neurons", *Pharmacol. Rev.*, vol. **35**, no. 1, pp. 53–68.

Bantick, R. A., De Vries, M. H., & Grasby, P. M. 2005, "The effect of a 5-HT1A receptor agonist on striatal dopamine release", *Synapse*, vol. **57**, no. 2, pp. 67–75.

Baran, H. & Jellinger, K. 1992, "Human brain phenolsulfotransferase. Regional distribution in Parkinson's disease", *J. Neural. Transm. Park. Dis. Dement. Sect.*, vol. **4**, pp. 267–276.

Barbeau, A., Sourkes, T. L., & Murphy, G. F. 1962, "[Les catécholamines dans la maladie to Parkinson]," in *Monoamines et système nerveux central*, J. de Ajuriaguerra, ed., Georg & Cie SA, Geneva, pp. 247–262.

Barbier, P., Colelli, A., Maggio, R., Bravi, D., & Corsini, G. U. 1997, "Pergolide binds tightly to dopamine D2 short receptors and induces receptor sequestration", *J. Neural. Transm.*, vol. **104**, no. 8–9, pp. 867–874.

Barnes, J. M., Barnes, N. M., Costall, B., & Naylor, R. J. 1990, "The actions of (-)N-n-propylnorapomorphine and selective dopamine D1 and D2 receptor agonists to modify the release of [3H]dopamine from the rat nucleus accumbens", *Neuropharmacology*, vol. **29**, no. 4, pp. 327–336.

Baron, J. C., Maziere, B., Loc'h, C., Cambon, H., Sgouropoulos, P., Bonnet, A. M., & Agid, Y. 1986, "Loss of striatal [76Br]bromospiperone binding sites demonstrated by positron tomography in progressive supranuclear palsy", *J. Cereb. Blood Flow Metab.*, vol. **6**, no. 2, pp. 131–136.

Barrett, S. P., Boileau, I., Okker, J., Pihl, R. O., & Dagher, A. 2004, "The hedonic response to cigarette smoking is proportional to dopamine release in the human striatum as measured by positron emission tomography and [11C]raclopride", *Synapse*, vol. **54**, no. 2, pp. 65–71.

Barrio, J. R., Huang, S. C., & Phelps, M. E. 1997, "Biological imaging and the molecular basis of dopaminergic diseases", *Biochem. Pharmacol.*, vol. **54**, no. 3, pp. 341–348.

Bart, J., Willemsen, A. T., Groen, H. J., van der Graaf, W. T., Wegman, T. D., Vaalburg, W., de Vries, E. G., & Hendriikse, N. H. 2003, "Quantitative assessment of P-glycoprotein function in the rat blood-brain barrier by distribution volume of [11C]verapamil measured with PET", *Neuroimage*, vol. **20**, no. 3, pp. 1775–1782.

Baumann, M. H., Raley, T. J., Partilla, J. S., & Rothman, R. B. 1993, "Biosynthesis of dopamine and serotonin in the rat brain after repeated cocaine injections: a microdissection mapping study", *Synapse*, vol. **14**, no. 1, pp. 40–50.

Bean, A. J., Shepard, P. D., Bunney, B. S., Nestler, E. J., & Roth, R. H. 1988, "The effects of pertussis toxin on autoreceptor-mediated inhibition of dopamine synthesis in the rat striatum", *Mol. Pharmacol.*, vol. **34**, no. 6, pp. 715–718.

Bench, C. J., Price, G. W., Lammertsma, A. A., Cremer, J. C., Luthra, S. K., Turton, D., Dolan, R. J., Kettler, R., Dingemanse, J., Da Prada, M., *et al.* 1991, "Measurement of human cerebral monoamine oxidase type B (MAO-B) activity with positron emission tomography (PET): a dose ranging study with the reversible inhibitor Ro 19-6327", *Eur. J. Clin. Pharmacol.*, vol. **40**, no. 2, pp. 169–173.

Bendayan, R., Ronaldson, P. T., Gingras, D., & Bendayan, M. 2006, "In situ localization of P-glycoprotein (ABCB1) in human and rat brain", *J. Histochem. Cytochem.*, vol. **54**, no. 10, pp. 1159–1167.

Bennett, B. A. & Freed, C. R. 1986, "Mobilization of storage pool dopamine and late ipsilateral augmentation of striatal dopamine synthesis in the trained circling rat", *J. Neurochem.*, vol. **47**, no. 2, pp. 472–476.

Benveniste, H., Hansen, A. J., & Ottosen, N. S. 1989, "Determination of brain interstitial concentrations by microdialysis", *J. Neurochem.*, vol. **52**, no. 6, pp. 1741–1750.

Benwell, M. E. & Balfour, D. J. 1992, "The effects of acute and repeated nicotine treatment on nucleus accumbens dopamine and locomotor activity", *Br. J. Pharmacol.*, vol. **105**, no. 4, pp. 849–856.

Berding, G., Brucke, T., Odin, P., Brooks, D. J., Kolbe, H., Gielow, P., Harke, H., Knoop, B. O., Dengler, R., & Knapp, W. H. 2003, "[123I]beta-CIT SPECT imaging of dopamine and serotonin transporters in Parkinson's disease and multiple system atrophy", *Nuklearmedizin*, vol. **42**, no. 1, pp. 31–38.

Bergstrom, M., Kumlien, E., Lilja, A., Tyrefors, N., Westerberg, G., & Langstrom, B. 1998, "Temporal lobe epilepsy visualized with PET with 11C-L-deuterium-deprenyl – analysis of kinetic data", *Acta Neurol. Scand.*, vol. **98**, no. 4, pp. 224–231.

Bergstrom, M., Westerberg, G., & Langstrom, B. 1997, "11C-harmine as a tracer for monoamine oxidase A (MAO-A): in vitro and in vivo studies", *Nucl. Med. Biol.*, vol. **24**, no. 4, pp. 287–293.

Bergstrom, M., Westerberg, G., Nemeth, G., Traut, M., Gross, G., Greger, G., Muller-Peltzer, H., Safer, A., Eckernas, S. A., Grahner, A., & Langstrom, B. 1997, "MAO-A inhibition in brain after dosing with esuprone, moclobemide and placebo in healthy volunteers: in vivo studies with positron emission tomography", *Eur. J. Clin. Pharmacol.*, vol. **52**, no. 2, pp. 121–128.

Berretta, S., Sachs, Z., & Graybiel, A. M. 1999, "Cortically driven Fos induction in the striatum is amplified by local dopamine D2-class receptor blockade", *Eur. J. Neurosci.*, vol. **11**, no. 12, pp. 4309–4319.

Best, S. E., Sarrel, P. M., Malison, R. T., Laruelle, M., Zoghbi, S. S., Baldwin, R. M., Seibyl, J. P., Innis, R. B., & van Dyck, C. H. 2005, "Striatal dopamine transporter availability with [123I]beta-CIT SPECT is unrelated to gender or menstrual cycle", *Psychopharmacology (Berl)*, vol. **183**, no. 2, pp. 181–189.

Bezin, L., Marcel, D., Garcia, C., Blum, D., Lafargue, P., Lellouche, J. P., Pujol, J. F., & Weissmann, D. 2000, "In situ examination of tyrosine hydroxylase activity in the rat locus coeruleus using (3',5')-[(3)H(2)]-alpha-fluoromethyl-tyrosine as substrate of the enzyme", *Synapse*, vol. **35**, no. 3, pp. 201–211.

Bibb, J. A., Snyder, G. L., Nishi, A., Yan, Z., Meijer, L., Fienberg, A. A., Tsai, L. H., Kwon, Y. T., Girault, J. A., Czernik, A. J., Huganir, R. L., Hemmings, H. C., Jr., Nairn, A. C., & Greengard, P. 1999, "Phosphorylation of DARPP-32 by Cdk5 modulates dopamine signalling in neurons", *Nature*, vol. **402**, no. 6762, pp. 669–671.

Birrell, C. E. & Balfour, D. J. 1998, "The influence of nicotine pretreatment on mesoaccumbens dopamine overflow and locomotor responses to D-amphetamine", *Psychopharmacology (Berl)*, vol. **140**, no. 2, pp. 142–149.

Biswas, B. & Carlsson, A. 1978, "On the mode of action of diazepam on brain catecholamine metabolism", *Naunyn Schmiedebergs Arch. Pharmacol.*, vol. **303**, no. 1, pp. 73–78.

Blennow, K., Wallin, A., Gottfries, C. G., Karlsson, I., Mansson, J. E., Skoog, I., Wikkelso, C., & Svennerholm, L. 1993, "Cerebrospinal fluid monoamine metabolites in 114 healthy individuals 18–88 years of age", *Eur. Neuropsychopharmacol.*, vol. **3**, no. 1, pp. 55–61.

Blomqvist, O., Engel, J. A., Nissbrandt, H., & Soderpalm, B. 1993, "The mesolimbic dopamine-activating properties of ethanol are antagonized by mecamylamine", *Eur. J. Pharmacol.*, vol. **249**, no. 2, pp. 207–213.

Bohnen, N. I., Albin, R. L., Frey, K. A., & Fink, J. K. 1999, "(+)-alpha-[11C]dihydrotetrabenazine PET imaging in familial paroxysmal dystonic choreoathetosis", *Neurology*, vol. **52**, no. 5, pp. 1067–1069.

Bohnen, N. I., Albin, R. L., Koeppe, R. A., Wernette, K. A., Kilbourn, M. R., Minoshima, S., & Frey, K. A. 2006, "Positron emission tomography of monoaminergic vesicular binding in aging and Parkinson disease", *J. Cereb. Blood Flow Metab.*, vol. **26**, no. 9, pp. 1198–1212.

Bohnen, N. I., Koeppe, R. A., Meyer, P., Ficaro, E., Wernette, K., Kilbourn, M. R., Kuhl, D. E., Frey, K. A., & Albin, R. L. 2000, "Decreased striatal monoaminergic terminals in Huntington disease", *Neurology*, vol. **54**, no. 9, pp. 1753–1759.

Bohnen, N. I., Kuwabara, H., Constantine, G. M., Mathis, C. A., & Moore, R. Y. 2007, "Grooved pegboard test as a biomarker of nigrostriatal denervation in Parkinson's disease", *Neurosci. Lett.*, vol. **424**, no. 3, pp. 185–189.

Boileau, I., Assaad, J. M., Pihl, R. O., Benkelfat, C., Leyton, M., Diksic, M., Tremblay, R. E., & Dagher, A. 2003, "Alcohol promotes dopamine release in the human nucleus accumbens", *Synapse*, vol. **49**, no. 4, pp. 226–231.

Boileau, I., Dagher, A., Leyton, M., Gunn, R. N., Baker, G. B., Diksic, M., & Benkelfat, C. 2006, "Modeling sensitization to stimulants in humans: an [11C]raclopride/positron emission tomography study in healthy men", *Arch. Gen. Psychiatry*, vol. **63**, no. 12, pp. 1386–1395.

Boileau, I., Dagher, A., Leyton, M., Welfeld, K., Booij, L., Diksic, M., & Benkelfat, C. 2007, "Conditioned dopamine release in humans: a positron emission tomography [11C]raclopride study with amphetamine", *J. Neurosci.*, vol. **27**, no. 15, pp. 3998–4003.

Booij, J., Bergmans, P., Winogrodzka, A., Speelman, J. D., & Wolters, E. C. 2001, "Imaging of dopamine transporters with [123I]FP-CIT SPECT does not suggest a significant effect of age on the symptomatic threshold of disease in Parkinson's disease", *Synapse*, vol. **39**, no. 2, pp. 101–108.

Booij, J., de Bruin, K., & Gunning, W. B. 2006, "Repeated administration of D-amphetamine induces loss of [123I]FP-CIT binding to striatal dopamine transporters in rat brain: a validation study", *Nucl. Med. Biol.*, vol. **33**, no. 3, pp. 409–411.

Booij, J., de Jong, J., de Bruin, K., Knol, R., de Win, M. M., & van Eck-Smit, B. L. 2007, "Quantification of striatal dopamine transporters with 123I-FP-CIT SPECT is influenced by the selective serotonin reuptake inhibitor paroxetine: a double-blind, placebo-controlled, crossover study in healthy control subjects", *J. Nucl. Med.*, vol. **48**, no. 3, pp. 359–366.

Borbely, K., Brooks, R. A., Wong, D. F., Burns, R. S., Cumming, P., Gjedde, A., & Di, C. G. 1999, "NMSP binding to dopamine and serotonin receptors in MPTP-induced parkinsonism: relation to dopa therapy", *Acta Neurol. Scand.*, vol. **100**, no. 1, pp. 42–52.

Borghammer, P., Kumakura, Y., & Cumming, P. 2005, "Fluorodopa F 18 positron emission tomography and the progression of Parkinson disease", *Arch. Neurol.*, vol. **62**, no. 9, pp. 1480–1481.

Bottlaender, M., Dolle, F., Guenther, I., Roumenov, D., Fuseau, C., Bramoulle, Y., Curet, O., Jegham, J., Pinquier, J. L., George, P., & Valette, H. 2003, "Mapping the cerebral monoamine oxidase type A: positron emission tomography characterization of the reversible selective inhibitor [11C]befloxatone", *J. Pharmacol. Exp. Ther.*, vol. **305**, no. 2, pp. 467–473.

Bouchard, S. & Roberge, A. G. 1979, "Biochemical properties and kinetic parameters of dihydroxyphenylalanine – 5-hydroxytryptophan decarboxylase in brain, liver, and adrenals of cat", *Can. J. Biochem.*, vol. **57**, no. 7, pp. 1014–1018.

Boulton, A. A. & Juorio, A. V. 1983, "Cerebral decarboxylation of meta- and para-tyrosine", *Experientia*, vol. **39**, no. 2, pp. 130–134.

Bouthenet, M. L., Souil, E., Martres, M. P., Sokoloff, P., Giros, B., & Schwartz, J. C. 1991, "Localization of dopamine D3 receptor mRNA in the rat brain using in situ hybridization histochemistry: comparison with dopamine D2 receptor mRNA", *Brain Res.*, vol. **564**, no. 2, pp. 203–219.

Bowers, M. B., Jr., Heninger, G. R., & Gerbode, F. 1969, "Cerebrospinal fluid 5-hydroxyindoleacetic acid and homovanillic acid in psychiatric patients", *Int. J. Neuropharmacol.*, vol. **8**, no. 3, pp. 255–262.

Boyes, B. E., Cumming, P., Martin, W. R., & McGeer, E. G. 1986, "Determination of plasma [18F]-6-fluorodopa during positron emission tomography: elimination and metabolism in carbidopa treated subjects", *Life Sci.*, vol. **39**, no. 23, pp. 2243–2252.

Bracha, H. S., Seitz, D. J., Otemaa, J., & Glick, S. D. 1987, "Rotational movement (circling) in normal humans: sex difference and relationship to hand, foot and eye preference", *Brain Res.*, vol. **411**, no. 2, pp. 231–235.

Brake, W. G., Zhang, T. Y., Diorio, J., Meaney, M. J., & Gratton, A. 2004, "Influence of early postnatal rearing conditions on mesocorticolimbic dopamine and behavioural responses to psychostimulants and stressors in adult rats", *Eur. J. Neurosci.*, vol. **19**, no. 7, pp. 1863–1874.

Breier, A., Kestler, L., Adler, C., Elman, I., Wiesenfeld, N., Malhotra, A., & Pickar, D. 1998, "Dopamine D2 receptor density and personal detachment in healthy subjects", *Am. J. Psychiatry*, vol. **155**, no. 10, pp. 1440–1442.

Breier, A., Su, T. P., Saunders, R., Carson, R. E., Kolachana, B. S., de Bartolomeis, A., Weinberger, D. R., Weisenfeld, N., Malhotra, A. K., Eckelman, W. C., & Pickar, D. 1997, "Schizophrenia is associated with elevated amphetamine-induced synaptic dopamine concentrations: evidence from a novel positron emission tomography method", *Proc. Natl. Acad. Sci. USA*, vol. **94**, no. 6, pp. 2569–2574.

Bressan, R. A., Erlandsson, K., Jones, H. M., Mulligan, R., Flanagan, R. J., Ell, P. J., & Pilowsky, L. S. 2003, "Is regionally selective D2/D3 dopamine occupancy sufficient for atypical antipsychotic effect? An in vivo quantitative [123I]epidepride SPET study of amisulpride-treated patients", *Am. J. Psychiatry*, vol. **160**, no. 8, pp. 1413–1420.

Brodie, B. B., Costa, E., Dlabac, A., Neff, N. H., & Smookler, H. H. 1966, "Application of steady state kinetics to the estimation of synthesis rate and turnover time of tissue catecholamines", *J. Pharmacol. Exp. Ther.*, vol. **154**, no. 3, pp. 493–498.

Brody, A. L., Mandelkern, M. A., Olmstead, R. E., Allen-Martinez, Z., Scheibal, D., Abrams, A. L., Costello, M. R., Farahi, J., Saxena, S., Monterosso, J., & London, E. D. 2008, "Ventral striatal dopamine release in response to smoking a regular vs a denicotinized cigarette", *Neuropsychopharmacology* [Epub ahead of print].

Brody, A. L., Mandelkern, M. A., Olmstead, R. E., Scheibal, D., Hahn, E., Shiraga, S., Zamora-Paja, E., Farahi, J., Saxena, S., London, E. D., & McCracken, J. T. 2006, "Gene variants of brain dopamine pathways and smoking-induced dopamine release in the ventral caudate/nucleus accumbens", *Arch. Gen. Psychiatry*, vol. **63**, no. 7, pp. 808–816.

Brody, A. L., Olmstead, R. E., London, E. D., Farahi, J., Meyer, J. H., Grossman, P., Lee, G. S., Huang, J., Hahn, E. L., & Mandelkern, M. A. 2004, "Smoking-induced ventral striatum dopamine release", *Am. J. Psychiatry*, vol. **161**, no. 7, pp. 1211–1218.

Broussolle, E., Dentresangle, C., Landais, P., Garcia-Larrea, L., Pollak, P., Croisile, B., Hibert, O., Bonnefoi, F., Galy, G., Froment, J. C., & Comar, D. 1999, "The relation of putamen and caudate nucleus 18F-Dopa uptake to motor and cognitive performances in Parkinson's disease", *J. Neurol. Sci.*, vol. **166**, no. 2, pp. 141–151.

Brown, E. E., Damsma, G., Cumming, P., & Fibiger, H. C. 1991, "Interstitial 3-methoxytyramine reflects striatal dopamine release: an in vivo microdialysis study", *J. Neurochem.*, vol. **57**, no. 2, pp. 701–707.

Brown, W. D., DeJesus, O. T., Pyzalski, R. W., Malischke, L., Roberts, A. D., Shelton, S. E., Uno, H., Houser, W. D., Nickles, R. J., & Holden, J. E. 1999, "Localization of trapping of 6-[(18)F]fluoro-L-m-tyrosine, an aromatic L-amino acid decarboxylase tracer for PET", *Synapse*, vol. **34**, no. 2, pp. 111–123.

Bruck, A., Aalto, S., Nurmi, E., Bergman, J., & Rinne, J. O. 2005, "Cortical 6-[18F]fluoro-L-dopa uptake and frontal cognitive functions in early Parkinson's disease", *Neurobiol. Aging*, vol. **26**, no. 6, pp. 891–898.

Bruck, A., Aalto, S., Nurmi, E., Vahlberg, T., Bergman, J., & Rinne, J. O. 2006, "Striatal subregional 6-[18F]fluoro-L-dopa uptake in early Parkinson's disease: a two-year follow-up study", *Mov. Disord.*, vol. **21**, no. 7, pp. 958–963.

Brunswick, D. J., Amsterdam, J. D., Mozley, P. D., & Newberg, A. 2003, "Greater availability of brain dopamine transporters in major depression shown by [99m Tc]TRODAT-1 SPECT imaging", *Am. J. Psychiatry*, vol. **160**, no. 10, pp. 1836–1841.

Buckland, P. R., Spurlock, G., & McGuffin, P. 1996, "Amphetamine and vigabatrin down regulate aromatic L-amino acid decarboxylase mRNA levels", *Brain Res. Mol. Brain Res.*, vol. **35**, no. 1–2, pp. 69–76.

Budygin, E. A., Brodie, M. S., Sotnikova, T. D., Mateo, Y., John, C. E., Cyr, M., Gainetdinov, R. R., & Jones, S. R. 2004, "Dissociation of rewarding and dopamine transporter-mediated properties of amphetamine", *Proc. Natl. Acad. Sci. USA*, vol. **101**, no. 20, pp. 7781–7786.

Budygin, E. A., Gainetdinov, R. R., Kilpatrick, M. R., Rayevsky, K. S., Mannisto, P. T., & Wightman, R. M. 1999, "Effect of tolcapone, a catechol-O-methyltransferase inhibitor, on striatal dopaminergic transmission during blockade of dopamine uptake", *Eur. J. Pharmacol.*, vol. **370**, no. 2, pp. 125–131.

Budygin, E. A., John, C. E., Mateo, Y., & Jones, S. R. 2002, "Lack of cocaine effect on dopamine clearance in the core and shell of the nucleus accumbens of dopamine transporter knock-out mice", *J. Neurosci.*, vol. **22**, no. 10, p. RC222.

Bullard, W. P. & Capson, T. L. 1983, "Steady-state kinetics of bovine striatal tyrosine hydroxylase", *Mol. Pharmacol.*, vol. **23**, no. 1, pp. 104–111.

Bunney, B. S., Aghajanian, G. K., & Roth, R. H. 1973, "Comparison of effects of L-dopa, amphetamine and apomorphine on firing rate of rat dopaminergic neurones", *Nat. New Biol.*, vol. **245**, no. 143, pp. 123–125.

Burger, L. Y. & Martin-Iverson, M. T. 1994, "Increased occupation of D1 and D2 dopamine receptors accompanies cocaine-induced behavioral sensitization", *Brain Res.*, vol. **639**, no. 2, pp. 228–232.

Burns, R. S., Chiueh, C. C., Markey, S. P., Ebert, M. H., Jacobowitz, D. M., & Kopin, I. J. 1983, "A primate model of parkinsonism: selective destruction of dopaminergic neurons in the pars compacta of the substantia nigra by N-methyl-4-phenyl-1,2,3,6-tetrahydropyridine", *Proc. Natl. Acad. Sci. USA*, vol. **80**, no. 14, pp. 4546–4550.

Buu, N. T. 1989, "Vesicular accumulation of dopamine following L-DOPA administration", *Biochem. Pharmacol.*, vol. **38**, no. 11, pp. 1787–1792.

Buyukuysal, R. L. & Mogol, E. 2000, "Synthesis and release of dopamine in rat striatal slices: requirement for exogenous tyrosine in the medium", *Neurochem. Res.*, vol. **25**, no. 4, pp. 533–540.

Cabello, C. R., Thune, J. J., Pakkenberg, H., & Pakkenberg, B. 2002, "Ageing of substantia nigra in humans: cell loss may be compensated by hypertrophy", *Neuropathol. Appl. Neurobiol.*, vol. **28**, no. 4, pp. 283–291.

Cadoni, C., Solinas, M., & Di Chiara, G. 2000, "Psychostimulant sensitization: differential changes in accumbal shell and core dopamine", *Eur. J. Pharmacol.*, vol. **388**, no. 1, pp. 69–76.

Campbell, I. C., Murphy, D. L., Walker, M. N., Lovenberg, W., & Robinson, D. S. 1980, "Monoamine oxidase inhibitors (MAOI) increase rat brain aromatic amino acid decarboxylase activity", *Br. J. Clin. Pharmacol.*, vol. **9**, no. 4, pp. 431–432.

Canesi, M., Benti, R., Marotta, G., Cilia, R., Isaias, I. U., Gerundini, P., Pezzoli, G., & Antonini, A. 2007, "Striatal dopamine transporter binding in patients with Parkinson's disease and severe occupational hydrocarbon exposure", *Eur. J. Neurol.*, vol. **14**, no. 3, pp. 297–299.

Cardenas, L., Houle, S., Kapur, S., & Busto, U. E. 2004, "Oral D-amphetamine causes prolonged displacement of [11C]raclopride as measured by PET", *Synapse*, vol. **51**, no. 1, pp. 27–31.

Carey, M. P., Diewald, L. M., Esposito, F. J., Pellicano, M. P., Gironi Carnevale, U. A., Sergeant, J. A., Papa, M., & Sadile, A. G. 1998, "Differential distribution, affinity and plasticity of dopamine D-1 and D-2 receptors in the target sites of the mesolimbic system in an animal model of ADHD", *Behav.Brain Res.*, vol. **94**, no. 1, pp. 173–185.

Carlsson, A. 1966, "Physiological and pharmacological release of monoamines in the central nervous system," in *Mechanisms of Release of Biogenic Amines*, U. S. von Euler, S. Rosell, & B. Unyäs, eds., Pergamon Press, Oxford, pp. 331–346.

Carlsson, A., Davis, J. N., Kehr, W., Lindqvist, M., & Atack, C. V. 1972, "Simultaneous measurement of tyrosine and tryptophan hydroxylase activities in brain in vivo using an inhibitor of the aromatic amino acid decarboxylase", *Naunyn Schmiedebergs Arch. Pharmacol.*, vol. **275**, no. 2, pp. 153–168.

Carlsson, A., Falck, B., & Hillarp, N. A. 1962, "Cellular localization of brain monoamines", *Acta Physiol. Scand. Suppl.*, vol. **56**, no. 196, pp. 1–28.

Carlsson, A., Kehr, W., & Lindqvist, M. 1976, "The role of intraneuronal amine levels in the feedback control of dopamine, noradrenaline and 5-hydroxytryptamine synthesis in rat brain", *J. Neural Transm.*, vol. **39**, no. 1–2, pp. 1–19.

Carlsson, A., Kehr, W., & Lindqvist, M. 1977, "Agonist – antagonist interaction on dopamine receptors in brain, as reflected in the rates of tyrosine and tryptophan hydroxylation", *J. Neural Transm.*, vol. **40**, no. 2, pp. 99–113.

Carlsson, A. & Lindqvist, M. 1963, "Effect of chlorpromazine or haloperidol on formation of 3methoxytyramine and normetanephrine in mouse brain", *Acta Pharmacol. Toxicol. (Copenh)*, vol. **20**, pp. 140–144.

Carlsson, A., Lindqvist, M., & Magnusson, T. 1957, "3,4-Dihydroxyphenylalanine and 5-hydroxytryptophan as reserpine antagonists", *Nature*, vol. **180**, no. 4596, p. 1200.

Carson, R. E., Breier, A., de Bartolomeis, A., Saunders, R. C., Su, T. P., Schmall, B., Der, M. G., Pickar, D., & Eckelman, W. C. 1997, "Quantification of amphetamine-induced changes in [11C]raclopride binding with continuous infusion", *J. Cereb. Blood Flow Metab.*, vol. **17**, no. 4, pp. 437–447.

Caspi, A., Moffitt, T. E., Cannon, M., McClay, J., Murray, R., Harrington, H., Taylor, A., Arseneault, L., Williams, B., Braithwaite, A., Poulton, R., & Craig, I. W. 2005, "Moderation of the effect of adolescent-onset cannabis use on adult psychosis by a functional polymorphism in the catechol-O-methyltransferase gene:

longitudinal evidence of a gene X environment interaction", *Biol. Psychiatry*, vol. **57**, no. 10, pp. 1117–1127.

Cassel, G. & Persson, S. A. 1992, "Effects of acute lethal cyanide intoxication on central dopaminergic pathways", *Pharmacol. Toxicol.*, vol. **70**, no. 2, pp. 148–151.

Caviness, J. N. & Wightman, R. M. 1982, "Use of rapid superfusion to differentiate the release of dopamine from striatal tissue induced by sympathomimetic amines from release induced by potassium", *J. Pharmacol. Exp. Ther.*, vol. **223**, no. 1, pp. 90–96.

Centonze, D., Gubellini, P., Bernardi, G., & Calabresi, P. 1999, "Permissive role of interneurons in corticostriatal synaptic plasticity", *Brain Res. Brain Res. Rev.*, vol. **31**, no. 1, pp. 1–5.

Cervenka, S., Bäckman, L., Cselényi, Z., Halldin, C., & Farde, L. 2008, "Associations between dopamine D2-receptor binding and cognitive performance indicate functional compartmentalization of the human striatum", *Neuroimage*, vol. **40**, no. 3, pp. 1287–1295.

Cervenka, S., Palhagen, S. E., Comley, R. A., Panagiotidis, G., Cselenyi, Z., Matthews, J. C., Lai, R. Y., Halldin, C., & Farde, L. 2006, "Support for dopaminergic hypoactivity in restless legs syndrome: a PET study on D2-receptor binding", *Brain*, vol. **129** (Pt 8), pp. 2017–2028.

Chalon, S., Emond, P., Bodard, S., Vilar, M. P., Thiercelin, C., Besnard, J. C., & Guilloteau, D. 1999, "Time course of changes in striatal dopamine transporters and D2 receptors with specific iodinated markers in a rat model of Parkinson's disease", *Synapse*, vol. **31**, no. 2, pp. 134–139.

Chalon, S., Hall, H., Saba, W., Garreau, L., Dolle, F., Halldin, C., Emond, P., Bottlaender, M., Deloye, J. B., Helfenbein, J., Madelmont, J. C., Bodard, S., Mincheva, Z., Besnard, J. C., & Guilloteau, D. 2006, "Pharmacological characterization of (E)-N-(4-fluorobut-2-enyl)-2beta-carbomethoxy-3beta-(4'-tolyl) nortropane (LBT-999) as a highly promising fluorinated ligand for the dopamine transporter", *J. Pharmacol. Exp. Ther.*, vol. **317**, no. 1, pp. 147–152.

Chan, G. L., Holden, J. E., Stoessl, A. J., Samii, A., Doudet, D. J., Dobko, T., Morrison, K. S., Adam, M., Schulzer, M., Calne, D. B., & Ruth, T. J. 1999, "Reproducibility studies with 11C-DTBZ, a monoamine vesicular transporter inhibitor in healthy human subjects", *J. Nucl. Med.*, vol. **40**, no. 2, pp. 283–289.

Checkoway, H., Powers, K., Smith-Weller, T., Franklin, G. M., Longstreth, W. T., Jr., & Swanson, P. D. 2002, "Parkinson's disease risks associated with cigarette smoking, alcohol consumption, and caffeine intake", *Am. J. Epidemiol.*, vol. **155**, no. 8, pp. 732–738.

Chen, G. & Ewing, A. G. 1995, "Multiple classes of catecholamine vesicles observed during exocytosis from the Planorbis cell body", *Brain Res.*, vol. **701**, no. 1–2, pp. 167–174.

Chen, L., He, M., Sibille, E., Thompson, A., Sarnyai, Z., Baker, H., Shippenberg, T., & Toth, M. 1999, "Adaptive changes in postsynaptic dopamine receptors despite unaltered dopamine dynamics in mice lacking monoamine oxidase B", *J. Neurochem.*, vol. **73**, no. 2, pp. 647–655.

Chen, M. K., Lee, J. S., McGlothan, J. L., Furukawa, E., Adams, R. J., Alexander, M., Wong, D. F., & Guilarte, T. R. 2006, "Acute manganese administration alters dopamine transporter levels in the non-human primate striatum", *Neurotoxicology*, vol. **27**, no. 2, pp. 229–236.

Chen, N. H., Lai, Y. J., & Pan, W. H. 1997, "Effects of different perfusion medium on the extracellular basal concentration of dopamine in striatum and medial prefrontal cortex: a zero-net flux microdialysis study", *Neurosci. Lett.*, vol. **225**, no. 3, pp. 197–200.

Chen, Y., Hillefors-Berglund, M., Herrera-Marschitz, M., Bjelke, B., Gross, J., Andersson, K., & von Euler, G. 1997, "Perinatal asphyxia induces long-term changes in dopamine D1, D2, and D3 receptor binding in the rat brain", *Exp. Neurol.*, vol. **146**, no. 1, pp. 74–80.

Cheon, K. A., Ryu, Y. H., Kim, Y. K., Namkoong, K., Kim, C. H., & Lee, J. D. 2003, "Dopamine transporter density in the basal ganglia assessed with [123I]IPT SPET in children with attention deficit hyperactivity disorder", *Eur. J. Nucl. Med. Mol. Imaging*, vol. **30**, no. 2, pp. 306–311.

Cheon, K. A., Ryu, Y. H., Namkoong, K., Kim, C. H., Kim, J. J., & Lee, J. D. 2004, "Dopamine transporter density of the basal ganglia assessed with [123I]IPT SPECT in drug-naive children with Tourette's disorder", *Psychiatry Res.*, vol. **130**, no. 1, pp. 85–95.

Chien, J. B., Wallingford, R. A., & Ewing, A. G. 1990, "Estimation of free dopamine in the cytoplasm of the giant dopamine cell of Planorbis corneus by voltammetry and capillary electrophoresis", *J. Neurochem.*, vol. **54**, no. 2, pp. 633–638.

Chiodo, L. A., Bannon, M. J., Grace, A. A., Roth, R. H., & Bunney, B. S. 1984, "Evidence for the absence of impulse-regulating somatodendritic and synthesis-modulating nerve terminal autoreceptors on subpopulations of mesocortical dopamine neurons", *Neuroscience*, vol. **12**, no. 1, pp. 1–16.

Cho, S., Duchemin, A. M., Neff, N. H., & Hadjiconstantinou, M. 1996, "Modulation of tyrosine hydroxylase and aromatic L-amino acid decarboxylase after inhibiting monoamine oxidase-A", *Eur. J. Pharmacol.*, vol. **314**, no. 1–2, pp. 51–59.

Chou, Y. H., Karlsson, P., Halldin, C., Olsson, H., & Farde, L. 1999, "A PET study of D(1)-like dopamine receptor ligand binding during altered endogenous dopamine levels in the primate brain", *Psychopharmacology (Berl)*, vol. **146**, no. 2, pp. 220–227.

Christenson, J. G., Dairman, W., & Udenfriend, S. 1970, "Preparation and properties of a homogeneous aromatic L-amino acid decarboxylase from hog kidney", *Arch. Biochem. Biophys.*, vol. **141**, no. 1, pp. 356–367.

Chugani, D. C., Ackermann, R. F., & Phelps, M. E. 1988, "In vivo [3H]spiperone binding: evidence for accumulation in corpus striatum by agonist-mediated receptor internalization", *J. Cereb. Blood Flow Metab.*, vol. **8**, no. 3, pp. 291–303.

Ciliax, B. J., Nash, N., Heilman, C., Sunahara, R., Hartney, A., Tiberi, M., Rye, D. B., Caron, M. G., Niznik, H. B., & Levey, A. I. 2000, "Dopamine D(5) receptor immunolocalization in rat and monkey brain", *Synapse*, vol. **37**, no. 2, pp. 125–145.

Clarke, P. B. & Pert, A. 1985, "Autoradiographic evidence for nicotine receptors on nigrostriatal and mesolimbic dopaminergic neurons", *Brain Res.*, vol. **348**, no. 2, pp. 355–358.

Cline, E. J., Adams, C. E., Larson, G. A., Gerhardt, G. A., & Zahniser, N. R. 1995, "Medial dorsal striatum is more sensitive than lateral dorsal striatum to cocaine inhibition of exogenous dopamine clearance: relation to [3H]mazindol binding, but not striosome/matrix", *Exp. Neurol.*, vol. **134**, no. 1, pp. 135–149.

Cohen, G., Heikkila, R. E., Allis, B., Cabbat, F., Dembiec, D., MacNamee, D., Mytilineou, C., & Winston, B. 1976, "Destruction of sympathetic nerve terminals by 6-hydroxydopamine: protection by 1-phenyl-3-(2-thiazolyl)-2-thiourea, diethyldithiocarbamate, methimazole, cysteamine, ethanol and n-butanol", *J. Pharmacol. Exp. Ther.*, vol. **199**, no. 2, pp. 336–352.

Collins, F. A., Murphy, D. L., Reiss, A. L., Sims, K. B., Lewis, J. G., Freund, L., Karoum, F., Zhu, D., Maumenee, I. H., & Antonarakis, S. E. 1992, "Clinical, biochemical, and neuropsychiatric evaluation of a patient with a contiguous gene syndrome due to a microdeletion Xp11.3 including the Norrie disease locus and monoamine oxidase (MAOA and MAOB) genes", *Am. J. Med. Genet.*, vol. **42**, no. 1, pp. 127–134.

Commissiong, J. W. 1985, "Monoamine metabolites: their relationship and lack of relationship to monoaminergic neuronal activity", *Biochem. Pharmacol.*, vol. **34**, no. 8, pp. 1127–1131.

Cools, R., Gibbs, S. E., Miyakawa, A., Jagust, W., & D'Esposito, M. 2008, "Working memory capacity predicts dopamine synthesis capacity in the human stratum", *J. Neurosci.*, vol. **28**, no. 5, pp. 1208–1212.

Copeland, B. J., Vogelsberg, V., Neff, N. H., & Hadjiconstantinou, M. 1996, "Protein kinase C activators decrease dopamine uptake into striatal synaptosomes", *J. Pharmacol. Exp. Ther.*, vol. **277**, no. 3, pp. 1527–1532.

Corrigall, W. A., Franklin, K. B., Coen, K. M., & Clarke, P. B. 1992, "The mesolimbic dopaminergic system is implicated in the reinforcing effects of nicotine", *Psychopharmacology (Berl)*, vol. **107**, no. 2–3, pp. 285–289.

Corvol, J. C., Muriel, M. P., Valjent, E., Feger, J., Hanoun, N., Girault, J. A., Hirsch, E. C., & Herve, D. 2004, "Persistent increase in olfactory type G-protein alpha subunit levels may underlie D1 receptor functional hypersensitivity in Parkinson disease", *J. Neurosci.*, vol. **24**, no. 31, pp. 7007–7014.

Cowell, R. M., Kantor, L., Hewlett, G. H., Frey, K. A., & Gnegy, M. E. 2000, "Dopamine transporter antagonists block phorbol ester-induced dopamine release and dopamine transporter phosphorylation in striatal synaptosomes", *Eur. J. Pharmacol.*, vol. **389**, no. 1, pp. 59–65.

Crawford, C. A., McDougall, S. A., & Bardo, M. T. 1994, "Effects of EEDQ on the synthesis and metabolism of dopamine in preweanling and adult rats", *Neuropharmacology*, vol. **33**, no. 12, pp. 1559–1565.

Crossman, A. R., Sambrook, M. A., Gergies, S. W., & Slater, P. 1977, "The neurological basis of motor asymmetry following unilateral 6-hydroxydopamine brain lesions in the rat: the effect of motor decortication", *J. Neurol. Sci.*, vol. **34**, no. 3, pp. 407–414.

Cumming, P., Ase, A., Diksic, M., Harrison, J., Jolly, D., Kuwabara, H., Laliberte, C., & Gjedde, A. 1995a, "Metabolism and blood-brain clearance of L-3,4-dihydroxy-[3H]phenylalanine ([3H]DOPA) and 6-[18F]fluoro-L-DOPA in the rat", *Biochem. Pharmacol.*, vol. **50**, no. 7, pp. 943–946.

Cumming, P., Ase, A., Kuwabara, H., & Gjedde, A. 1998, "[3H]DOPA formed from [3H]tyrosine in living rat brain is not committed to dopamine synthesis", *J. Cereb. Blood Flow Metab.*, vol. **18**, no. 5, pp. 491–499.

Cumming, P., Ase, A., Laliberte, C., Kuwabara, H., & Gjedde, A. 1997a, "In vivo regulation of DOPA decarboxylase by dopamine receptors in rat brain", *J. Cereb. Blood Flow Metab.*, vol. **17**, no. 11, pp. 1254–1260.

Cumming, P., Boyes, B. E., Martin, W. R., Adam, M., Grierson, J., Ruth, T., & McGeer, E. G. 1987a, "The metabolism of [18F]6-fluoro-L-3,4-dihydroxyphenylalanine in the hooded rat", *J. Neurochem.*, vol. **48**, no. 2, pp. 601–608.

Cumming, P., Boyes, B. E., Martin, W. R., Adam, M., Ruth, T. J., & McGeer, E. G. 1987b, "Altered metabolism of [18F]-6-fluorodopa in the hooded rat following inhibition of catechol-O-methyltransferase with U-0521", *Biochem. Pharmacol.*, vol. **36**, no. 15, pp. 2527–2531.

Cumming, P., Brown, E., Damsma, G., & Fibiger, H. 1992, "Formation and clearance of interstitial metabolites of dopamine and serotonin in the rat striatum: an in vivo microdialysis study", *J. Neurochem.*, vol. **59**, no. 5, pp. 1905–1914.

Cumming, P., Danielsen, E. H., Vafaee, M., Falborg, L., Steffensen, E., Sorensen, J. C., Gillings, N., Bender, D., Marthi, K., Andersen, F., Munk, O., Smith, D., Moller, A., & Gjedde, A. 2001, "Normalization of markers for dopamine innervation in striatum of MPTP-lesioned miniature pigs with intrastriatal grafts", *Acta Neurol. Scand.*, vol. **103**, no. 5, pp. 309–315.

Cumming, P., Gillings, N. M., Jensen, S. B., Bjarkam, C., & Gjedde, A. 2003a, "Kinetics of the uptake and distribution of the dopamine D(2,3) agonist (R)-N-[1-(11)C]n-propylnorapomorphine in brain of healthy and MPTP-treated Gottingen miniature pigs", *Nucl. Med. Biol.*, vol. **30**, no. 5, pp. 547–553.

Cumming, P. & Gjedde, A. 1998, "Compartmental analysis of dopa decarboxylation in living brain from dynamic positron emission tomograms", *Synapse*, vol. **29**, no. 1, pp. 37–61.

Cumming, P., Hausser, M., Martin, W. R., Grierson, J., Adam, M. J., Ruth, T. J., & McGeer, E. G. 1988, "Kinetics of in vitro decarboxylation and the in vivo metabolism of 2-18F- and 6-18F-fluorodopa in the hooded rat", *Biochem. Pharmacol.*, vol. **37**, no. 2, pp. 247–250.

Cumming, P., Kuwabara, H., Ase, A., & Gjedde, A. 1995b, "Regulation of DOPA decarboxylase activity in brain of living rat", *J. Neurochem.*, vol. **65**, no. 3, pp. 1381–1390.

Cumming, P., Kuwabara, H., & Gjedde, A. 1994, "A kinetic analysis of 6-[18F] fluoro-L-dihydroxyphenylalanine metabolism in the rat", *J. Neurochem.*, vol. **63**, no. 5, pp. 1675–1682.

Cumming, P., Leger, G. C., Kuwabara, H., & Gjedde, A. 1993, "Pharmacokinetics of plasma 6-[18F]fluoro-L-3,4-dihydroxyphenylalanine ([18F]fdopa) in humans", *J. Cereb. Blood Flow Metab.*, vol. **13**, no. 4, pp. 668–675.

Cumming, P., Ljubic-Thibal, V., Laliberte, C., & Diksic, M. 1997b, "The effect of unilateral neurotoxic lesions to serotonin fibres in the medial forebrain bundle on the metabolism of [3H]DOPA in the telencephalon of the living rat", *Brain Res.*, vol. **747**, no. 1, pp. 60–69.

Cumming, P., Munk, O. L., & Doudet, D. 2001, "Loss of metabolites from monkey striatum during PET with FDOPA", *Synapse*, vol. **41**, no. 3, pp. 212–218.

Cumming, P., Rosa-Neto, P., Watanabe, H., Smith, D., Bender, D., Clarke, P. B., & Gjedde, A. 2003b, "Effects of acute nicotine on hemodynamics and binding of [11C]raclopride to dopamine D2,3 receptors in pig brain", *Neuroimage*, vol. **19**, no. 3, pp. 1127–1136.

Cumming, P., Venkatachalam, T. K., Rajagopal, S., Diksic, M., & Gjedde, A. 1994, "Brain uptake of alpha-[14C]methyl-para-tyrosine in the rat", *Synapse*, vol. **17**, no. 2, pp. 125–128.

Cumming, P., Wong, D. F., Gillings, N., Hilton, J., Scheffel, U., & Gjedde, A. 2002, "Specific binding of [(11)C]raclopride and N-[(3)H]propyl-norapomorphine to dopamine receptors in living mouse striatum: occupancy by endogenous dopamine and guanosine triphosphate-free G protein", *J. Cereb. Blood Flow Metab.*, vol. **22**, no. 5, pp. 596–604.

Cumming, P., Yokoi, F., Chen, A., Deep, P., Dagher, A., Reutens, D., Kapczinski, F., Wong, D. F., & Gjedde, A. 1999, "Pharmacokinetics of radiotracers in human plasma during positron emission tomography", *Synapse*, vol. **34**, no. 2, pp. 124–134.

Curzon, G., Hutson, P. H., Kantamaneni, B. D., Sahakian, B. J., & Sarna, G. S. 1985, "3,4-Dihydroxyphenylethylamine and 5-hydroxytryptamine metabolism in the rat: acidic metabolites in cisternal cerebrospinal fluid before and after giving probenecid", *J. Neurochem.*, vol. **45**, no. 2, pp. 508–513.

Curzon, G., Hutson, P. H., Kennett, G. A., Marcou, M., & Sarna, G. S. 1986, "Monitoring dopamine metabolism in the brain of the freely moving rat", *Ann. N.Y. Acad. Sci.*, vol. **473**, pp. 224–238.

Czoty, P. W., Gage, H. D., & Nader, M. A. 2005, "PET imaging of striatal dopamine D2 receptors in nonhuman primates: increases in availability produced by chronic raclopride treatment", *Synapse*, vol. **58**, no. 4, pp. 215–219.

Dagher, A., Bleicher, C., Aston, J. A., Gunn, R. N., Clarke, P. B., & Cumming, P. 2001, "Reduced dopamine D1 receptor binding in the ventral striatum of cigarette smokers", *Synapse*, vol. **42**, no. 1, pp. 48–53.

Dall, A. M., Danielsen, E. H., Sorensen, J. C., Andersen, F., Moller, A., Zimmer, J., Gjedde, A. H., & Cumming, P. 2002, "Quantitative [18F]fluorodopa/PET and histology of fetal mesencephalic dopaminergic grafts to the striatum of MPTP-poisoned minipigs", *Cell Transplant.*, vol. **11**, no. 8, pp. 733–746.

Dalley, J. W., Fryer, T. D., Brichard, L., Robinson, E. S., Theobald, D. E., Laane, K., Pena, Y., Murphy, E. R., Shah, Y., Probst, K., Abakumova, I., Aigbirhio, F. I., Richards, H. K., Hong, Y., Baron, J. C., Everitt, B. J., & Robbins, T. W. 2007, "Nucleus accumbens D2/3 receptors predict trait impulsivity and cocaine reinforcement", *Science*, vol. **315**, no. 5816, pp. 1267–1270.

Daniels, A. J. & Reinhard, J. F., Jr. 1988, "Energy-driven uptake of the neurotoxin 1-methyl-4-phenylpyridinium into chromaffin granules via the catecholamine transporter", *J. Biol. Chem.*, vol. **263**, no. 11, pp. 5034–5036.

Danielsen, E. H., Smith, D. F., Gee, A. D., Venkatachalam, T. K., Hansen, S. B., Hermansen, F., Gjedde, A., & Cumming, P. 1999, "Cerebral 6-[(18)F]fluoro-L-DOPA (FDOPA) metabolism in pig studied by positron emission tomography", *Synapse*, vol. **33**, no. 4, pp. 247–258.

Darchen, F., Masuo, Y., Vial, M., Rostene, W., & Scherman, D. 1989, "Quantitative autoradiography of the rat brain vesicular monoamine transporter using the binding of [3H]dihydrotetrabenazine and 7-amino-8-[125I]iodoketanserin", *Neuroscience*, vol. **33**, no. 2, pp. 341–349.

de la Fuente-Fernandez, R., Furtado, S., Guttman, M., Furukawa, Y., Lee, C. S., Calne, D. B., Ruth, T. J., & Stoessl, A. J. 2003, "VMAT2 binding is elevated in dopa-responsive dystonia: visualizing empty vesicles by PET", *Synapse*, vol. **49**, no. 1, pp. 20–28.

de la Fuente-Fernandez, R., Lim, A. S., Sossi, V., Holden, J. E., Calne, D. B., Ruth, T. J., Stoessl, A. J. 2001, "Apomorphine-induced changes in synaptic dopamine levels: positron emission tomography evidence for presynaptic inhibition", *J. Cereb. Blood Flow Metab.*, vol. **21**, no. 10, pp. 1151–1159.

de la Fuente-Fernandez, R., Ruth, T. J., Sossi, V., Schulzer, M., Calne, D. B., & Stoessl, A. J. 2001, "Expectation and dopamine release: mechanism of the placebo effect in Parkinson's disease", *Science*, vol. **293**, no. 5532, pp. 1164–1166.

de la Fuente-Fernandez, Sossi, V., Huang, Z., Furtado, S., Lu, J. Q., Calne, D. B., Ruth, T. J., & Stoessl, A. J. 2004, "Levodopa-induced changes in synaptic dopamine levels increase with progression of Parkinson's disease: implications for dyskinesias", *Brain*, vol. **127** (Pt 12), pp. 2747–2754.

de Win, M. M., Habraken, J. B., Reneman, L., van den Brink, W., den Heeten, G. J., & Booij, J. 2005, "Validation of [(123)I]beta-CIT SPECT to assess serotonin transporters in vivo in humans: a double-blind, placebo-controlled, crossover study with the selective serotonin reuptake inhibitor citalopram", *Neuropsychopharmacology*, vol. **30**, no. 5, pp. 996–1005.

Decamp, E., Wade, T., & Schneider, J. S. 1999, "Differential regulation of striatal dopamine D(1) and D(2) receptors in acute and chronic parkinsonian monkeys", *Brain Res.*, vol. **847**, no. 1, pp. 134–138.

Dedek, J., Baumes, R., Tien-Duc, N., Gomeni, R., & Korf, J. 1979, "Turnover of free and conjugated (sulphonyloxy) dihydroxyphenylacetic acid and homovanillic acid in rat striatum", *J. Neurochem.*, vol. **33**, no. 3, pp. 687–695.

Dedek, J., Gomeni, R., & Korf, J. 1979, "A model of dopamine metabolism in rat brain, assessed by the influence of drugs [proceedings]", *Arch. Int. Physiol Biochim.*, vol. **87**, no. 4, pp. 794–795.

Deep, P., Gjedde, A., & Cumming, P. 1997, "On the accuracy of an [18F]FDOPA compartmental model: evidence for vesicular storage of [18F]fluorodopamine in vivo", *J. Neurosci. Methods*, vol. **76**, no. 2, pp. 157–165.

Deep, P., Kuwabara, H., Gjedde, A., & Cumming, P. 1997, "The kinetic behaviour of [3H] DOPA in living rat brain investigated by compartmental modelling of static autoradiograms", *J. Neurosci. Methods*, vol. **78**, no. 1–2, pp. 157–168.

Dekker, M. C., Eshuis, S. A., Maguire, R. P., van der Veenma, D. L., Pruim, J., Snijders, P. J., Oostra, B. A., van Duijn, C. M., & Leenders, K. L. 2004, "PET neuroimaging and mutations in the DJ-1 gene", *J. Neural Transm.*, vol. **111**, no. 12, pp. 1575–1581.

Del Zompo M., Piccardi, M. P., Ruiu, S., Corsini, G. U., & Vaccari, A. 1992, "Characterization of a putatively vesicular binding site for [3H]MPP+ in mouse striatal membranes", *Brain Res.*, vol. **571**, no. 2, pp. 354–357.

Demarest, K. T. & Moore, K. E. 1979, "Comparison of dopamine synthesis regulation in the terminals of nigrostriatal, mesolimbic, tuberoinfundibular and tuberohypophyseal neurons", *J. Neural Transm.*, vol. **46**, no. 4, pp. 263–277.

Demarest, K. T., Smith, D. J., & Azzaro, A. J. 1980, "The presence of the type A form of monoamine oxidase within nigrostriatal dopamine-containing neurons", *J. Pharmacol. Exp. Ther.*, vol. **215**, no. 2, pp. 461–468.

Desnos, C., Laran, M. P., Langley, K., Aunis, D., & Henry, J. P. 1995, "Long term stimulation changes the vesicular monoamine transporter content of chromaffin granules", *J. Biol. Chem.*, vol. **270**, no. 27, pp. 16030–16038.

Dewey, S. L., Brodie, J. D., Gerasimov, M., Horan, B., Gardner, E. L., & Ashby, C. R., Jr. 1999, "A pharmacologic strategy for the treatment of nicotine addiction", *Synapse*, vol. **31**, no. 1, pp. 76–86.

Dewey, S. L., Logan, J., Wolf, A. P., Brodie, J. D., Angrist, B., Fowler, J. S., & Volkow, N. D. 1991, "Amphetamine induced decreases in (18F)-N-methylspiroperidol binding in the baboon brain using positron emission tomography (PET)", *Synapse*, vol. **7**, no. 4, pp. 324–327.

Dewey, S. L., Smith, G. S., Logan, J., Brodie, J. D., Yu, D. W., Ferrieri, R. A., King, P. T., MacGregor, R. R., Martin, T. P., Wolf, A. P., & *et al.* 1992, "GABAergic inhibition of endogenous dopamine release measured in vivo with 11C-raclopride and positron emission tomography", *J. Neurosci.*, vol. **12**, no. 10, pp. 3773–3780.

Di Chiara G., Bassareo, V., Fenu, S., De Luca, M. A., Spina, L., Cadoni, C., Acquas, E., Carboni, E., Valentini, V., & Lecca, D. 2004, "Dopamine and drug addiction: the nucleus accumbens shell connection", *Neuropharmacology*, vol. **47** (Suppl. 1), pp. 227–241.

Di Chiara G. & Imperato, A. 1988, "Drugs abused by humans preferentially increase synaptic dopamine concentrations in the mesolimbic system of freely moving rats", *Proc. Natl. Acad. Sci. USA*, vol. **85**, no. 14, pp. 5274–5278.

Di Giulio, A. M., Groppetti, A., Cattabeni, F., Galli, C. L., Maggi, A., Algeri, S., & Ponzio, F. 1978, "Significance of dopamine metabolites in the evaluation of drugs acting on dopaminergic neurons", *Eur. J. Pharmacol.*, vol. **52**, no. 2, pp. 201–207.

Dickinson, S. D., Sabeti, J., Larson, G. A., Giardina, K., Rubinstein, M., Kelly, M. A., Grandy, D. K., Low, M. J., Gerhardt, G. A., & Zahniser, N. R. 1999, "Dopamine D2 receptor-deficient mice exhibit decreased dopamine transporter function but no changes in dopamine release in dorsal striatum", *J. Neurochem.*, vol. **72**, no. 1, pp. 148–156.

Ding, Y. S., Logan, J., Gatley, S. J., Fowler, J. S., & Volkow, N. D. 1998, "PET studies of peripheral catechol-O-methyltransferase in non-human primates using [18F]Ro41-0960", *J. Neural Transm.*, vol. **105**, no. 10–12, pp. 1199–1211.

Dluzen, D., Reddy, A., & McDermott, J. 1992, "The aromatic amino acid decarboxylase inhibitor, NSD-1015, increases release of dopamine: response characteristics", *Neuropharmacology*, vol. **31**, no. 12, pp. 1223–1229.

Dominici, P., Filipponi, P., Schinina, M. E., Barra, D., & Borri, V. C. 1990, "Pig kidney dopa decarboxylase. Structure and function", *Ann. N.Y. Acad. Sci.*, vol. **585**, pp. 162–172.

Donaldson, I., Dolphin, A., Jenner, P., Marsden, C. D., & Pycock, C. 1976, "The roles of noradrenaline and dopamine in contraversive circling behaviour seen after unilateral electrolytic lesions of the locus coeruleus", *Eur. J. Pharmacol.*, vol. **39**, no. 2, pp. 179–191.

Doteuchi, M., Wang, C., & Costa, E. 1974, "Compartmentation of dopamine in rat striatum", *Mol. Pharmacol.*, vol. **10**, no. 2, pp. 225–234.

Doudet, D. J. & Holden, J. E. 2003, "Sequential versus nonsequential measurement of density and affinity of dopamine D2 receptors with [11C]raclopride: effect of methamphetamine", *J. Cereb. Blood Flow Metab.*, vol. **23**, no. 12, pp. 1489–1494.

Doudet, D. J., Jivan, S., Ruth, T. J., & Wyatt, R. J. 2002, "In vivo PET studies of the dopamine D1 receptors in rhesus monkeys with long-term MPTP-induced Parkinsonism", *Synapse*, vol. **44**, no. 2, pp. 111–115.

Doudet, D. J., Rosa-Neto, P., Munk, O. L., Ruth, T. J., Jivan, S., & Cumming, P. 2006, "Effect of age on markers for monoaminergic neurons of normal and MPTP-lesioned rhesus monkeys: a multi-tracer PET study", *Neuroimage*, vol. **30**, no. 1, pp. 26–35.

Doudet, D. J., Ruth, T. J., & Holden, J. E. 2006, "Sequential versus nonsequential measurement of density and affinity of dopamine D2 receptors with [11C]raclopride: 2: effects of DAT inhibitors", *J. Cereb. Blood Flow Metab.*, vol. **26**, no. 1, pp. 28–37.

Dougherty, D. D., Bonab, A. A., Ottowitz, W. E., Livni, E., Alpert, N. M., Rauch, S. L., Fava, M., & Fischman, A. J. 2006, "Decreased striatal D1 binding as measured using PET and [11C]SCH 23,390 in patients with major depression with anger attacks", *Depress Anxiety*, vol. **23**, no. 3, pp. 175–177.

Dresel, S., Krause, J., Krause, K. H., LaFougere, C., Brinkbaumer, K., Kung, H. F., Hahn, K., & Tatsch, K. 2000, "Attention deficit hyperactivity disorder: binding of [99mTc]TRODAT-1 to the dopamine transporter before and after methylphenidate treatment", *Eur. J. Nucl. Med.*, vol. **27**, no. 10, pp. 1518–1524.

Dresel, S. H., Kung, M. P., Huang, X., Plossl, K., Hou, C., Shiue, C. Y., Karp, J., & Kung, H. F. 1999, "In vivo imaging of serotonin transporters with [99mTc]TRODAT-1 in nonhuman primates", *Eur. J. Nucl. Med.*, vol. **26**, no. 4, pp. 342–347.

Drevets, W. C., Gautier, C., Price, J. C., Kupfer, D. J., Kinahan, P. E., Grace, A. A., Price, J. L., & Mathis, C. A. 2001, "Amphetamine-induced dopamine release in human ventral striatum correlates with euphoria", *Biol. Psychiatry*, vol. **49**, no. 2, pp. 81–96.

Dugast, C., Brun, P., Sotty, F., Renaud, B., & Suaud-Chagny, M. F. 1997, "On the involvement of a tonic dopamine D2-autoinhibition in the regulation of pulse-to-pulse-evoked dopamine release in the rat striatum in vivo", *Naunyn Schmiedebergs Arch. Pharmacol.*, vol. **355**, no. 6, pp. 716–719.

Dumartin, B., Caille, I., Gonon, F., & Bloch, B. 1998, "Internalization of D1 dopamine receptor in striatal neurons in vivo as evidence of activation by dopamine agonists", *J. Neurosci.*, vol. **18**, no. 5, pp. 1650–1661.

Durden, D. A. & Philips, S. R. 1980, "Kinetic measurements of the turnover rates of phenylethylamine and tryptamine in vivo in the rat brain", *J. Neurochem.*, vol. **34**, no. 6, pp. 1725–1732.

During, M. J., Acworth, I. N., & Wurtman, R. J. 1988a, "Effects of systemic L-tyrosine on dopamine release from rat corpus striatum and nucleus accumbens", *Brain Res.*, vol. **452**, no. 1–2, pp. 378–380.

During, M. J., Acworth, I. N., & Wurtman, R. J. 1988b, "Phenylalanine administration influences dopamine release in the rat's corpus striatum", *Neurosci. Lett.*, vol. **93**, no. 1, pp. 91–95.

During, M. J., Acworth, I. N., & Wurtman, R. J. 1989, "Dopamine release in rat striatum: physiological coupling to tyrosine supply", *J. Neurochem.*, vol. **52**, no. 5, pp. 1449–1454.

Dyck, L. E. 1987, "Effect of decarboxylase inhibitors on brain p-tyrosine levels", *Biochem. Pharmacol.*, vol. **36**, no. 8, pp. 1373–1376.

Ebadi, M. & Simonneaux, V. 1991, "Ambivalence on the multiplicity of mammalian aromatic L-amino acid decarboxylase", *Adv. Exp. Med. Biol.*, vol. **294**, pp. 115–125.

Ebert, D., Feistel, H., Kaschka, W., Barocka, A., & Pirner, A. 1994, "Single photon emission computerized tomography assessment of cerebral dopamine D2 receptor blockade in depression before and after sleep deprivation – preliminary results", *Biol. Psychiatry*, vol. **35**, no. 11, pp. 880–885.

Ebinger, M. & Uhr, M. 2006, "ABC drug transporter at the blood-brain barrier: effects on drug metabolism and drug response", *Eur. Arch. Psychiatry Clin. Neurosci.*, vol. **256**, no. 5, pp. 294–298.

Ehringer, H. & Hornykiewicz, O. 1960, "[Distribution of noradrenaline and dopamine (3-hydroxytyramine) in the human brain and their behavior in diseases of the extrapyramidal system]", *Klin. Wochenschr.*, vol. **38**, pp. 1236–1239.

Ekelund, J., Slifstein, M., Narendran, R., Guillin, O., Belani, H., Guo, N. N., Hwang, Y., Hwang, D. R., Abi-Dargham, A., & Laruelle, M. 2007, "In vivo DA D(1) receptor selectivity of NNC 112 and SCH 23390", *Mol. Imaging Biol.*, vol. **9**, no. 3, pp. 117–125.

Elazar, Z. & Fuchs, S. 1991, "Phosphorylation by cyclic AMP-dependent protein kinase modulates agonist binding to the D2 dopamine receptor", *J. Neurochem.*, vol. **56**, no. 1, pp. 75–80.

Elghozi, J. L., Mignot, E., & Le Quan-Bui, K. H. 1983, "Probenecid sensitive pathway of elimination of dopamine and serotonin metabolites in CSF of the rat", *J. Neural Transm.*, vol. **57**, no. 1–2, pp. 85–94.

Elsworth, J. D., Brittan, M. S., Taylor, J. R., Sladek, J. R., Jr., Redmond, D. E., Jr., Innis, R. B., Zea-Ponce, Y., & Roth, R. H. 1998, "Upregulation of striatal D2 receptors in the MPTP-treated vervet monkey is reversed by grafts of fetal ventral mesencephalon: an autoradiographic study", *Brain Res.*, vol. **795**, no. 1–2, pp. 55–62.

Elverfors, A., Pileblad, E., Lagerkvist, S., Bergquist, F., Jonason, J., & Nissbrandt, H. 1997, "3-Methoxytyramine formation following monoamine oxidase inhibition is a poor index of dendritic dopamine release in the substantia nigra", *J. Neurochem.*, vol. **69**, no. 4, pp. 1684–1692.

Endres, C. J., Kolachana, B. S., Saunders, R. C., Su, T., Weinberger, D., Breier, A., Eckelman, W. C., & Carson, R. E. 1997a, "Kinetic modeling of [11C]raclopride: combined PET-microdialysis studies", *J. Cereb. Blood Flow Metab.*, vol. **17**, no. 9, pp. 932–942.

Endres, C. J., Swaminathan, S., DeJesus, O. T., Sievert, M., Ruoho, A. E., Murali, D., Rommelfanger, S. G., & Holden, J. E. 1997b, "Affinities of dopamine analogs for monoamine granular and plasma membrane transporters: implications for PET dopamine studies", *Life Sci.*, vol. **60**, no. 26, pp. 2399–2406.

Erickson, J. D. & Eiden, L. E. 1993, "Functional identification and molecular cloning of a human brain vesicle monoamine transporter", *J. Neurochem.*, vol. **61**, no. 6, pp. 2314–2317.

Erickson, J. D., Eiden, L. E., & Hoffman, B. J. 1992, "Expression cloning of a reserpine-sensitive vesicular monoamine transporter", *Proc. Natl. Acad. Sci. USA*, vol. **89**, no. 22, pp. 10993–10997.

Ernst, M., Zametkin, A. J., Matochik, J. A., Pascualvaca, D., Jons, P. H., Hardy, K., Hankerson, J. G., Doudet, D. J., & Cohen, R. M. 1996, "Presynaptic dopaminergic deficits in Lesch-Nyhan disease", *N Engl. J. Med.*, vol. **334**, no. 24, pp. 1568–1572.

Evans, A. H., Pavese, N., Lawrence, A. D., Tai, Y. F., Appel, S., Doder, M., Brooks, D. J., Lees, A. J., & Piccini, P. 2006, "Compulsive drug use linked to sensitized ventral striatal dopamine transmission", *Ann. Neurol.*, vol. **59**, no. 5, pp. 852–858.

Fairbrother, I. S., Arbuthnott, G. W., Kelly, J. S., & Butcher, S. P. 1990, "In vivo mechanisms underlying dopamine release from rat nigrostriatal terminals: II. Studies using potassium and tyramine", *J. Neurochem.*, vol. **54**, no. 6, pp. 1844–1851.

Falany, C. N., Vazquez, M. E., Heroux, J. A., & Roth, J. A. 1990, "Purification and characterization of human liver phenol-sulfating phenol sulfotransferase", *Arch. Biochem. Biophys.*, vol. **278**, no. 2, pp. 312–318.

Fan, J. B., Zhang, C. S., Gu, N. F., Li, X. W., Sun, W. W., Wang, H. Y., Feng, G. Y., St. Clair, D., & He, L. 2005, "Catechol-O-methyltransferase gene Val/Met functional polymorphism and risk of schizophrenia: a large-scale association study plus meta-analysis", *Biol. Psychiatry*, vol. **57**, no. 2, pp. 139–144.

Farde, L., Hall, H., Ehrin, E., & Sedvall, G. 1986, "Quantitative analysis of D2 dopamine receptor binding in the living human brain by PET", *Science*, vol. **231**, no. 4735, pp. 258–261.

Farde, L., Hall, H., Pauli, S., & Halldin, C. 1995, "Variability in D2-dopamine receptor density and affinity: a PET study with [11C]raclopride in man", *Synapse*, vol. **20**, no. 3, pp. 200–208.

Farde, L., Halldin, C., Muller, L., Suhara, T., Karlsson, P., & Hall, H. 1994, "PET study of [11C]beta-CIT binding to monoamine transporters in the monkey and human brain", *Synapse*, vol. **16**, no. 2, pp. 93–103.

Farde, L., Suhara, T., Nyberg, S., Karlsson, P., Nakashima, Y., Hietala, J., & Halldin, C. 1997, "A PET-study of [11C]FLB 457 binding to extrastriatal D2-dopamine receptors in healthy subjects and antipsychotic drug-treated patients", *Psychopharmacology (Berl)*, vol. **133**, no. 4, pp. 396–404.

Farde, L., Wiesel, F. A., Stone-Elander, S., Halldin, C., Nordstrom, A. L., Hall, H., & Sedvall, G. 1990, "D2 dopamine receptors in neuroleptic-naive schizophrenic patients. A positron emission tomography study with [11C]raclopride", *Arch. Gen. Psychiatry*, vol. **47**, no. 3, pp. 213–219.

Fedi, M., Berkovic, S. F., Scheffer, I. E., O'Keefe G., Marini, C., Mulligan, R., Gong, S., Tochon-Danguy, H., & Reutens, D. C. 2008, "Reduced striatal D1 receptor binding in autosomal dominant nocturnal frontal lobe epilepsy", *Neurology*, vol. **71**, no. 11, pp. 795–798.

Fernstrom, M. H., Baker, R. L., & Fernstrom, J. D. 1989, "In vivo tyrosine hydroxylation rate in retina: effects of phenylalanine and tyrosine administration in rats pretreated with p-chlorophenylalanine", *Brain Res.*, vol. **499**, no. 2, pp. 291–298.

Ferre, S., von Euler, G., Johansson, B., Fredholm, B. B., & Fuxe, K. 1991, "Stimulation of high-affinity adenosine A2 receptors decreases the affinity of dopamine D2 receptors in rat striatal membranes", *Proc. Natl. Acad. Sci. USA*, vol. **88**, no. 16, pp. 7238–7241.

Fiedler, J. & Daniels, A. J. 1984, "Uptake of magnesium by chromaffin granules in vitro: role of the proton electrochemical gradient", *J. Neurochem.*, vol. **42**, no. 5, pp. 1291–1297.

Filloux, F., Wagster, M. V., Folstein, S., Price, D. L., Hedreen, J. C., Dawson, T. M., & Wamsley, J. K. 1990, "Nigral dopamine type-1 receptors are reduced in Huntington's disease: a postmortem autoradiographic study using [3H]SCH 23390 and correlation with [3H]forskolin binding", *Exp. Neurol.*, vol. **110**, no. 2, pp. 219–227.

Fine, M. I., Masserano, J. M., & Weiner, N. 1986, "The effects of reserpine and haloperidol on tyrosine hydroxylase activity in the brains of aged rats", *Life Sci.*, vol. **39**, no. 3, pp. 235–241.

Finnema, S. J., Seneca, N., Farde, L., Shchukin, E., Sovago, J., Gulyas, B., Wikstrom, H. V., Innis, R. B., Neumeyer, J. L., & Halldin, C. 2005, "A preliminary PET evaluation of the new dopamine D2 receptor agonist [11C]MNPA in cynomolgus monkey", *Nucl. Med. Biol.*, vol. **32**, no. 4, pp. 353–360.

Firnau, G., Sood, S., Chirakal, R., Nahmias, C., & Garnett, E. S. 1987, "Cerebral metabolism of 6-[18F]fluoro-L-3,4-dihydroxyphenylalanine in the primate", *J. Neurochem.*, vol. **48**, no. 4, pp. 1077–1082.

Fischer, J. F. & Cho, A. K. 1979, "Chemical release of dopamine from striatal homogenates: evidence for an exchange diffusion model", *J. Pharmacol. Exp. Ther.*, vol. **208**, no. 2, pp. 203–209.

Fischman, A. J., Bonab, A. A., Babich, J. W., Livni, E., Alpert, N. M., Meltzer, P. C., & Madras, B. K. 2001, "[(11)C, (127)I] Altropane: a highly selective ligand for PET imaging of dopamine transporter sites", *Synapse*, vol. **39**, no. 4, pp. 332–342.

Fischman, A. J., Bonab, A. A., Babich, J. W., Palmer, E. P., Alpert, N. M., Elmaleh, D. R., Callahan, R. J., Barrow, S. A., Graham, W., Meltzer, P. C., Hanson, R. N., & Madras, B. K. 1998, "Rapid detection of Parkinson's disease by SPECT with altropane: a selective ligand for dopamine transporters", *Synapse*, vol. **29**, no. 2, pp. 128–141.

Fishburn, C. S., Elazar, Z., & Fuchs, S. 1995, "Differential glycosylation and intracellular trafficking for the long and short isoforms of the D2 dopamine receptor", *J. Biol. Chem.*, vol. **270**, no. 50, pp. 29819–29824.

Floel, A., Garraux, G., Xu, B., Breitenstein, C., Knecht, S., Herscovitch, P., & Cohen, L. G. 2008, "Levodopa increases memory encoding and dopamine release in the striatum in the elderly", *Neurobiol. Aging.*, vol. **29**, no. 2, pp. 267–279.

Fornai, F., Chen, K., Giorgi, F. S., Gesi, M., Alessandri, M. G., & Shih, J. C. 1999, "Striatal dopamine metabolism in monoamine oxidase B-deficient mice: a brain dialysis study", *J. Neurochem.*, vol. **73**, no. 6, pp. 2434–2440.

Fowler, C. J. & Benedetti, M. S. 1983, "The metabolism of dopamine by both forms of monoamine oxidase in the rat brain and its inhibition by cimoxatone", *J. Neurochem.*, vol. **40**, no. 6, pp. 1534–1541.

Fowler, C. J. & Tipton, K. F. 1982, "Deamination of 5-hydroxytryptamine by both forms of monoamine oxidase in the rat brain", *J. Neurochem.*, vol. **38**, no. 3, pp. 733–736.

Fowler, J. S., Alia-Klein, N., Kriplani, A., Logan, J., Williams, B., Zhu, W., Craig, I. W., Telang, F., Goldstein, R., Volkow, N. D., Vaska, P., & Wang, G. J. 2007, "Evidence that brain MAO A activity does not correspond to MAO A genotype in healthy male subjects", *Biol. Psychiatry*, vol. **62**, no. 4, pp. 355–358.

Fowler, J. S., Logan, J., Ding, Y. S., Franceschi, D., Wang, G. J., Volkow, N. D., Pappas, N., Schlyer, D., Gatley, S. J., Alexoff, D., Felder, C., Biegon, A., & Zhu, W. 2001, "Non-MAO A binding of clorgyline in white matter in human brain", *J. Neurochem.*, vol. **79**, no. 5, pp. 1039–1046.

Fowler, J. S., MacGregor, R. R., Wolf, A. P., Arnett, C. D., Dewey, S. L., Schlyer, D., Christman, D., Logan, J., Smith, M., Sachs, H., & *et al.* 1987, "Mapping human brain monoamine oxidase A and B with 11C-labeled suicide inactivators and PET", *Science*, vol. **235**, no. 4787, pp. 481–485.

Fowler, J. S., Volkow, N. D., Logan, J., Gatley, S. J., Pappas, N., King, P., Ding, Y. S., & Wang, G. J. 1998a, "Measuring dopamine transporter occupancy by cocaine in vivo: radiotracer considerations", *Synapse*, vol. **28**, no. 2, pp. 111–116.

Fowler, J. S., Volkow, N. D., Logan, J., Schlyer, D. J., MacGregor, R. R., Wang, G. J., Wolf, A. P., Pappas, N., Alexoff, D., Shea, C., *et al.* 1993, "Monoamine oxidase B (MAO B) inhibitor therapy in Parkinson's disease: the degree and reversibility of human brain MAO B inhibition by Ro 19 6327", *Neurology*, vol. **43**, no. 10, pp. 1984–1992.

Fowler, J. S., Volkow, N. D., Wang, G. J., Pappas, N., Logan, J., MacGregor, R., Alexoff, D., Wolf, A. P., Warner, D., Cilento, R., & Zezulkova, I. 1998b, "Neuropharmacological actions of cigarette smoke: brain monoamine oxidase B (MAO B) inhibition", *J. Addict. Dis.*, vol. **17**, no. 1, pp. 23–34.

Fowler, J. S., Volkow, N. D., Wang, G. J., Pappas, N., Logan, J., Shea, C., Alexoff, D., MacGregor, R. R., Schlyer, D. J., Zezulkova, I., & Wolf, A. P. 1996, "Brain monoamine oxidase A inhibition in cigarette smokers", *Proc. Natl. Acad. Sci. USA*, vol. **93**, no. 24, pp. 14065–14069.

Fowler, J. S., Wang, G. J., Volkow, N. D., Franceschi, D., Logan, J., Pappas, N., Shea, C., MacGregor, R. R., & Garza, V. 1999, "Smoking a single cigarette does not produce a measurable reduction in brain MAO B in non-smokers", *Nicotine. Tob. Res.*, vol. **1**, no. 4, pp. 325–329.

Fowler, J. S., Wang, G. J., Volkow, N. D., Logan, J., Franceschi, D., Franceschi, M., MacGregor, R., Shea, C., Garza, V., Liu, N., & Ding, Y. S. 2000, "Evidence that gingko biloba extract does not inhibit MAO A and B in living human brain", *Life Sci.*, vol. **66**, no. 9, pp. L141–L146.

Fowler, J. S., Wolf, A. P., MacGregor, R. R., Dewey, S. L., Logan, J., Schlyer, D. J., & Langstrom, B. 1988, "Mechanistic positron emission tomography studies: demonstration of a deuterium isotope effect in the monoamine oxidase-catalyzed binding of [11C]L-deprenyl in living baboon brain", *J. Neurochem.*, vol. **51**, no. 5, pp. 1524–1534.

Francis, L. P., Broch, O. J., Monge, P., & Solheim, E. 1980, "Subcellular distribution of dopamine metabolites and their elimination from the rat brain", *Neuropharmacology*, vol. **19**, no. 3, pp. 269–276.

Frank, G. K., Bailer, U. F., Henry, S. E., Drevets, W., Meltzer, C. C., Price, J. C., Mathis, C. A., Wagner, A., Hoge, J., Ziolko, S., Barbarich-Marsteller, N., Weissfeld, L., & Kaye, W. H. 2005, "Increased dopamine D2/D3 receptor binding after recovery from anorexia nervosa measured by positron emission tomography and [11C]raclopride", *Biol. Psychiatry*, vol. **58**, no. 11, pp. 908–912.

Freedman, N. M., Mishani, E., Krausz, Y., Weininger, J., Lester, H., Blaugrund, E., Ehrlich, D., & Chisin, R. 2005, "In vivo measurement of brain monoamine oxidase B occupancy by rasagiline, using (11)C-l-deprenyl and PET", *J. Nucl. Med.*, vol. **46**, no. 10, pp. 1618–1624.

Freedman, S. B., Patel, S., Marwood, R., Emms, F., Seabrook, G. R., Knowles, M. R., & McAllister, G. 1994, "Expression and pharmacological characterization of the human D3 dopamine receptor", *J. Pharmacol. Exp. Ther.*, vol. **268**, no. 1, pp. 417–426.

Freeman, A. S. & Bunney, B. S. 1987, "Activity of A9 and A10 dopaminergic neurons in unrestrained rats: further characterization and effects of apomorphine and cholecystokinin", *Brain Res.*, vol. **405**, no. 1, pp. 46–55.

Frei, B. & Richter, C. 1986, "N-methyl-4-phenylpyridine (MMP+) together with 6-hydroxydopamine or dopamine stimulates Ca2+ release from mitochondria", *FEBS Lett.*, vol. **198**, no. 1, pp. 99–102.

Frost, J. J., Rosier, A. J., Reich, S. G., Smith, J. S., Ehlers, M. D., Snyder, S. H., Ravert, H. T., & Dannals, R. F. 1993, "Positron emission tomographic imaging of the dopamine transporter with 11C-WIN 35,428 reveals marked declines in mild Parkinson's disease", *Ann. Neurol.*, vol. **34**, no. 3, pp. 423–431.

Frost, J. J., Smith, A. C., Kuhar, M. J., Dannals, R. F., & Wagner, H. N., Jr. 1987, "In vivo binding of 3H-N-methylspiperone to dopamine and serotonin receptors", *Life Sci.*, vol. **40**, no. 10, pp. 987–995.

Fujita, M., Verhoeff, N. P., Varrone, A., Zoghbi, S. S., Baldwin, R. M., Jatlow, P. A., Anderson, G. M., Seibyl, J. P., & Innis, R. B. 2000, "Imaging extrastriatal dopamine D(2) receptor occupancy by endogenous dopamine in healthy humans", *Eur. J. Pharmacol.*, vol. **387**, no. 2, pp. 179–188.

Fuller, R. W. & Snoddy, H. D. 1982, "L-Tyrosine enhancement of the elevation of 3,4-dihydroxyphenylacetic acid concentration in rat brain by spiperone and amfonelic acid", *J. Pharm. Pharmacol.*, vol. **34**, no. 2, pp. 117–118.

Fuxe, K., Ferre, S., Canals, M., Torvinen, M., Terasmaa, A., Marcellino, D., Goldberg, S. R., Staines, W., Jacobsen, K. X., Lluis, C., Woods, A. S., Agnati, L. F., & Franco, R. 2005, "Adenosine A2A and dopamine D2 heteromeric receptor complexes and their function", *J. Mol. Neurosci.*, vol. **26**, no. 2–3, pp. 209–220.

Gaig, C., Marti, M. J., Tolosa, E., Valldeoriola, F., Paredes, P., Lomena, F. J., & Nakamae, F. 2006, "123I-Ioflupane SPECT in the diagnosis of suspected psychogenic Parkinsonism", *Mov. Disord.*, vol. **21**, no. 11, pp. 1994–1998.

Gal, E. M., & Whitacre, D. H. 1982, "Mechanism of irreversible inactivation of phenylalanine-4- and tryptophan-5-hydroxylases by [4-36Cl, 2-14C]p-chlorophenylalanine: a revision", *Neurochem. Res.*, vol. **7**, no. 1, pp. 13–26.

Gale, K., Costa, E., Toffano, G., Hong, J. S., & Guidotti, A. 1978, "Evidence for a role of nigral gamma-aminobutyric acid and substance P in the haloperidol-induced activation of striatal tyrosine hydroxylase", *J. Pharmacol. Exp. Ther.*, vol. **206**, no. 1, pp. 29–37.

Galloway, M. P., Wolf, M. E., & Roth, R. H. 1986, "Regulation of dopamine synthesis in the medial prefrontal cortex is mediated by release modulating autoreceptors: studies in vivo", *J. Pharmacol. Exp. Ther.*, vol. **236**, no. 3, pp. 689–698.

Gatley, S. J., Ding, Y. S., Volkow, N. D., Chen, R., Sugano, Y., & Fowler, J. S. 1995a, "Binding of d-threo-[11C]methylphenidate to the dopamine transporter in vivo: insensitivity to synaptic dopamine", *Eur. J. Pharmacol.*, vol. **281**, no. 2, pp. 141–149.

Gatley, S. J., MacGregor, R. R., Fowler, J. S., Wolf, A. P., Dewey, S. L., & Schlyer, D. J. 1990, "Rapid stereoselective hydrolysis of (+)-cocaine in baboon plasma prevents its uptake in the brain: implications for behavioral studies", *J. Neurochem.*, vol. **54**, no. 2, pp. 720–723.

Gatley, S. J., Volkow, N. D., Fowler, J. S., Dewey, S. L., & Logan, J. 1995b, "Sensitivity of striatal [11C]cocaine binding to decreases in synaptic dopamine", *Synapse*, vol. **20**, no. 2, pp. 137–144.

Gefvert, O., Lindstrom, L. H., Waters, N., Waters, S., Carlsson, A., & Tedroff, J. 2003, "Different corticostriatal patterns of L-DOPA utilization in patients with untreated schizophrenia and patients treated with classical antipsychotics or clozapine", *Scand. J. Psychol.*, vol. **44**, no. 3, pp. 289–292.

Gerasimov, M. R., Ashby, C. R., Jr., Gardner, E. L., Mills, M. J., Brodie, J. D., & Dewey, S. L. 1999, "Gamma-vinyl GABA inhibits methamphetamine, heroin, or ethanol-induced increases in nucleus accumbens dopamine", *Synapse*, vol. **34**, no. 1, pp. 11–19.

Gerfen, C. R. 1992, "The neostriatal mosaic: multiple levels of compartmental organization", *Trends Neurosci.*, vol. **15**, no. 4, pp. 133–139.

Geurts, M., Hermans, E., & Maloteaux, J. M. 1999, "Enhanced striatal dopamine D(2) receptor-induced [35S]GTPgammaS binding after haloperidol treatment", *Eur. J. Pharmacol.*, vol. **382**, no. 2, pp. 119–127.

Giardino, L. 1996, "Right-left asymmetry of D1- and D2-receptor density is lost in the basal ganglia of old rats", *Brain Res.*, vol. **720**, no. 1–2, pp. 235–238.

Gibson, C. J. 1992, "Tyrosine augments dopamine release in stimulated rat retina", *Brain Res.*, vol. **595**, no. 2, pp. 201–205.

Gifford, A. N., Gatley, S. J., & Ashby, C. R., Jr. 1996, "Endogenously released dopamine inhibits the binding of dopaminergic PET and SPECT ligands in superfused rat striatal slices", *Synapse*, vol. **22**, no. 3, pp. 232–238.

Gilman, S., Frey, K. A., Koeppe, R. A., Junck, L., Little, R., Vander Borght, T. M., Lohman, M., Martorello, S., Lee, L. C., Jewett, D. M., & Kilbourn, M. R. 1996, "Decreased striatal monoaminergic terminals in olivopontocerebellar atrophy and multiple system atrophy demonstrated with positron emission tomography", *Ann. Neurol.*, vol. **40**, no. 6, pp. 885–892.

Gilman, S., Koeppe, R. A., Adams, K. M., Junck, L., Kluin, K. J., Johnson-Greene, D., Martorello, S., Heumann, M., & Bandekar, R. 1998, "Decreased striatal monoaminergic terminals in severe chronic alcoholism demonstrated with (+) [11C]dihydrotetrabenazine and positron emission tomography", *Ann. Neurol.*, vol. **44**, no. 3, pp. 326–333.

Gilman, S., Koeppe, R. A., Junck, L., Little, R., Kluin, K. J., Heumann, M., Martorello, S., & Johanns, J. 1999, "Decreased striatal monoaminergic terminals in multiple system atrophy detected with positron emission tomography", *Ann. Neurol.*, vol. **45**, no. 6, pp. 769–777.

Gilman, S., Koeppe, R. A., Little, R., An, H., Junck, L., Giordani, B., Persad, C., Heumann, M., & Wernette, K. 2004, "Striatal monoamine terminals in Lewy body dementia and Alzheimer's disease", *Ann. Neurol.*, vol. **55**, no. 6, pp. 774–780.

Ginovart, N., Farde, L., Halldin, C., & Swahn, C. G. 1997a, "Effect of reserpine-induced depletion of synaptic dopamine on [11C]raclopride binding to D2-dopamine receptors in the monkey brain", *Synapse*, vol. **25**, no. 4, pp. 321–325.

Ginovart, N., Galineau, L., Willeit, M., Mizrahi, R., Bloomfield, P. M., Seeman, P., Houle, S., Kapur, S., & Wilson, A. A. 2006, "Binding characteristics and sensitivity to endogenous dopamine of [11C]-(+)-PHNO, a new agonist radiotracer for imaging the high-affinity state of D2 receptors in vivo using positron emission tomography", *J. Neurochem.*, vol. **97**, no. 4, pp. 1089–1103.

Ginovart, N., Lundin, A., Farde, L., Halldin, C., Backman, L., Swahn, C. G., Pauli, S., & Sedvall, G. 1997b, "PET study of the pre- and post-synaptic dopaminergic markers for the neurodegenerative process in Huntington's disease", *Brain*, vol. **120** (Pt 3), pp. 503–514.

Ginovart, N., Willeit, M., Rusjan, P., Graff, A., Bloomfield, P. M., Houle, S., Kapur, S., & Wilson, A. A. 2007, "Positron emission tomography quantification of [(11)C]-(+)-PHNO binding in the human brain", *J. Cereb. Blood Flow Metab.*, vol. **27**, no. 4, pp. 857–871.

Ginovart, N., Wilson, A. A., Houle, S., & Kapur, S. 2004, "Amphetamine pretreatment induces a change in both D2-Receptor density and apparent affinity: a

[11C]raclopride positron emission tomography study in cats", *Biol. Psychiatry*, vol. **55**, no. 12, pp. 1188–1194.

Giros, B., el Mestikawy, S., Bertrand, L., & Caron, M. G. 1991, "Cloning and functional characterization of a cocaine-sensitive dopamine transporter", *FEBS Lett.*, vol. **295**, no. 1–3, pp. 149–154.

Giros, B., el Mestikawy, S., Godinot, N., Zheng, K., Han, H., Yang-Feng, T., & Caron, M. G. 1992, "Cloning, pharmacological characterization, and chromosome assignment of the human dopamine transporter", *Mol. Pharmacol.*, vol. **42**, no. 3, pp. 383–390.

Giros, B., Jaber, M., Jones, S. R., Wightman, R. M., & Caron, M. G. 1996, "Hyperlocomotion and indifference to cocaine and amphetamine in mice lacking the dopamine transporter", *Nature*, vol. **379**, no. 6566, pp. 606–612.

Giros, B., Sokoloff, P., Martres, M. P., Riou, J. F., Emorine, L. J., & Schwartz, J. C. 1989, "Alternative splicing directs the expression of two D2 dopamine receptor isoforms", *Nature*, vol. **342**, no. 6252, pp. 923–926.

Gjedde, A. 1981, "High- and low-affinity transport of D-glucose from blood to brain", *J. Neurochem.*, vol. **36**, no. 4, pp. 1463–1471.

Gjedde, A., Leger, G. C., Cumming, P., Yasuhara, Y., Evans, A. C., Guttman, M., & Kuwabara, H. 1993, "Striatal L-dopa decarboxylase activity in Parkinson's disease in vivo: implications for the regulation of dopamine synthesis", *J. Neurochem.*, vol. **61**, no. 4, pp. 1538–1541.

Gjedde, A., Reith, J., Dyve, S., Leger, G., Guttman, M., Diksic, M., Evans, A., & Kuwabara, H. 1991, "Dopa decarboxylase activity of the living human brain", *Proc. Natl. Acad. Sci. USA*, vol. **88**, no. 7, pp. 2721–2725.

Glenthoj, B. Y., Mackeprang, T., Svarer, C., Rasmussen, H., Pinborg, L. H., Friberg, L., Baare, W., Hemmingsen, R., & Videbaek, C. 2006, "Frontal dopamine D(2/3) receptor binding in drug-naive first-episode schizophrenic patients correlates with positive psychotic symptoms and gender", *Biol. Psychiatry*, vol. **60**, no. 6, pp. 621–629.

Gonzalez-Quevedo, A., Garcia, J. C., Fernandez, R., & Fernandez, C. L. 1993, "Monoamine metabolites in normal human cerebrospinal fluid and in degenerative diseases of the central nervous system", *Bol. Estud. Med. Biol.*, vol. **41**, no. 1–4, pp. 13–19.

Gordon, I., Rehavi, M., & Mintz, M. 1994, "Bilateral imbalance in striatal DA-uptake controls rotation behavior", *Brain Res.*, vol. **646**, no. 2, pp. 207–210.

Goridis, C. & Neff, N. H. 1971, "Monoamine oxidase: an approximation of turnover rates", *J. Neurochem.*, vol. **18**, no. 9, pp. 1673–1682.

Grace, A. A. 1991, "Phasic versus tonic dopamine release and the modulation of dopamine system responsivity: a hypothesis for the etiology of schizophrenia", *Neuroscience*, vol. **41**, no. 1, pp. 1–24.

Grace, A. A. & Bunney, B. S. 1983, "Intracellular and extracellular electrophysiology of nigral dopaminergic neurons – 3. Evidence for electrotonic coupling", *Neuroscience*, vol. **10**, no. 2, pp. 333–348.

Grace, A. A., Bunney, B. S., Moore, H., & Todd, C. L. 1997, "Dopamine-cell depolarization block as a model for the therapeutic actions of antipsychotic drugs", *Trends Neurosci.*, vol. **20**, no. 1, pp. 31–37.

Graff-Guerrero, A., Willeit, M., Ginovart, N., Mamo, D., Mizrahi, R., Rusjan, P., Vitcu, I., Seeman, P., Wilson, A. A., & Kapur, S. 2008, "Brain region binding of the D(2/3) agonist [(11)C]-(+)-PHNO and the D(2/3) antagonist [(11)C]raclopride in healthy humans", *Hum. Brain Mapp.*, vol. **29**, no. 4, pp. 400–410.

Graham, R. C., Jr. & Karnovsky, M. J. 1965, "The histochemical demonstration of monoamine oxidase activity by coupled peroxidatic oxidation", *J. Histochem. Cytochem.*, vol. **13**, no. 7, pp. 604–605.

Graham, W. C., Clarke, C. E., Boyce, S., Sambrook, M. A., Crossman, A. R., & Woodruff, G. N. 1990, "Autoradiographic studies in animal models of hemi-parkinsonism reveal dopamine D2 but not D1 receptor supersensitivity. II. Unilateral intra-carotid infusion of MPTP in the monkey (Macaca fascicularis)", *Brain Res.*, vol. **514**, no. 1, pp. 103–110.

Graham, W. C., Sambrook, M. A., & Crossman, A. R. 1993, "Differential effect of chronic dopaminergic treatment on dopamine D1 and D2 receptors in the monkey brain in MPTP-induced parkinsonism", *Brain Res.*, vol. **602**, no. 2, pp. 290–303.

Grima, B., Lamouroux, A., Boni, C., Julien, J. F., Javoy-Agid, F., & Mallet, J. 1987, "A single human gene encoding multiple tyrosine hydroxylases with different predicted functional characteristics", *Nature*, vol. **326**, no. 6114, pp. 707–711.

Grimsby, J., Chen, K., Wang, L. J., Lan, N. C., & Shih, J. C. 1991, "Human monoamine oxidase A and B genes exhibit identical exon-intron organization", *Proc. Natl. Acad. Sci. USA*, vol. **88**, no. 9, pp. 3637–3641.

Grimsby, J., Toth, M., Chen, K., Kumazawa, J., Klaidman, L., Adams, J. D., Karoum, J., Gal, J., & Shih, J. C. 1997, "Increased stress response and beta-phenylethylamine in MAOB-deficient mice", *Nat. Genet.*, vol. **17**, no. 2, pp. 206–210.

Groppetti, A., Algeri, S., Cattabeni, F., Di Giulio, A. M., Galli, C. L., Ponzio, F., & Spano, P. F. 1977, "Changes in specific activity of dopamine metabolites as evidence of a multiple compartmentation of dopamine in striatal neurons", *J. Neurochem.*, vol. **28**, no. 1, pp. 193–197.

Grunder, G., Landvogt, C., Vernaleken, I., Buchholz, H. G., Ondracek, J., Siessmeier, T., Hartter, S., Schreckenberger, M., Stoeter, P., Hiemke, C., Rosch, F., Wong, D. F., & Bartenstein, P. 2006, "The striatal and extrastriatal D2/D3 receptor-binding profile of clozapine in patients with schizophrenia", *Neuropsychopharmacology*, vol. **31**, no. 5, pp. 1027–1035.

Grunder, G., Vernaleken, I., Muller, M. J., Davids, E., Heydari, N., Buchholz, H. G., Bartenstein, P., Munk, O. L., Stoeter, P., Wong, D. F., Gjedde, A., & Cumming, P. 2003, "Subchronic haloperidol downregulates dopamine synthesis capacity in the brain of schizophrenic patients in vivo", *Neuropsychopharmacology*, vol. **28**, no. 4, pp. 787–794.

Guigoni, C., Aubert, I., Li, Q., Gurevich, V. V., Benovic, J. L., Ferry, S., Mach, U., Stark, H., Leriche, L., Hakansson, K., Bioulac, B. H., Gross, C. E., Sokoloff, P., Fisone, G., Gurevich, E. V., Bloch, B., & Bezard, E. 2005, "Pathogenesis of levodopa-induced dyskinesia: focus on D1 and D3 dopamine receptors", *Parkinsonism. Relat. Disord.*, vol. **11** (Suppl. 1), pp. S25–S29.

Guivarc'h, D., Vernier, P., & Vincent, J. D. 1995, "Sex steroid hormones change the differential distribution of the isoforms of the D2 dopamine receptor messenger RNA in the rat brain", *Neuroscience*, vol. **69**, no. 1, pp. 159–166.

Guo, N., Hwang, D. R., Lo, E. S., Huang, Y. Y., Laruelle, M., & Abi-Dargham, A. 2003, "Dopamine depletion and in vivo binding of PET D1 receptor radioligands: implications for imaging studies in schizophrenia", *Neuropsychopharmacology*, vol. **28**, no. 9, pp. 1703–1711.

Hadjiconstantinou, M., Neff, N. H., Zhou, L. W., & Weiss, B. 1996, "D2 dopamine receptor antisense increases the activity and mRNA of tyrosine hydroxylase and aromatic L-amino acid decarboxylase in mouse brain", *Neurosci. Lett.*, vol. **217**, no. 2–3, pp. 105–108.

Hadjiconstantinou, M., Rossetti, Z., Silvia, C., Krajnc, D., & Neff, N. H. 1988, "Aromatic L-amino acid decarboxylase activity of the rat retina is modulated in vivo by environmental light", *J. Neurochem.*, vol. **51**, no. 5, pp. 1560–1564.

Hadjiconstantinou, M., Wemlinger, T. A., Sylvia, C. P., Hubble, J. P., & Neff, N. H. 1993, "Aromatic L-amino acid decarboxylase activity of mouse striatum is modulated via dopamine receptors", *J. Neurochem.*, vol. **60**, no. 6, pp. 2175–2180.

Hagberg, G. E., Torstenson, R., Marteinsdottir, I., Fredrikson, M., Langstrom, B., & Blomqvist, G. 2002, "Kinetic compartment modeling of [11C]-5-hydroxy-L-tryptophan for positron emission tomography assessment of serotonin synthesis in human brain", *J. Cereb. Blood Flow Metab.*, vol. **22**, no. 11, pp. 1352–1366.

Hagelberg, N., Aalto, S., Kajander, J., Oikonen, V., Hinkka, S., Nagren, K., Hietala, J., & Scheinin, H. 2004, "Alfentanil increases cortical dopamine D2/D3 receptor binding in healthy subjects", *Pain*, vol. **109**, no. 1–2, pp. 86–93.

Hagelberg, N., Kajander, J. K., Nagren, K., Hinkka, S., Hietala, J., & Scheinin, H. 2002, "Mu-receptor agonism with alfentanil increases striatal dopamine D2 receptor binding in man", *Synapse*, vol. **45**, no. 1, pp. 25–30.

Hajnal, A. & Lenard, L. 1997, "Feeding-related dopamine in the amygdala of freely moving rats", *Neuroreport*, vol. **8**, no. 12, pp. 2817–2820.

Hakyemez, H. S., Dagher, A., Smith, S. D., & Zald, D. H. 2008, "Striatal dopamine transmission in healthy humans during a passive monetary reward task", *Neuroimage*, vol. **39**, no. 4, pp. 2058–2065.

Hall, H., Wedel, I., Halldin, C., Kopp, J., & Farde, L. 1990, "Comparison of the in vitro receptor binding properties of N-[3H]methylspiperone and [3H]raclopride to rat and human brain membranes", *J. Neurochem.*, vol. **55**, no. 6, pp. 2048–2057.

Hall, M. D., Jenner, P., & Marsden, C. D. 1983, "Turnover of specific [3H]spiperone and [3H]N, n-propylnorapomorphine binding sites in rat striatum following phenoxybenzamine administration", *Biochem. Pharmacol.*, vol. **32**, no. 19, pp. 2973–2977.

Halldin, C., Foged, C., Chou, Y. H., Karlsson, P., Swahn, C. G., Sandell, J., Sedvall, G., & Farde, L. 1998, "Carbon-11-NNC 112: a radioligand for PET examination of striatal and neocortical D1-dopamine receptors", *J. Nucl. Med.*, vol. **39**, no. 12, pp. 2061–2068.

Halliwell, J. V. & Horne, A. L. 1998, "Evidence for enhancement of gap junctional coupling between rat island of Calleja granule cells in vitro by the activation of dopamine D3 receptors", *J. Physiol.*, vol. **506** (Pt 1), pp. 175–194.

Hamblin, M. W., Leff, S. E., & Creese, I. 1984, "Interactions of agonists with D-2 dopamine receptors: evidence for a single receptor population existing in multiple agonist affinity-states in rat striatal membranes", *Biochem. Pharmacol.*, vol. **33**, no. 6, pp. 877–887.

Han, S., Rowell, P. P., & Carr, L. A. 1999, "D2 autoreceptors are not involved in the down-regulation of the striatal dopamine transporter caused by alpha-methyl-p-tyrosine", *Res. Commun. Mol. Pathol. Pharmacol.*, vol. **104**, no. 3, pp. 331–338.

Harada, N., Nishiyama, S., Ohba, H., Sato, K., Kakiuchi, T., & Tsukada, H. 2002, "Age differences in phosphodiesterase type-IV and its functional response to dopamine D1 receptor modulation in the living brain: a PET study in conscious monkeys", *Synapse*, vol. **44**, no. 3, pp. 139–145.

Harrington, C. A., Lewis, E. J., Krzemien, D., & Chikaraishi, D. M. 1987, "Identification and cell type specificity of the tyrosine hydroxylase gene promoter", *Nucleic Acids Res.*, vol. **15**, no. 5, pp. 2363–2384.

Harrington, K. A., Augood, S. J., Kingsbury, A. E., Foster, O. J., & Emson, P. C. 1996, "Dopamine transporter (Dat) and synaptic vesicle amine transporter (VMAT2) gene expression in the substantia nigra of control and Parkinson's disease", *Brain Res. Mol. Brain Res.*, vol. **36**, no. 1, pp. 157–162.

Harris, G. C. & Aston-Jones, G. 1994, "Involvement of D2 dopamine receptors in the nucleus accumbens in the opiate withdrawal syndrome", *Nature*, vol. **371**, no. 6493, pp. 155–157.

Hartvig, P., Lindner, K. J., Bjurling, P., Laengstrom, B., & Tedroff, J. 1995, "Pyridoxine effect on synthesis rate of serotonin in the monkey brain measured with positron emission tomography", *J. Neural Transm. Gen. Sect.*, vol. **102**, no. 2, pp. 91–97.

Hartvig, P., Tedroff, J., Lindner, K. J., Bjurling, P., Chang, C. W., Tsukada, H., Watanabe, Y., & Langstrom, B. 1993, "Positron emission tomographic studies on aromatic L-amino acid decarboxylase activity in vivo for L-dopa and 5-hydroxy-L-tryptophan in the monkey brain", *J. Neural Transm. Gen. Sect.*, vol. **94**, no. 2, pp. 127–135.

Hassoun, W., Le Cavorsin, M., Ginovart, N., Zimmer, L., Gualda, V., Bonnefoi, F., & Leviel, V. 2003, "PET study of the [11C]raclopride binding in the striatum of the awake cat: effects of anaesthetics and role of cerebral blood flow", *Eur. J. Nucl. Med. Mol. Imaging*, vol. **30**, no. 1, pp. 141–148.

Hassoun, W., Thobois, S., Ginovart, N., Garcia-Larrea, L., Cavorsin, M. L., Guillouet, S., Bonnefoi, F., Costes, N., Lavenne, F., Martin, J. P., Broussolle, E., & Leviel, V. 2005, "Striatal dopamine during sensorial stimulations: a [18F]FDOPA PET study in human and cats", *Neurosci. Lett.*, vol. **383**, no. 1–2, pp. 63–67.

Hattori, S., Naoi, M., & Nishino, H. 1994, "Striatal dopamine turnover during treadmill running in the rat: relation to the speed of running", *Brain Res. Bull.*, vol. **35**, no. 1, pp. 41–49.

Hauptmann, N., Grimsby, J., Shih, J. C., & Cadenas, E. 1996, "The metabolism of tyramine by monoamine oxidase A/B causes oxidative damage to mitochondrial DNA", *Arch. Biochem. Biophys.*, vol. **335**, no. 2, pp. 295–304.

Haycock, J. W. 1987, "Stimulation-dependent phosphorylation of tyrosine hydroxylase in rat corpus striatum", *Brain Res. Bull.*, vol. **19**, no. 6, pp. 619–622.

Hedner, T. & Lundborg, P. 1985, "Development of dopamine autoreceptors in the postnatal rat brain", *J. Neural Transm.*, vol. **62**, no. 1–2, pp. 53–63.

Heffner, T. G. & Seiden, L. S. 1980, "Synthesis of catecholamines from [3H]tyrosine in brain during the performance of operant behavior", *Brain Res.*, vol. **183**, no. 2, pp. 403–419.

Heinz, A., Goldman, D., Jones, D. W., Palmour, R., Hommer, D., Gorey, J. G., Lee, K. S., Linnoila, M., & Weinberger, D. R. 2000, "Genotype influences in vivo dopamine transporter availability in human striatum", *Neuropsychopharmacology*, vol. **22**, no. 2, pp. 133–139.

Heinz, A., Siessmeier, T., Wrase, J., Buchholz, H. G., Grunder, G., Kumakura, Y., Cumming, P., Schreckenberger, M., Smolka, M. N., Rosch, F., Mann, K., & Bartenstein, P. 2005, "Correlation of alcohol craving with striatal dopamine synthesis capacity and D2/3 receptor availability: a combined [18F]DOPA and [18F]DMFP PET study in detoxified alcoholic patients", *Am. J. Psychiatry*, vol. **162**, no. 8, pp. 1515–1520.

Henry, J. P. & Scherman, D. 1989, "Radioligands of the vesicular monoamine transporter and their use as markers of monoamine storage vesicles", *Biochem. Pharmacol.*, vol. **38**, no. 15, pp. 2395–2404.

Hernandez-Lopez, S., Gongora-Alfaro, J. L., Martinez-Fong, D., Rosales, M. G., & Aceves, J. 1994, "Cholinergic stimulation of rostral and caudal substantia nigra pars compacta produces opposite effects on circling behavior and striatal dopamine release measured by brain microdialysis", *Neuroscience*, vol. **62**, no. 2, pp. 441–447.

Herraiz, T. & Chaparro, C. 2005, "Human monoamine oxidase is inhibited by tobacco smoke: beta-carboline alkaloids act as potent and reversible inhibitors", *Biochem. Biophys. Res. Commun.*, vol. **326**, no. 2, pp. 378–386.

Herve, D., Trovero, F., Blanc, G., Glowinski, J., & Tassin, J. P. 1992, "Autoradiographic identification of D1 dopamine receptors labelled with [3H]dopamine: distribution, regulation and relationship to coupling", *Neuroscience*, vol. **46**, no. 3, pp. 687–700.

Hess, E. J., Battaglia, G., Norman, A. B., Iorio, L. C., & Creese, I. 1986, "Guanine nucleotide regulation of agonist interactions at [3H]SCH23390-labeled D1 dopamine receptors in rat striatum", *Eur. J. Pharmacol.*, vol. **121**, no. 1, pp. 31–38.

Hietala, J., Syvalahti, E., Vilkman, H., Vuorio, K., Rakkolainen, V., Bergman, J., Haaparanta, M., Solin, O., Kuoppamaki, M., Eronen, E., Ruotsalainen, U., & Salokangas, R. K. 1999, "Depressive symptoms and presynaptic dopamine function in neuroleptic-naive schizophrenia", *Schizophr. Res.*, vol. **35**, no. 1, pp. 41–50.

Hietala, J., West, C., Syvalahti, E., Nagren, K., Lehikoinen, P., Sonninen, P., & Ruotsalainen, U. 1994, "Striatal D2 dopamine receptor binding characteristics in vivo in patients with alcohol dependence", *Psychopharmacology (Berl)*, vol. **116**, no. 3, pp. 285–290.

Hilker, R., Klein, C., Hedrich, K., Ozelius, L. J., Vieregge, P., Herholz, K., Pramstaller, P. P., & Heiss, W. D. 2002, "The striatal dopaminergic deficit is dependent on the number of mutant alleles in a family with mutations in the parkin gene: evidence for enzymatic parkin function in humans", *Neurosci. Lett.*, vol. **323**, no. 1, pp. 50–54.

Hilker, R., Schweitzer, K., Coburger, S., Ghaemi, M., Weisenbach, S., Jacobs, A. H., Rudolf, J., Herholz, K., & Heiss, W. D. 2005, "Nonlinear progression of Parkinson disease as determined by serial positron emission tomographic imaging of striatal fluorodopa F 18 activity", *Arch. Neurol.*, vol. **62**, no. 3, pp. 378–382.

Hilker, R., Voges, J., Ghaemi, M., Lehrke, R., Rudolf, J., Koulousakis, A., Herholz, K., Wienhard, K., Sturm, V., & Heiss, W. D. 2003, "Deep brain stimulation of the subthalamic nucleus does not increase the striatal dopamine concentration in parkinsonian humans", *Mov. Disord.*, vol. **18**, no. 1, pp. 41–48.

Hillefors, M., von Euler, M., Hedlund, P. B., & von Euler, G. 1999, "Prominent binding of the dopamine D3 agonist [3H]PD 128907 in the caudate-putamen of the adult rat", *Brain Res.*, vol. **822**, no. 1–2, pp. 126–131.

Hilton, M. A., Fonda, M. L., & Hilton, F. K. 1998, "The effect of tyrosine-deficient total parenteral nutrition on the synthesis of dihydroxyphenylalanine in neural tissue and the activities of tyrosine and branched-chain aminotransferases", *Metabolism*, vol. **47**, no. 2, pp. 168–176.

Hirvonen, J., van Erp, T. G., Huttunen, J., Aalto, S., Nagren, K., Huttunen, M., Lonnqvist, J., Kaprio, J., Cannon, T. D., & Hietala, J. 2006, "Brain dopamine d1 receptors in twins discordant for schizophrenia", *Am. J. Psychiatry*, vol. **163**, no. 10, pp. 1747–1753.

Hirvonen, J., van Erp, T. G., Huttunen, J., Aalto, S., Nagren, K., Huttunen, M., Lonnqvist, J., Kaprio, J., Hietala, J., & Cannon, T. D. 2005, "Increased caudate dopamine D2 receptor availability as a genetic marker for schizophrenia", *Arch. Gen. Psychiatry*, vol. **62**, no. 4, pp. 371–378.

Holden, J. E., Doudet, D., Endres, C. J., Chan, G. L., Morrison, K. S., Vingerhoets, F. J., Snow, B. J., Pate, B. D., Sossi, V., Buckley, K. R., & Ruth, T. J. 1997, "Graphical analysis of 6-fluoro-L-dopa trapping: effect of inhibition of catechol-O-methyltransferase", *J. Nucl. Med.*, vol. **38**, no. 10, pp. 1568–1574.

Hollerman, J. R. & Schultz, W. 1998, "Dopamine neurons report an error in the temporal prediction of reward during learning", *Nat. Neurosci.*, vol. **1**, no. 4, pp. 304–309.

Holtje, M., von Jagow, B., Pahner, I., Lautenschlager, M., Hortnagl, H., Nurnberg, B., Jahn, R., & Ahnert-Hilger, G. 2000, "The neuronal monoamine transporter VMAT2 is regulated by the trimeric GTPase Go(2)", *J. Neurosci.*, vol. **20**, no. 6, pp. 2131–2141.

Hong, J., Shu-Leong, H., Tao, X., & Lap-Ping, Y. 1998, "Distribution of catechol-O-methyltransferase expression in human central nervous system", *Neuroreport*, vol. **9**, no. 12, pp. 2861–2864.

Hope, B. T., Michael, G. J., Knigge, K. M., & Vincent, S. R. 1991, "Neuronal NADPH diaphorase is a nitric oxide synthase", *Proc. Natl. Acad. Sci. USA*, vol. **88**, no. 7, pp. 2811–2814.

Horie, C., Suzuki, Y., Kiyosawa, M., Mochizuki, M., Wakakura, M., Oda, K., Ishiwata, K., & Ishii, K. 2008, "Decreased dopamine, D.(2) receptor binding in essential blepharospasm", *Acta Neurol. Scand.* [Epub ahead of print].

Horne, M. K., Cheng, C. H., & Wooten, G. F. 1984, "The cerebral metabolism of L-dihydroxyphenylalanine. An autoradiographic and biochemical study", *Pharmacology*, vol. **28**, no. 1, pp. 12–26.

Hoshi, H., Kuwabara, H., Leger, G., Cumming, P., Guttman, M., & Gjedde, A. 1993, "6-[18F]fluoro-L-dopa metabolism in living human brain: a comparison of six analytical methods", *J. Cereb. Blood Flow Metab.*, vol. **13**, no. 1, pp. 57–69.

Hoshiga, M., Hatakeyama, K., Watanabe, M., Shimada, M., & Kagamiyama, H. 1993, "Autoradiographic distribution of [14C]tetrahydrobiopterin and its developmental change in mice", *J. Pharmacol. Exp. Ther.*, vol. **267**, no. 2, pp. 971–978.

Hosoi, R., Ishikawa, M., Kobayashi, K., Gee, A., Yamaguchi, M., & Inoue, O. 2002, "Effects of rolipram on in vivo dopamine receptor binding", *J. Neural Transm.*, vol. **109**, no. 9, pp. 1139–1149.

Hsiao, M. C., Lin, K. J., Liu, C. Y., Tzen, K. Y., & Yen, T. C. 2003, "Dopamine transporter change in drug-naive schizophrenia: an imaging study with 99mTc-TRODAT-1", *Schizophr. Res.*, vol. **65**, no. 1, pp. 39–46.

Huang, C. C., Weng, Y. H., Lu, C. S., Chu, N. S., & Yen, T. C. 2003, "Dopamine transporter binding in chronic manganese intoxication", *J. Neurol.*, vol. **250**, no. 11, pp. 1335–1339.

Huang, J. T. & Wajda, I. J. 1977, "The influence of 3,4-dihydroxyphenylacetic acid on the accumulation of 5-hydroxyindoleacetic acid in the choroid plexus and kidney cortex slices of rats", *Res. Commun. Chem. Pathol. Pharmacol.*, vol. **16**, no. 4, pp. 649–668.

Huang, N., Ase, A. R., Hebert, C., van Gelder, N. M., & Reader, T. A. 1997, "Effects of chronic neuroleptic treatments on dopamine D1 and D2 receptors: homogenate binding and autoradiographic studies", *Neurochem. Int.*, vol. **30**, no. 3, pp. 277–290.

Huang, S. C., Stout, D. B., Yee, R. E., Satyamurthy, N., & Barrio, J. R. 1998, "Distribution volume of radiolabeled large neutral amino acids in brain tissue", *J. Cereb. Blood Flow Metab.*, vol. **18**, no. 12, pp. 1288–1293.

Huang, S. C., Yu, D. C., Barrio, J. R., Grafton, S., Melega, W. P., Hoffman, J. M., Satyamurthy, N., Mazziotta, J. C., & Phelps, M. E. 1991, "Kinetics and modeling of L-6-[18F]fluoro-dopa in human positron emission tomographic studies", *J. Cereb. Blood Flow Metab.*, vol. **11**, no. 6, pp. 898–913.

Hunter, L. W., Rorie, D. K., & Tyce, G. M. 1993, "Inhibition of aromatic L-amino acid decarboxylase under physiological conditions: optimization of 3-hydroxybenzylhydrazine concentration to prevent concurrent inhibition of monoamine oxidase", *Biochem. Pharmacol.*, vol. **45**, no. 6, pp. 1363–1366.

Hurd, Y. L. & Ungerstedt, U. 1989, "Cocaine: an in vivo microdialysis evaluation of its acute action on dopamine transmission in rat striatum", *Synapse*, vol. **3**, no. 1, pp. 48–54.

Hutson, P. H. & Curzon, G. 1986, "Dopamine metabolites in rat cisternal cerebrospinal fluid: major contribution from extrastriatal dopamine neurones", *J. Neurochem.*, vol. **46**, no. 1, pp. 186–190.

Huttunen, J., Heinimaa, M., Svirskis, T., Nyman, M., Kajander, J., Forsback, S., Solin, O., Ilonen, T., Korkeila, J., Ristkari, T., McGlashan, T., Salokangas, R. K., & Hietala, J. 2008, "Striatal dopamine synthesis in first-degree relatives of patients with schizophrenia", *Biol. Psychiatry.*, vol. **63**, no. 1, pp. 114–117.

Hwang, D. R., Kegeles, L. S., & Laruelle, M. 2000, "(-)-N-[(11)C]propyl-norapomorphine: a positron-labeled dopamine agonist for PET imaging of D(2) receptors", *Nucl. Med. Biol.*, vol. **27**, no. 6, pp. 533–539.

Hwang, W. J., Yao, W. J., Wey, S. P., Shen, L. H., & Ting, G. 2002, "Downregulation of striatal dopamine D2 receptors in advanced Parkinson's disease contributes to the development of motor fluctuation", *Eur. Neurol.*, vol. **47**, no. 2, pp. 113–117.

Ichinose, H., Kojima, K., Togari, A., Kato, Y., Parvez, S., Parvez, H., & Nagatsu, T. 1985, "Simple purification of aromatic L-amino acid decarboxylase from human pheochromocytoma using high-performance liquid chromatography", *Anal. Biochem.*, vol. **150**, no. 2, pp. 408–414.

Ichinose, H., Ohye, T., Takahashi, E., Seki, N., Hori, T., Segawa, M., Nomura, Y., Endo, K., Tanaka, H., Tsuji, S., *et al.* 1994, "Hereditary progressive dystonia with marked diurnal fluctuation caused by mutations in the GTP cyclohydrolase I gene", *Nat. Genet.*, vol. **8**, no. 3, pp. 236–242.

Ikeda, M., Levitt, M., & Udenfriend, S. 1967, "Phenylalanine as substrate and inhibitor of tyrosine hydroxylase", *Arch. Biochem. Biophys.*, vol. **120**, no. 2, pp. 420–427.

Ikemoto, K., Kitahama, K., Maeda, T., Tokunaga, Y., Valatx, J. L., De, M. E., & Seif, I. 1997, "Electron-microscopic study of MAOB-containing structures in the nucleus accumbens shell: using MAOA-deficient transgenic mice", *Brain Res.*, vol. **771**, no. 1, pp. 163–166.

Imperato, A., Angelucci, L., Casolini, P., Zocchi, A., & Puglisi-Allegra, S. 1992, "Repeated stressful experiences differently affect limbic dopamine release during and following stress", *Brain Res.*, vol. **577**, no. 2, pp. 194–199.

Inaji, M., Okauchi, T., Ando, K., Maeda, J., Nagai, Y., Yoshizaki, T., Okano, H., Nariai, T., Ohno, K., Obayashi, S., Higuchi, M., & Suhara, T. 2005a, "Correlation between quantitative imaging and behavior in unilaterally 6-OHDA-lesioned rats", *Brain Res.*, vol. **1064**, no. 1–2, pp. 136–145.

Inaji, M., Yoshizaki, T., Okauchi, T., Maeda, J., Nagai, Y., Nariai, T., Ohno, K., Ando, K., Okano, H., Obayashi, S., & Suhara, T. 2005b, "In vivo PET measurements with [11C]PE2I to evaluate fetal mesencephalic transplantations to unilateral 6-OHDA-lesioned rats", *Cell Transplant.*, vol. **14**, no. 9, pp. 655–663.

Innis, R. B., Marek, K. L., Sheff, K., Zoghbi, S., Castronuovo, J., Feigin, A., & Seibyl, J. P. 1999, "Effect of treatment with L-dopa/carbidopa or L-selegiline on striatal dopamine transporter SPECT imaging with [123I]beta-CIT", *Mov. Disord.*, vol. **14**, no. 3, pp. 436–442.

Innis, R. B., Seibyl, J. P., Scanley, B. E., Laruelle, M., Abi-Dargham, A., Wallace, E., Baldwin, R. M., Zea-Ponce, Y., Zoghbi, S., Wang, S., *et al.* 1993, "Single photon emission computed tomographic imaging demonstrates loss of striatal dopamine transporters in Parkinson disease", *Proc. Natl. Acad. Sci. USA*, vol. **90**, no. 24, pp. 11965–11969.

Inoue, M., Katsumi, Y., Hayashi, T., Mukai, T., Ishizu, K., Hashikawa, K., Saji, H., & Fukuyama, H. 2004, "Sensory stimulation accelerates dopamine release in the basal ganglia", *Brain Res.*, vol. **1026**, no. 2, pp. 179–184.

Inoue, O., Kobayashi, K., Hosoi, R., Yamaguchi, M., & Gee, A. 1999, "Discrepancies in apparent dopamine D2 receptor occupancy between 3H-raclopride and 3H-N-methylspiperone", *J. Neural Transm.*, vol. **106**, no. 11–12, pp. 1099–1104.

Inoue, O., Tsukada, H., Yonezawa, H., Suhara, T., & Langstrom, B. 1991, "Reserpine-induced reduction of in vivo binding of SCH 23390 and N-methylspiperone and its reversal by d-amphetamine", *Eur. J. Pharmacol.*, vol. **197**, no. 2–3, pp. 143–149.

Ishikawa, T., Dhawan, V., Chaly, T., Robeson, W., Belakhlef, A., Mandel, F., Dahl, R., Margouleff, C., & Eidelberg, D. 1996, "Fluorodopa positron emission tomography with an inhibitor of catechol-O-methyltransferase: effect of the plasma 3-O-methyldopa fraction on data analysis", *J. Cereb. Blood Flow Metab.*, vol. **16**, no. 5, pp. 854–863.

Ishiwata, K., Kawamura, K., Yanai, K., & Hendrikse, N. H. 2007, "In vivo evaluation of P-glycoprotein modulation of 8 PET radioligands used clinically", *J. Nucl. Med.*, vol. **48**, no. 1, pp. 81–87.

Ito, K., Haga, T., Lameh, J., & Sadee, W. 1999, "Sequestration of dopamine D2 receptors depends on coexpression of G-protein-coupled receptor kinases 2 or 5", *Eur. J. Biochem.*, vol. **260**, no. 1, pp. 112–119.

Iurlo, M., Leone, G., Schilstrom, B., Linner, L., Nomikos, G., Hertel, P., Silvestrini, B., & Svensson, H. 2001, "Effects of harmine on dopamine output and metabolism in rat striatum: role of monoamine oxidase-A inhibition", *Psychopharmacology (Berl)*, vol. **159**, no. 1, pp. 98–104.

Iuvone, P. M. 1984, "Calcium, ATP, and magnesium activate soluble tyrosine hydroxylase from rat striatum", *J. Neurochem.*, vol. **43**, no. 5, pp. 1359–1368.

Iuvone, P. M., Rauch, A. L., Marshburn, P. B., Glass, D. B., & Neff, N. H. 1982, "Activation of retinal tyrosine hydroxylase in vitro by cyclic AMP-dependent protein kinase: characterization and comparison to activation in vivo by photic stimulation", *J. Neurochem.*, vol. **39**, no. 6, pp. 1632–1640.

Jahng, J. W., Houpt, T. A., Wessel, T. C., Chen, K., Shih, J. C., & Joh, T. H. 1997, "Localization of monoamine oxidase A and B mRNA in the rat brain by in situ hybridization", *Synapse*, vol. **25**, no. 1, pp. 30–36.

Janson, A. M., Hedlund, P. B., Hillefors, M., & von Euler, G. 1992, "Chronic nicotine treatment decreases dopamine D2 agonist binding in the rat basal ganglia", *Neuroreport*, vol. **3**, no. 12, pp. 1117–1120.

Javoy, F. & Glowinski, J. 1971, "Dynamic characteristic of the 'functional compartment' of dopamine in dopaminergic terminals of the rat striatum", *J. Neurochem.*, vol. **18**, no. 7, pp. 1305–1311.

Javoy, F., Sotelo, C., Herbet, A., & Agid, Y. 1976, "Specificity of dopaminergic neuronal degeneration induced by intracerebral injection of 6-hydroxydopamine in the nigrostriatal dopamine system", *Brain Res.*, vol. **102**, no. 2, pp. 201–215.

Jeffery, D. R. & Roth, J. A. 1984, "Characterization of membrane-bound and soluble catechol-O-methyltransferase from human frontal cortex", *J. Neurochem.*, vol. **42**, no. 3, pp. 826–832.

Jeffery, D. R. & Roth, J. A. 1987, "Kinetic reaction mechanism for magnesium binding to membrane-bound and soluble catechol O-methyltransferase", *Biochemistry*, vol. **26**, no. 10, pp. 2955–2958.

Jensen, S. B., Olsen, A. K., Pedersen, K., & Cumming, P. 2006, "Effect of monoamine oxidase inhibition on amphetamine-evoked changes in dopamine receptor availability in the living pig: a dual tracer PET study with [11C]harmine and [11C]raclopride", *Synapse*, vol. **59**, no. 7, pp. 427–434.

Jensen, S. B., Di Santo, R., Olsen, A. K., Pedersen, K., Costi, R., Cirilli, R., & Cumming, P. 2008, "Synthesis and cerebral uptake of 1-(1-[(11C)]methyl-1H-pyrrol-2-yl)-2-phenyl-2-(1-pyrrolidinyl)ethanone, a novel tracer for positron emission tomography studies of monoamine oxidase type A", *J. Med. Chem.*, vol. **51**, no. 6, pp. 1617–1622.

Johansson, A., Engler, H., Blomquist, G., Scott, B., Wall, A., Aquilonius, S. M., Langstrom, B., & Askmark, H. 2007, "Evidence for astrocytosis in ALS demonstrated by [11C](L)-deprenyl-D2 PET", *J. Neurol. Sci.*, vol. **255**, no. 1–2, pp. 17–22.

Johnson, E. A., Tsai, C. E., Shahan, Y. H., & Azzaro, A. J. 1993, "Serotonin 5-HT1A receptors mediate inhibition of tyrosine hydroxylation in rat striatum", *J. Pharmacol. Exp. Ther.*, vol. **266**, no. 1, pp. 133–141.

Johnson, L. A., Furman, C. A., Zhang, M., Guptaroy, B., & Gnegy, M. E. 2005, "Rapid delivery of the dopamine transporter to the plasmalemmal membrane upon amphetamine stimulation", *Neuropharmacology*, vol. **49**, no. 6, pp. 750–758.

Johnson, R. G., Carty, S., & Scarpa, A. 1982, "A model of biogenic amine accumulation into chromaffin granules and ghosts based on coupling to the electrochemical proton gradient", *Fed. Proc.*, vol. **41**, no. 11, pp. 2746–2754.

Johnson, R. G., Carty, S. E., & Scarpa, A. 1981, "Proton: substrate stoichiometries during active transport of biogenic amines in chromaffin ghosts", *J. Biol. Chem.*, vol. **256**, no. 11, pp. 5773–5780.

Jones, S. R., Gainetdinov, R. R., Jaber, M., Giros, B., Wightman, R. M., & Caron, M. G. 1998a, "Profound neuronal plasticity in response to inactivation of the dopamine transporter", *Proc. Natl. Acad. Sci. USA*, vol. **95**, no. 7, pp. 4029–4034.

Jones, S. R., Gainetdinov, R. R., Wightman, R. M., & Caron, M. G. 1998b, "Mechanisms of amphetamine action revealed in mice lacking the dopamine transporter", *J. Neurosci.*, vol. **18**, no. 6, pp. 1979–1986.

Jones, S. R., Garris, P. A., Kilts, C. D., & Wightman, R. M. 1995, "Comparison of dopamine uptake in the basolateral amygdaloid nucleus, caudate-putamen, and nucleus accumbens of the rat", *J. Neurochem.*, vol. **64**, no. 6, pp. 2581–2589.

Jones, S. R., Joseph, J. D., Barak, L. S., Caron, M. G., & Wightman, R. M. 1999, "Dopamine neuronal transport kinetics and effects of amphetamine", *J. Neurochem.*, vol. **73**, no. 6, pp. 2406–2414.

Jonsson, E. G., Nothen, M. M., Grunhage, F., Farde, L., Nakashima, Y., Propping, P., & Sedvall, G. C. 1999, "Polymorphisms in the dopamine D2 receptor gene and their relationships to striatal dopamine receptor density of healthy volunteers", *Mol. Psychiatry*, vol. **4**, no. 3, pp. 290–296.

Jordan, S., Bankiewicz, K. S., Eberling, J. L., VanBrocklin, H. F., O'Neil, J. P., & Jagust, W. J. 1998, "An in vivo microdialysis study of striatal 6-[18F]fluoro-L-m-tyrosine metabolism", *Neurochem. Res.*, vol. **23**, no. 4, pp. 513–517.

Jucaite, A., Fernell, E., Halldin, C., Forssberg, H., & Farde, L. 2005, "Reduced midbrain dopamine transporter binding in male adolescents with attention-deficit/hyperactivity disorder: association between striatal dopamine markers and motor hyperactivity", *Biol. Psychiatry*, vol. **57**, no. 3, pp. 229–238.

Juorio, A. V. & Yu, P. H. 1985, "Effects of benzene and other organic solvents on the decarboxylation of some brain aromatic-L-amino acids", *Biochem. Pharmacol.*, vol. **34**, no. 9, pp. 1381–1387.

Kaasinen, V., Aalto, S., Nagren, K., Hietala, J., Sonninen, P., & Rinne, J. O. 2003, "Extrastriatal dopamine D(2) receptors in Parkinson's disease: a longitudinal study", *J. Neural Transm.*, vol. **110**, no. 6, pp. 591–601.

Kaasinen, V., Aalto, S., Nagren, K., & Rinne, J. O. 2004a, "Dopaminergic effects of caffeine in the human striatum and thalamus", *Neuroreport*, vol. **15**, no. 2, pp. 281–285.

Kaasinen, V., Aalto, S., Nagren, K., & Rinne, J. O. 2004b, "Expectation of caffeine induces dopaminergic responses in humans", *Eur. J. Neurosci.*, vol. **19**, no. 8, pp. 2352–2356.

Kaasinen, V., Aalto, S., Nagren, K., & Rinne, J. O. 2004c, "Insular dopamine D2 receptors and novelty seeking personality in Parkinson's disease", *Mov. Disord.*, vol. **19**, no. 11, pp. 1348–1351.

Kaasinen, V., Kemppainen, N., Nagren, K., Helenius, H., Kurki, T., & Rinne, J. O. 2002a, "Age-related loss of extrastriatal dopamine D(2)-like receptors in women", *J. Neurochem.*, vol. **81**, no. 5, pp. 1005–1010.

Kaasinen, V., Nagren, K., Hietala, J., Farde, L., & Rinne, J. O. 2001a, "Sex differences in extrastriatal dopamine D(2)-like receptors in the human brain", *Am. J. Psychiatry*, vol. **158**, no. 2, pp. 308–311.

Kaasinen, V., Nurmi, E., Bergman, J., Eskola, O., Solin, O., Sonninen, P., & Rinne, J. O. 2001b, "Personality traits and brain dopaminergic function in Parkinson's disease", *Proc. Natl. Acad. Sci. USA*, vol. **98**, no. 23, pp. 13272–13277.

Kaasinen, V., Nurmi, E., Bergman, J., Solin, O., Kurki, T., & Rinne, J. O. 2002b, "Personality traits and striatal 6-[18F]fluoro-L-dopa uptake in healthy elderly subjects", *Neurosci. Lett.*, vol. **332**, no. 1, pp. 61–64.

Kaasinen, V., Nurmi, E., Bruck, A., Eskola, O., Bergman, J., Solin, O., & Rinne, J. O. 2001c, "Increased frontal [(18)F]fluorodopa uptake in early Parkinson's disease: sex differences in the prefrontal cortex", *Brain*, vol. **124** (Pt 6), pp. 1125–1130.

Kaasinen, V., Ruottinen, H. M., Nagren, K., Lehikoinen, P., Oikonen, V., & Rinne, J. O. 2000, "Upregulation of putaminal dopamine D2 receptors in early Parkinson's disease: a comparative PET study with [11C] raclopride and [11C]N-methylspiperone", *J. Nucl. Med.*, vol. **41**, no. 1, pp. 65–70.

Kafetzopoulos, E. & Papadopoulos, G. 1983, "Turning behavior after unilateral lesion of the subthalamic nucleus in the rat", *Behav. Brain Res.*, vol. **8**, no. 2, pp. 217–223.

Kahlig, K. M., Javitch, J. A., & Galli, A. 2004, "Amphetamine regulation of dopamine transport. Combined measurements of transporter currents and transporter imaging support the endocytosis of an active carrier", *J. Biol. Chem.*, vol. **279**, no. 10, pp. 8966–8975.

Kanai, Y., Segawa, H., Miyamoto, K., Uchino, H., Takeda, E., & Endou, H. 1998, "Expression cloning and characterization of a transporter for large neutral amino acids activated by the heavy chain of 4F2 antigen (CD98)", *J. Biol. Chem.*, vol. **273**, no. 37, pp. 23629–23632.

Kaneda, N., Kobayashi, K., Ichinose, H., Kishi, F., Nakazawa, A., Kurosawa, Y., Fujita, K., & Nagatsu, T. 1987, "Isolation of a novel cDNA clone for human tyrosine hydroxylase: alternative RNA splicing produces four kinds of mRNA from a single gene", *Biochem. Biophys. Res. Commun.*, vol. **146**, no. 3, pp. 971–975.

Kang, S. J., Scott, W. K., Li, Y. J., Hauser, M. A., van der Walt, J. M., Fujiwara, K., Mayhew, G. M., West, S. G., Vance, J. M., & Martin, E. R. 2006, "Family-based case-control study of MAOA and MAOB polymorphisms in Parkinson disease", *Mov. Disord.*, vol. **21**, no. 12, pp. 2175–2180.

Kao, P. F., Tzen, K. Y., Yen, T. C., Lu, C. S., Weng, Y. H., Wey, S. P., & Ting, G. 2001, "The optimal imaging time for [99Tcm]TRODAT-1/SPET in normal subjects and patients with Parkinson's disease", *Nucl. Med. Commun.*, vol. **22**, no. 2, pp. 151–154.

Kapatos, G. & Kaufman, S. 1981, "Peripherally administered reduced pterins do enter the brain", *Science*, vol. **212**, no. 4497, pp. 955–956.

Kapatos, G. & Zigmond, M. 1977, "Dopamine biosynthesis from L-tyrosine and L-phenylalanine in rat brain synaptosomes: preferential use of newly accumulated precursors", *J. Neurochem.*, vol. **28**, no. 5, pp. 1109–1119.

Karhunen, T., Tilgmann, C., Ulmanen, I., & Panula, P. 1995, "Catechol-O-methyltransferase (COMT) in rat brain: immunoelectron microscopic study with an antiserum against rat recombinant COMT protein", *Neurosci. Lett.*, vol. **187**, no. 1, pp. 57–60.

Karlsson, P., Farde, L., Halldin, C., & Sedvall, G. 2002, "PET study of D(1) dopamine receptor binding in neuroleptic-naive patients with schizophrenia", *Am. J. Psychiatry*, vol. **159**, no. 5, pp. 761–767.

Karoum, F., Chrapusta, S. J., & Egan, M. F. 1994, "3-Methoxytyramine is the major metabolite of released dopamine in the rat frontal cortex: reassessment of the effects of antipsychotics on the dynamics of dopamine release and metabolism in the frontal cortex, nucleus accumbens, and striatum by a simple two pool model", *J. Neurochem.*, vol. **63**, no. 3, pp. 972–979.

Karoum, F., Neff, N. H., & Wyatt, R. J. 1977, "The dynamics of dopamine metabolism in various regions of rat brain", *Eur. J. Pharmacol.*, vol. **44**, no. 4, pp. 311–318.

Kashihara, K., Ishihara, T., Akiyama, K., & Abe, K. 1999, "D1/D2 receptor synergism on CREB DNA-binding activities in the caudate-putamen of rat", *Neurol. Res.*, vol. **21**, no. 8, pp. 781–784.

Katoh, A., Nabeshima, T., Kuno, A., Wada, M., Ukai, R., & Kameyama, T. 1996, "Changes in striatal dopamine release in stress-induced conditioned suppression of motility in rats", *Behav. Brain Res.*, vol. **77**, no. 1–2, pp. 219–221.

Katz, I., Lloyd, T., & Kaufman, S. 1976, "Studies on phenylalanine and tyrosine hydroxylation by rat brain tyrosine hydroxylase", *Biochim. Biophys. Acta*, vol. **445**, no. 3, pp. 567–578.

Kaufman, S. 1987, "Tetrahyrdobiopterin and hydroxylation systems in health and disease," in *Unconjugated Pterins in Neurobiology: Basic and Clinical Aspects*, W. Lovenberg & R. A. Levine, eds., Taylor and Francis, London, pp. 1–28.

Kawasaki, Y., Hayashi, H., Hatakeyama, K., & Kagamiyama, H. 1992, "Evaluation of the holoenzyme content of aromatic L-amino acid decarboxylase in brain and liver tissues", *Biochem. Biophys. Res. Commun.*, vol. **186**, no. 3, pp. 1242–1248.

Kebabian, J. W. & Calne, D. B. 1979, "Multiple receptors for dopamine", *Nature*, vol. **277**, no. 5692, pp. 93–96.

Keefe, K. A. & Gerfen, C. R. 1995, "D1-D2 dopamine receptor synergy in striatum: effects of intrastriatal infusions of dopamine agonists and antagonists on immediate early gene expression", *Neuroscience*, vol. **66**, no. 4, pp. 903–913.

Kegeles, L. S., Abi-Dargham, A., Zea-Ponce, Y., Rodenhiser-Hill, J., Mann, J. J., Van Heertum, R. L., Cooper, T. B., Carlsson, A., & Laruelle, M. 2000, "Modulation of amphetamine-induced striatal dopamine release by ketamine in humans: implications for schizophrenia", *Biol. Psychiatry*, vol. **48**, no. 7, pp. 627–640.

Kegeles, L. S., Martinez, D., Kochan, L. D., Hwang, D. R., Huang, Y., Mawlawi, O., Suckow, R. F., Van Heertum, R. L., & Laruelle, M. 2002, "NMDA antagonist effects on striatal dopamine release: positron emission tomography studies in humans", *Synapse*, vol. **43**, no. 1, pp. 19–29.

Kehr, W. 1974, "Temporal changes in catecholamine synthesis of rat forebrain structures after axotomy", *J. Neural Transm.*, vol. **35**, no. 4, pp. 307–317.

Kemppainen, N., Laine, M., Laakso, M. P., Kaasinen, V., Nagren, K., Vahlberg, T., Kurki, T., & Rinne, J. O. 2003, "Hippocampal dopamine D2 receptors correlate with memory functions in Alzheimer's disease", *Eur. J. Neurosci.*, vol. **18**, no. 1, pp. 149–154.

Kemppainen, N., Ruottinen, H., Nagren, K., & Rinne, J. O. 2000, "PET shows that striatal dopamine D1 and D2 receptors are differentially affected in AD", *Neurology*, vol. **55**, no. 2, pp. 205–209.

Kessler, R. M., Ansari, M. S., Riccardi, P., Li, R., Jayathilake, K., Dawant, B., & Meltzer, H. Y. 2005, "Occupancy of striatal and extrastriatal dopamine D2/D3 receptors by olanzapine and haloperidol", *Neuropsychopharmacology*, vol. **30**, no. 12, pp. 2283–2289.

Kestler, L. P., Malhotra, A. K., Finch, C., Adler, C., & Breier, A. 2000, "The relation between dopamine D2 receptor density and personality: preliminary evidence from the NEO personality inventory-revised", *Neuropsychiatry Neuropsychol. Behav. Neurol.*, vol. **13**, no. 1, pp. 48–52.

Khan, N. L., Brooks, D. J., Pavese, N., Sweeney, M. G., Wood, N. W., Lees, A. J., & Piccini, P. 2002, "Progression of nigrostriatal dysfunction in a parkin kindred: an [18F]dopa PET and clinical study", *Brain*, vol. **125** (Pt 10), pp. 2248–2256.

Khan, Z. U., Mrzljak, L., Gutierrez, A., de la Calle, A., & Goldman-Rakic, P. S. 1998, "Prominence of the dopamine D2 short isoform in dopaminergic pathways", *Proc. Natl. Acad. Sci. USA*, vol. **95**, no. 13, pp. 7731–7736.

Kilbourn, M. & Sherman, P. 1997, "In vivo binding of (+)-alpha-[3H] dihydrotetrabenazine to the vesicular monoamine transporter of rat brain: bolus vs. equilibrium studies", *Eur. J. Pharmacol.*, vol. **331**, no. 2–3, pp. 161–168.

Kilbourn, M. R., DaSilva, J. N., Frey, K. A., Koeppe, R. A., & Kuhl, D. E. 1993, "In vivo imaging of vesicular monoamine transporters in human brain using [11C]tetrabenazine and positron emission tomography", *J. Neurochem.*, vol. **60**, no. 6, pp. 2315–2318.

Kilbourn, M. R., Hockley, B., Lee, L., Hou, C., Goswami, R., Ponde, D. E., Kung, M. P., & Kung, H. F. 2007, "Pharmacokinetics of [(18)F]fluoroalkyl derivatives of dihydrotetrabenazine in rat and monkey brain", *Nucl. Med. Biol.*, vol. **34**, no. 3, pp. 233–237.

Kilts, C. D., Anderson, C. M., Ely, T. D., & Nishita, J. K. 1987, "Absence of synthesis-modulating nerve terminal autoreceptors on mesoamygdaloid and other mesolimbic dopamine neuronal populations", *J. Neurosci.*, vol. **7**, no. 12, pp. 3961–3975.

Kim, C. H., Koo, M. S., Cheon, K. A., Ryu, Y. H., Lee, J. D., & Lee, H. S. 2003, "Dopamine transporter density of basal ganglia assessed with [123I]IPT SPET in obsessive-compulsive disorder", *Eur. J. Nucl. Med. Mol. Imaging*, vol. **30**, no. 12, pp. 1637–1643.

Kim, K. S., Lee, M. K., Carroll, J., & Joh, T. H. 1993, "Both the basal and inducible transcription of the tyrosine hydroxylase gene are dependent upon a cAMP response element", *J. Biol. Chem.*, vol. **268**, no. 21, pp. 15689–15695.

Kim, K. S., Tinti, C., Song, B., Cubells, J. F., & Joh, T. H. 1994, "Cyclic AMP-dependent protein kinase regulates basal and cyclic AMP-stimulated but not phorbol ester-stimulated transcription of the tyrosine hydroxylase gene", *J. Neurochem.*, vol. **63**, no. 3, pp. 834–842.

Kish, S. J., Robitaille, Y., el-Awar, M., Clark, B., Schut, L., Ball, M. J., Young, L. T., Currier, R., & Shannak, K. 1992a, "Striatal monoamine neurotransmitters and metabolites in dominantly inherited olivopontocerebellar atrophy", *Neurology*, vol. **42**, no. 8, pp. 1573–1577.

Kish, S. J., Shannak, K., Rajput, A., Deck, J. H., & Hornykiewicz, O. 1992b, "Aging produces a specific pattern of striatal dopamine loss: implications for the etiology of idiopathic Parkinson's disease", *J. Neurochem.*, vol. **58**, no. 2, pp. 642–648.

Kish, S. J., Zhong, X. H., Hornykiewicz, O., & Haycock, J. W. 1995, "Striatal 3,4-dihydroxyphenylalanine decarboxylase in aging: disparity between postmortem and positron emission tomography studies?", *Ann. Neurol.*, vol. **38**, no. 2, pp. 260–264.

Kishore, A., Nygaard, T. G., de la Fuente-Fernandez, R., Naini, A. B., Schulzer, M., Mak, E., Ruth, T. J., Calne, D. B., Snow, B. J., & Stoessl, A. J. 1998, "Striatal D2 receptors in symptomatic and asymptomatic carriers of dopa-responsive dystonia measured with [11C]-raclopride and positron-emission tomography", *Neurology*, vol. **50**, no. 4, pp. 1028–1032.

Klebaur, J. E., Bevins, R. A., Segar, T. M., & Bardo, M. T. 2001, "Individual differences in behavioral responses to novelty and amphetamine self-administration in male and female rats", *Behav. Pharmacol.*, vol. **12**, no. 4, pp. 267–275.

Klimke, A., Larisch, R., Janz, A., Vosberg, H., Muller-Gartner, H. W., & Gaebel, W. 1999, "Dopamine D2 receptor binding before and after treatment of major depression measured by [123I]IBZM SPECT", *Psychiatry Res.*, vol. **90**, no. 2, pp. 91–101.

Klint, T., Hillegaart, V., Edlund, P. O., Wijkstrom, A., & Ahlenius, S. 1988, "Effects of postpuberal castration on dopamine receptor sensitivity in the male rat brain", *Pharmacol. Toxicol.*, vol. **62**, no. 2, pp. 64–68.

Knable, M. B., Hyde, T. M., Murray, A. M., Herman, M. M., & Kleinman, J. E. 1996, "A postmortem study of frontal cortical dopamine D1 receptors in schizophrenics, psychiatric controls, and normal controls", *Biol. Psychiatry*, vol. **40**, no. 12, pp. 1191–1199.

Knoll, J., Miklya, I., Knoll, B., Marko, R., & Racz, D. 1996, "Phenylethylamine and tyramine are mixed-acting sympathomimetic amines in the brain", *Life Sci.*, vol. 58, no. 23, pp. 2101–2114.

Knoth, J., Peabody, J. O., Huettl, P., & Njus, D. 1984, "Kinetics of tyramine transport and permeation across chromaffin-vesicle membranes", *Biochemistry*, vol. **23**, no. 9, pp. 2011–2016.

Knudsen, G. M., Karlsborg, M., Thomsen, G., Krabbe, K., Regeur, L., Nygaard, T., Videbaek, C., & Werdelin, L. 2004, "Imaging of dopamine transporters and D2 receptors in patients with Parkinson's disease and multiple system atrophy", *Eur. J. Nucl. Med. Mol. Imaging*, vol. **31**, no. 12, pp. 1631–1638.

Kobayashi, K., Inoue, O., Watanabe, Y., Onoe, H., & Langstrom, B. 1995, "Difference in response of D2 receptor binding between 11C-N-methylspiperone and 11C-raclopride against anesthetics in rhesus monkey brain", *J. Neural Transm. Gen. Sect.*, vol. **100**, no. 2, pp. 147–151.

Kochersperger, L. M., Parker, E. L., Siciliano, M., Darlington, G. J., & Denney, R. M. 1986, "Assignment of genes for human monoamine oxidases A and B to the X chromosome", *J. Neurosci. Res.*, vol. **16**, no. 4, pp. 601–616.

Koe, B. K. & Weissman, A. 1968, "The pharmacology of para-chlorophenylalanine, a selective depletor of serotonin stores", *Adv. Pharmacol.*, vol. **6** (Pt B, Suppl.), p. 47.

Koepp, M. J., Gunn, R. N., Lawrence, A. D., Cunningham, V. J., Dagher, A., Jones, T., Brooks, D. J., Bench, C. J., & Grasby, P. M. 1998, "Evidence for striatal dopamine release during a video game", *Nature*, vol. **393**, no. 6682, pp. 266–268.

Koeppe, R. A., Frey, K. A., Kuhl, D. E., & Kilbourn, M. R. 1999, "Assessment of extrastriatal vesicular monoamine transporter binding site density using stereoisomers of [11C]dihydrotetrabenazine", *J. Cereb. Blood Flow Metab.*, vol. **19**, no. 12, pp. 1376–1384.

Koeppe, R. A., Frey, K. A., Kume, A., Albin, R., Kilbourn, M. R., & Kuhl, D. E. 1997, "Equilibrium versus compartmental analysis for assessment of the vesicular monoamine transporter using (+)-alpha-[11C]dihydrotetrabenazine (DTBZ) and positron emission tomography", *J. Cereb. Blood Flow Metab.*, vol. **17**, no. 9, pp. 919–931.

Koeppe, R. A., Frey, K. A., Vander Borght, T. M., Karlamangla, A., Jewett, D. M., Lee, L. C., Kilbourn, M. R., & Kuhl, D. E. 1996, "Kinetic evaluation of [11C] dihydrotetrabenazine by dynamic PET: measurement of vesicular monoamine transporter", *J. Cereb. Blood Flow Metab.*, vol. **16**, no. 6, pp. 1288–1299.

Koerts, J., Leenders, K. L., Koning, M., Portman, A. T., & van Beilen, M. 2007, "Striatal dopaminergic activity (FDOPA-PET) associated with cognitive items of a depression scale (MADRS) in Parkinson's disease", *Eur. J. Neurosci.*, vol. **25**, no. 10, pp. 3132–3136.

Kohler, C., Hall, H., Ogren, S. O., & Gawell, L. 1985, "Specific in vitro and in vivo binding of 3H-raclopride. A potent substituted benzamide drug with high affinity for dopamine D-2 receptors in the rat brain", *Biochem. Pharmacol.*, vol. **34**, no. 13, pp. 2251–2259.

Koochesfahani, K. M., de la Fuente-Fernandez, R., Sossi, V., Schulzer, M., Yatham, L. N., Ruth, T. J., Blinder, S., & Stoessl, A. J. 2006, "Oral methylphenidate fails to elicit significant changes in extracellular putaminal dopamine levels in Parkinson's disease patients: positron emission tomographic studies", *Mov. Disord.*, vol. **21**, no. 7, pp. 970–975.

Korotkova, T. M., Ponomarenko, A. A., Haas, H. L., & Sergeeva, O. A. 2005, "Differential expression of the homeobox gene Pitx3 in midbrain dopaminergic neurons", *Eur. J. Neurosci.*, vol. **22**, no. 6, pp. 1287–1293.

Kortekaas, R., Maguire, R. P., Cremers, T. I., Dijkstra, D., van Waarde A., & Leenders, K. L. 2004, "In vivo binding behavior of dopamine receptor agonist (+)-PD 128907 and implications for the 'ceiling effect' in endogenous competition studies with [(11)C]raclopride-a positron emission tomography study in Macaca mulatta", *J. Cereb. Blood Flow Metab.*, vol. **24**, no. 5, pp. 531–535.

Koshimura, K., Miwa, S., Lee, K., Fujiwara, M., & Watanabe, Y. 1990, "Enhancement of dopamine release in vivo from the rat striatum by dialytic perfusion of 6R-L-erythro-5,6,7,8-tetrahydrobiopterin", *J. Neurochem.*, vol. **54**, no. 4, pp. 1391–1397.

Koshimura, K., Takagi, Y., Miwa, S., Kido, T., Watanabe, Y., Murakami, Y., Kato, Y., & Masaki, T. 1995, "Characterization of a dopamine-releasing action of 6R-L-erythro-tetrahydrobiopterin: comparison with a 6S-form", *J. Neurochem.*, vol. **65**, no. 2, pp. 827–830.

Koulu, M., Pesonen, U., Koskinen, S., Scheinin, H., Virtanen, R., & Scheinin, M. 1993, "Reduced turnover of dopamine and 5-hydroxytryptamine in discrete dopaminergic, noradrenergic and serotonergic rat brain areas after acutely administered medetomidine, a selective alpha 2-adrenoceptor agonist", *Pharmacol. Toxicol.*, vol. **72**, no. 3, pp. 182–187.

Krantz, D. E., Peter, D., Liu, Y., & Edwards, R. H. 1997, "Phosphorylation of a vesicular monoamine transporter by casein kinase II", *J. Biol. Chem.*, vol. **272**, no. 10, pp. 6752–6759.

Krieger, M., Coge, F., Gros, F., & Thibault, J. 1991, "Different mRNAs code for dopa decarboxylase in tissues of neuronal and nonneuronal origin", *Proc. Natl. Acad. Sci. USA*, vol. **88**, no. 6, pp. 2161–2165.

Kuczenski, R. 1983, "Effects of phospholipases on the kinetic properties of rat striatal membrane-bound tyrosine hydroxylase", *J. Neurochem.*, vol. **40**, no. 3, pp. 821–829.

Kuczenski, R., Segal, D. S., & Manley, L. D. 1990, "Apomorphine does not alter amphetamine-induced dopamine release measured in striatal dialysates", *J. Neurochem.*, vol. **54**, no. 5, pp. 1492–1499.

Kugaya, A., Seneca, N. M., Snyder, P. J., Williams, S. A., Malison, R. T., Baldwin, R. M., Seibyl, J. P., & Innis, R. B. 2003, "Changes in human in vivo serotonin and dopamine transporter availabilities during chronic antidepressant administration", *Neuropsychopharmacology*, vol. **28**, no. 2, pp. 413–420.

Kumakura, Y., Cumming, P., Vernaleken, I., Buchholz, H. G., Siessmeier, T., Bartenstein, P., & Gründer, G. 2007a, "Elevated turnover of [^{18}F]dopamine formed in the basal ganglia of patients with schizophrenia; An [^{18}F]FDOPA/PET study", *J. Neurosci.*, vol. **25**, no. 30, pp. 8080–8087.

Kumakura, Y., Cumming, P., Vernaleken, I., Buchholz, H. G., Siessmeier, T., Heinz, A., Kienast, T., Bartenstein, P., & Grunder, G. 2007b, "Elevated [18F]fluorodopamine turnover in brain of patients with schizophrenia: an [18F]fluorodopa/positron emission tomography study", *J. Neurosci.*, vol. **27**, no. 30, pp. 8080–8087.

Kumakura, Y., Gjedde, A., Danielsen, E. H., Christensen, S., & Cumming, P. 2006, "Dopamine storage capacity in caudate and putamen of patients with early Parkinson's disease: correlation with asymmetry of motor symptoms", *J. Cereb. Blood Flow Metab.*, vol. **26**, no. 3, pp. 358–370.

Kumakura, Y., Vernaleken, I., Grunder, G., Bartenstein, P., Gjedde, A., & Cumming, P. 2005, "PET studies of net blood-brain clearance of FDOPA to human brain: age-dependent decline of [18F]fluorodopamine storage capacity", *J. Cereb. Blood Flow Metab.*, vol. **25**, no. 7, pp. 807–819.

Kumar, A., Mann, S., Sossi, V., Ruth, T. J., Stoessl, A. J., Schulzer, M., & Lee, C. S. 2003, "[11C]DTBZ-PET correlates of levodopa responses in asymmetric Parkinson's disease", vol. **126** (Pt 12), pp. 2648–2655.

Kumlien, E., Bergstrom, M., Lilja, A., Andersson, J., Szekeres, V., Westerberg, C. E., Westerberg, G., Antoni, G., & Langstrom, B. 1995, "Positron emission tomography with [11C]deuterium-deprenyl in temporal lobe epilepsy", *Epilepsia*, vol. **36**, no. 7, pp. 712–721.

Kumlien, E., Hilton-Brown, P., Spannare, B., & Gillberg, P. G. 1992, "In vitro quantitative autoradiography of [3H]-L-deprenyl and [3H]-PK 11195 binding sites in human epileptic hippocampus", *Epilepsia*, vol. **33**, no. 4, pp. 610–617.

Kung, M. P., Chumpradit, S., Frederick, D., Garner, S., Burris, K. D., Molinoff, P. B., & Kung, H. F. 1994, "Characterization of binding sites for [125I]R(+)trans-7-OH-PIPAT in rat brain", *Naunyn Schmiedebergs Arch. Pharmacol.*, vol. **350**, no. 6, pp. 611–617.

Kung, M. P., Hou, C., Goswami, R., Ponde, D. E., Kilbourn, M. R., & Kung, H. F. 2007, "Characterization of optically resolved 9-fluoropropyl-dihydrotetrabenazine as a potential PET imaging agent targeting vesicular monoamine transporters", *Nucl. Med. Biol.*, vol. **34**, no. 3, pp. 239–246.

Kung, M. P., Stevenson, D. A., Plossl, K., Meegalla, S. K., Beckwith, A., Essman, W. D., Mu, M., Lucki, I., & Kung, H. F. 1997, "[99mTc]TRODAT-1: a novel technetium-99m complex as a dopamine transporter imaging agent", *Eur. J. Nucl. Med.*, vol. **24**, no. 4, pp. 372–380.

Kuroda, Y., Motohashi, N., Ito, H., Ito, S., Takano, A., Nishikawa, T., & Suhara, T. 2006, "Effects of repetitive transcranial magnetic stimulation on [11C]raclopride binding and cognitive function in patients with depression", *J. Affect. Disord.*, vol. **95**, no. 1–3, pp. 35–42.

Kuwabara, H., Cumming, P., Yasuhara, Y., Leger, G. C., Guttman, M., Diksic, M., Evans, A. C., & Gjedde, A. 1995, "Regional striatal DOPA transport and decarboxylase activity in Parkinson's disease", *J. Nucl. Med.*, vol. **36**, no. 7, pp. 1226–1231.

Kwan, S. W., Bergeron, J. M., & Abell, C. W. 1992, "Molecular properties of monoamine oxidases A and B", *Psychopharmacology (Berl)*, vol. **106** (Suppl. 106), pp. S1–S5.

la Fougere C., Krause, J., Krause, K. H., Josef, G. F., Hacker, M., Koch, W., Hahn, K., Tatsch, K., & Dresel, S. 2006, "Value of 99mTc-TRODAT-1 SPECT to predict clinical response to methylphenidate treatment in adults with attention deficit hyperactivity disorder", *Nucl. Med. Commun.*, vol. **27**, no. 9, pp. 733–737.

Laakso, A., Bergman, J., Haaparanta, M., Vilkman, H., Solin, O., & Hietala, J. 1998, "[18F]CFT [(18F)WIN 35,428], a radioligand to study the dopamine transporter with PET: characterization in human subjects", *Synapse*, vol. **28**, no. 3, pp. 244–250.

Laakso, A., Bergman, J., Haaparanta, M., Vilkman, H., Solin, O., Syvalahti, E., & Hietala, J. 2001, "Decreased striatal dopamine transporter binding in vivo in chronic schizophrenia", *Schizophr. Res.*, vol. **52**, no. 1–2, pp. 115–120.

Laakso, A., Pohjalainen, T., Bergman, J., Kajander, J., Haaparanta, M., Solin, O., Syvalahti, E., & Hietala, J. 2005, "The A1 allele of the human D2 dopamine receptor gene is associated with increased activity of striatal L-amino acid decarboxylase in healthy subjects", *Pharmacogenet. Genomics*, vol. **15**, no. 6, pp. 387–391.

Laakso, A., Vilkman, H., Alakare, B., Haaparanta, M., Bergman, J., Solin, O., Peurasaari, J., Rakkolainen, V., Syvalahti, E., & Hietala, J. 2000a, "Striatal dopamine transporter binding in neuroleptic-naive patients with schizophrenia studied with positron emission tomography", *Am. J. Psychiatry*, vol. **157**, no. 2, pp. 269–271.

Laakso, A., Vilkman, H., Bergman, J., Haaparanta, M., Solin, O., Syvalahti, E., Salokangas, R. K., & Hietala, J. 2002, "Sex differences in striatal presynaptic dopamine synthesis capacity in healthy subjects", *Biol. Psychiatry*, vol. **52**, no. 7, pp. 759–763.

Laakso, A., Vilkman, H., Kajander, J., Bergman, J., Haaparanta, M., Solin, O., & Hietala, J. 2000b, "Prediction of detached personality in healthy subjects by low dopamine transporter binding", *Am. J. Psychiatry*, vol. **157**, no. 2, pp. 290–292.

Laakso, A., Wallius, E., Kajander, J., Bergman, J., Eskola, O., Solin, O., Ilonen, T., Salokangas, R. K., Syvalahti, E., & Hietala, J. 2003, "Personality traits and striatal dopamine synthesis capacity in healthy subjects", *Am. J. Psychiatry*, vol. **160**, no. 5, pp. 904–910.

Laine, T. P., Ahonen, A., Räsänen, P., Pohjalainen, T., Tiihonen, J., & Hietala, J. 2001, "The A1 allele of the D2 dopamine receptor gene is associated with high dopamine transporter density in detoxified alcoholics", *Alcohol Alcohol*, vol. **36**, no. 3, pp. 262–265.

Laine, T. P., Ahonen, A., Räsänen, P., & Tiihonen, J. 1999, "Dopamine transporter availability and depressive symptoms during alcohol withdrawal", *Psychiatry Res.*, vol. **90**, no. 3, pp. 153–157.

Lamensdorf, I. & Finberg, J. P. 1997, "Reduced striatal tyrosine hydroxylase activity is not accompanied by change in responsiveness of dopaminergic receptors following chronic treatment with deprenyl", *Neuropharmacology*, vol. **36**, no. 10, pp. 1455–1461.

Lammertsma, A. A., Bench, C. J., Price, G. W., Cremer, J. E., Luthra, S. K., Turton, D., Wood, N. D., & Frackowiak, R. S. 1991, "Measurement of cerebral monoamine oxidase B activity using L-[11C]deprenyl and dynamic positron emission tomography", *J. Cereb. Blood Flow Metab.*, vol. **11**, no. 4, pp. 545–556.

Lan, N. C., Heinzmann, C., Gal, A., Klisak, I., Orth, U., Lai, E., Grimsby, J., Sparkes, R. S., Mohandas, T., & Shih, J. C. 1989, "Human monoamine oxidase A and B genes map to Xp 11.23 and are deleted in a patient with Norrie disease", *Genomics*, vol. **4**, no. 4, pp. 552–559.

Landvogt, C., Mengel, E., Bartenstein, P., Buchholz, H. G., Schreckenberger, M., Siessmeier, T., Scheurich, A., Feldmann, R., Weglage, J., Cumming, P., Zepp, F., & Ullrich, K. 2007, "Reduced cerebral fluoro-L-dopamine uptake in adult patients suffering from phenylketonuria", *J. Cereb. Blood Flow Metab.*, vol. **28**, no. 4, pp. 824–831.

Langston, J. W., Ballard, P., Tetrud, J. W., & Irwin, I. 1983, "Chronic Parkinsonism in humans due to a product of meperidine-analog synthesis", *Science*, vol. **219**, no. 4587, pp. 979–980.

Larisch, R., Meyer, W., Klimke, A., Kehren, F., Vosberg, H., & Muller-Gartner, H. W. 1998, "Left-right asymmetry of striatal dopamine D2 receptors", *Nucl. Med. Commun.*, vol. **19**, no. 8, pp. 781–787.

Laruelle, M. 2000, "Imaging synaptic neurotransmission with in vivo binding competition techniques: a critical review", *J. Cereb. Blood Flow Metab.*, vol. **20**, no. 3, pp. 423–451.

Laruelle, M., Baldwin, R. M., Malison, R. T., Zea-Ponce, Y., Zoghbi, S. S., al-Tikriti, M. S., Sybirska, E. H., Zimmermann, R. C., Wisniewski, G., Neumeyer, J. L., *et al.* 1993, "SPECT imaging of dopamine and serotonin transporters with [123I] beta-CIT: pharmacological characterization of brain uptake in nonhuman primates", *Synapse*, vol. **13**, no. 4, pp. 295–309.

Laruelle, M., Abi-Dargham, A., Gil, R., Kegeles, L., & Innis, R. 1999, "Increased dopamine transmission in schizophrenia: relationship to illness phases", *Biol. Psychiatry*, vol. **46**, no. 1, pp. 56–72.

Laruelle, M., Abi-Dargham, A., van Dyck, C., Gil, R., D'Souza, D. C., Krystal, J., Seibyl, J., Baldwin, R., & Innis, R. 2000, "Dopamine and serotonin transporters in patients with schizophrenia: an imaging study with [(123)I]beta-CIT", *Biol. Psychiatry*, vol. **47**, no. 5, pp. 371–379.

Laruelle, M., D'Souza, C. D., Baldwin, R. M., Abi-Dargham, A., Kanes, S. J., Fingado, C. L., Seibyl, J. P., Zoghbi, S. S., Bowers, M. B., Jatlow, P., Charney, D. S., & Innis, R. B. 1997a, "Imaging D2 receptor occupancy by endogenous dopamine in humans", *Neuropsychopharmacology*, vol. **17**, no. 3, pp. 162–174.

Laruelle, M., Gelernter, J., & Innis, R. B. 1998, "D2 receptors binding potential is not affected by Taq1 polymorphism at the D2 receptor gene", *Mol. Psychiatry*, vol. **3**, no. 3, pp. 261–265.

Laruelle, M., Giddings, S. S., Zea-Ponce, Y., Charney, D. S., Neumeyer, J. L., Baldwin, R. M., & Innis, R. B. 1994, "Methyl 3 beta-(4-[125I]iodophenyl) tropane-2 beta-carboxylate in vitro binding to dopamine and serotonin transporters under 'physiological' conditions", *J. Neurochem.*, vol. **62**, no. 3, pp. 978–986.

Laruelle, M., Iyer, R. N., al-Tikriti, M. S., Zea-Ponce, Y., Malison, R., Zoghbi, S. S., Baldwin, R. M., Kung, H. F., Charney, D. S., Hoffer, P. B., Innis, R. B., & Bradberry, C. W. 1997b, "Microdialysis and SPECT measurements of amphetamine-induced dopamine release in nonhuman primates", *Synapse*, vol. **25**, no. 1, pp. 1–14.

Laschinski, G., Kittner, B., & Brautigam, M. 1986, "Direct inhibition of tyrosine hydroxylase from PC-12 cells by catechol derivatives", *Naunyn Schmiedebergs Arch. Pharmacol.*, vol. **332**, no. 4, pp. 346–350.

Lavalaye, J., Booij, J., Reneman, L., Habraken, J. B., & van Royen, E. A. 2000, "Effect of age and gender on dopamine transporter imaging with [123I]FP-CIT SPET in healthy volunteers", *Eur. J. Nucl. Med.*, vol. **27**, no. 7, pp. 867–869.

Lavigne, J. A., Helzlsouer, K. J., Huang, H. Y., Strickland, P. T., Bell, D. A., Selmin, O., Watson, M. A., Hoffman, S., Comstock, G. W., & Yager, J. D. 1997, "An association between the allele coding for a low activity variant of catechol-O-methyltransferase and the risk for breast cancer", *Cancer Res.*, vol. **57**, no. 24, pp. 5493–5497.

Lazar, M. A., Lockfeld, A. J., Truscott, R. J., & Barchas, J. D. 1982, "Tyrosine hydroxylase from bovine striatum: catalytic properties of the phosphorylated and nonphosphorylated forms of the purified enzyme", *J. Neurochem.*, vol. **39**, no. 2, pp. 409–422.

Lazar, M. A., Mefford, I. N., & Barchas, J. D. 1982, "Tyrosine hydroxylase activation. Comparison of in vitro phosphorylation and in vivo administration of haloperidol", *Biochem. Pharmacol.*, vol. **31**, no. 16, pp. 2599–2607.

Lazareno, S. & Nahorski, S. R. 1982, "Selective labelling of dopamine (D2) receptors in rat striatum by [3H]domperidone but not by [3H]spiperone", *Eur. J. Pharmacol.*, vol. **81**, no. 2, pp. 273–285.

Le Moine, C. & Bloch, B. 1995, "D1 and D2 dopamine receptor gene expression in the rat striatum: sensitive cRNA probes demonstrate prominent segregation of D1 and D2 mRNAs in distinct neuronal populations of the dorsal and ventral striatum", *J. Comp Neurol.*, vol. **355**, no. 3, pp. 418–426.

Le Moine, C. & Bloch, B. 1996, "Expression of the D3 dopamine receptor in peptidergic neurons of the nucleus accumbens: comparison with the D1 and D2 dopamine receptors", *Neuroscience*, vol. **73**, no. 1, pp. 131–143.

Le Moine C., Svenningsson, P., Fredholm, B. B., & Bloch, B. 1997, "Dopamine-adenosine interactions in the striatum and the globus pallidus: inhibition of striatopallidal neurons through either D2 or A2A receptors enhances D1 receptor-mediated effects on c-fos expression", *J. Neurosci.*, vol. **17**, no. 20, pp. 8038–8048.

Le Van Thai, A., Coste, E., Allen, J. M., Palmiter, R. D., & Weber, M. J. 1993, "Identification of a neuron-specific promoter of human aromatic L-amino acid decarboxylase gene", *Brain Res. Mol. Brain Res.*, vol. **17**, no. 3–4, pp. 227–238.

Lee, C. S., Samii, A., Sossi, V., Ruth, T. J., Schulzer, M., Holden, J. E., Wudel, J., Pal, P. K., de la Fuente-Fernandez, Calne, D. B., & Stoessl, A. J. 2000, "In vivo positron emission tomographic evidence for compensatory changes in presynaptic dopaminergic nerve terminals in Parkinson's disease", *Ann. Neurol.*, vol. **47**, no. 4, pp. 493–503.

Lee, S. P., O'Dowd, B. F., Rajaram, R. D., Nguyen, T., & George, S. R. 2003, "D2 dopamine receptor homodimerization is mediated by multiple sites of interaction, including an intermolecular interaction involving transmembrane domain 4", *Biochemistry*, vol. **42**, no. 37, pp. 11023–11031.

Leger, G., Gjedde, A., Kuwabara, H., Guttman, M., & Cumming, P. 1998, "Effect of catechol-O-methyltransferase inhibition on brain uptake of [18F]fluorodopa: implications for compartmental modelling and clinical usefulness", *Synapse*, vol. **30**, no. 4, pp. 351–361.

Lehericy, S., Brandel, J. P., Hirsch, E. C., Anglade, P., Villares, J., Scherman, D., Duyckaerts, C., Javoy-Agid, F., & Agid, Y. 1994, "Monoamine vesicular uptake sites in patients with Parkinson's disease and Alzheimer's disease, as measured by tritiated dihydrotetrabenazine autoradiography", *Brain Res.*, vol. **659**, no. 1–2, pp. 1–9.

Lenders, J. W., Eisenhofer, G., Abeling, N. G., Berger, W., Murphy, D. L., Konings, C. H., Wagemakers, L. M., Kopin, I. J., Karoum, F., van Gennip, A. H., & Brunner, H. G. 1996, "Specific genetic deficiencies of the A and B isoenzymes of monoamine oxidase are characterized by distinct neurochemical and clinical phenotypes", *J. Clin. Invest*, vol. **97**, no. 4, pp. 1010–1019.

Leroux-Nicollet, I. & Costentin, J. 1994, "Comparison of the subregional distributions of the monoamine vesicular transporter and dopamine uptake complex in the rat striatum and changes during aging", *J. Neural Transm. Gen. Sect.*, vol. **97**, no. 2, pp. 93–106.

Leroux-Nicollet, I., Darchen, F., Scherman, D., & Costentin, J. 1990, "Postnatal development of the monoamine vesicular transporter in mesencephalic and telencephalic regions of the rat brain: a quantitative autoradiographic study with [3H]dihydrotetrabenazine", *Neurosci. Lett.*, vol. **117**, no. 1–2, pp. 1–7.

Leslie, C. A. & Bennett, J. P., Jr. 1987, "[3H]spiperone binds selectively to rat striatal D2 dopamine receptors in vivo: a kinetic and pharmacological analysis", *Brain Res.*, vol. **407**, no. 2, pp. 253–262.

Leung, T. K., Lai, J. C., & Lim, L. 1981, "The regional distribution of monoamine oxidase activities towards different substrates: effects in rat brain of chronic administration of manganese chloride and of ageing", *J. Neurochem.*, vol. **36**, no. 6, pp. 2037–2043.

Levesque, D. & Di Paolo, T. 1993, "Modulation by estradiol and progesterone of the GTP effect on striatal D-2 dopamine receptors", *Biochem. Pharmacol.*, vol. **45**, no. 3, pp. 723–733.

Levesque, D., Gagnon, S., & Di Paolo, T. 1989, "Striatal D1 dopamine receptor density fluctuates during the rat estrous cycle", *Neurosci. Lett.*, vol. **98**, no. 3, pp. 345–350.

Leviel, V., Gobert, A., & Guibert, B. 1989, "Direct observation of dopamine compartmentation in striatal nerve terminal by 'in vivo' measurement of the specific activity of released dopamine", *Brain Res.*, vol. **499**, no. 2, pp. 205–213.

Leviel, V. & Guibert, B. 1987, "Involvement of intraterminal dopamine compartments in the amine release in the cat striatum", *Neurosci. Lett.*, vol. **76**, no. 2, pp. 197–202.

Levine, J., Martine, T., Feraro, R., Kimhi, R., & Bracha, H. S. 1997, "Medicated chronic schizophrenic patients do not demonstrate left turning asymmetry", *Neuropsychobiology*, vol. **36**, no. 1, pp. 22–24.

Levine, R. A., Kuhn, D. M., & Lovenberg, W. 1979, "The regional distribution of hydroxylase cofactor in rat brain", *J. Neurochem.*, vol. **32**, no. 5, pp. 1575–1578.

Levitt, P., Pintar, J. E., & Breakefield, X. O. 1982, "Immunocytochemical demonstration of monoamine oxidase B in brain astrocytes and serotonergic neurons", *Proc. Natl. Acad. Sci. USA*, vol. **79**, no. 20, pp. 6385–6389.

Lew, J. Y., Garcia-Espana, A., Lee, K. Y., Carr, K. D., Goldstein, M., Haycock, J. W., & Meller, E. 1999, "Increased site-specific phosphorylation of tyrosine hydroxylase accompanies stimulation of enzymatic activity induced by cessation of dopamine neuronal activity", *Mol. Pharmacol.*, vol. **55**, no. 2, pp. 202–209.

Leyton, M., Boileau, I., Benkelfat, C., Diksic, M., Baker, G., & Dagher, A. 2002, "Amphetamine-induced increases in extracellular dopamine, drug wanting, and novelty seeking: a PET/[11C]raclopride study in healthy men", *Neuropsychopharmacology*, vol. **27**, no. 6, pp. 1027–1035.

Leyton, M., Dagher, A., Boileau, I., Casey, K., Baker, G. B., Diksic, M., Gunn, R., Young, S. N., & Benkelfat, C. 2004, "Decreasing amphetamine-induced dopamine release by acute phenylalanine/tyrosine depletion: A PET/[11C]raclopride study in healthy men", *Neuropsychopharmacology*, vol. **29**, no. 2, pp. 427–432.

Li, P. P., Warsh, J. J., & Godse, D. D. 1984, "Formation and clearance of norepinephrine glycol metabolites in mouse brain", *J. Neurochem.*, vol. **43**, no. 5, pp. 1425–1433.

Li, T., Vallada, H., Curtis, D., Arranz, M., Xu, K., Cai, G., Deng, H., Liu, J., Murray, R., Liu, X., & Collier, D. A. 1997, "Catechol-O-methyltransferase Val158Met polymorphism: frequency analysis in Han Chinese subjects and allelic association of the low activity allele with bipolar affective disorder", *Pharmacogenetics*, vol. **7**, no. 5, pp. 349–353.

Li, X. M., Juorio, A. V., & Boulton, A. A. 1993, "NSD-1015 alters the gene expression of aromatic L-amino acid decarboxylase in rat PC12 pheochromocytoma cells", *Neurochem. Res.*, vol. **18**, no. 8, pp. 915–919.

Li, X. M., Juorio, A. V., Paterson, I. A., Zhu, M. Y., & Boulton, A. A. 1992, "Specific irreversible monoamine oxidase B inhibitors stimulate gene expression of aromatic L-amino acid decarboxylase in PC12 cells", *J. Neurochem.*, vol. **59**, no. 6, pp. 2324–2327.

Liang, N. Y. & Rutledge, C. O. 1982, "Evidence for carrier-mediated efflux of dopamine from corpus striatum", *Biochem. Pharmacol.*, vol. **31**, no. 15, pp. 2479–2484.

Linazasoro, G., Obeso, J. A., Gómez, J. C., Martínez, M., Antonini, A., & Leenders, K. L. 1999, "Modification of dopamine D2 receptor activity by pergolide in Parkinson's disease: an in vivo study by PET", *Clin Neuropharmacol.*, vol. **22**, no. 5, pp. 277–280.

Lind, N. M., Gjedde, A., Moustgaard, A., Olsen, A. K., Jensen, S. B., Jakobsen, S., Arnfred, S. M., Hansen, A. K., Hemmingsen, R. P., & Cumming, P. 2005, "Behavioral response to novelty correlates with dopamine receptor availability in striatum of Gottingen minipigs", *Behav. Brain Res.*, vol. **164**, no. 2, pp. 172–177.

Lindsey, K. P., Wilcox, K. M., Votaw, J. R., Goodman, M. M., Plisson, C., Carroll, F. I., Rice, K. C., & Howell, L. L. 2004, "Effects of dopamine transporter inhibitors on cocaine self-administration in rhesus monkeys: relationship to transporter occupancy determined by positron emission tomography neuroimaging", *J. Pharmacol. Exp. Ther.*, vol. **309**, no. 3, pp. 959–969.

Lindskog, M., Svenningsson, P., Fredholm, B. B., Greengard, P., & Fisone, G. 1999, "Activation of dopamine D2 receptors decreases DARPP-32 phosphorylation in striatonigral and striatopallidal projection neurons via different mechanisms", *Neuroscience*, vol. **88**, no. 4, pp. 1005–1008.

Lindstrom, L. H., Gefvert, O., Hagberg, G., Lundberg, T., Bergstrom, M., Hartvig, P., & Langstrom, B. 1999, "Increased dopamine synthesis rate in medial prefrontal cortex and striatum in schizophrenia indicated by L-(beta-11C) DOPA and PET", *Biol. Psychiatry*, vol. **46**, no. 5, pp. 681–688.

Lippens, F. J. P., van der Krogt, J. A., Noach, E. L., & van Valkenburg, C. F. M. 1988, "Monitoring the specific activities of dopamine and its metabolites in striatum and olfactory tubercle after intravenous administration of L-[^{3}H]tyrosine: complex relations, indicating more than two compartments", *Neurochem. Int*, vol. **12**, pp. 203–208.

Liskowsky, D. R. & Potter, L. T. 1985, "A pre-positron emission tomography study of L-3,4-dihydroxy-[3H]phenylalanine distribution in the rat", *Neurosci. Lett.*, vol. **53**, no. 2, pp. 161–167.

List, S. J. & Seeman, P. 1981, "Resolution of dopamine and serotonin receptor components of [3H]spiperone binding to rat brain regions", *Proc. Natl. Acad. Sci. USA*, vol. **78**, no. 4, pp. 2620–2624.

Liste, I., Rozas, G., Guerra, M. J., & Labandeira-Garcia, J. L. 1995, "Cortical stimulation induces Fos expression in striatal neurons via NMDA glutamate and dopamine receptors", *Brain Res.*, vol. **700**, no. 1–2, pp. 1–12.

Little, K. Y., Kirkman, J. A., Carroll, F. I., Clark, T. B., & Duncan, G. E. 1993, "Cocaine use increases [3H]WIN 35428 binding sites in human striatum", *Brain Res.*, vol. **628**, no. 1-2, pp. 17-25.

Liu, Y., Peter, D., Roghani, A., Schuldiner, S., Prive, G. G., Eisenberg, D., Brecha, N., & Edwards, R. H. 1992, "A cDNA that suppresses MPP+ toxicity encodes a vesicular amine transporter", *Cell*, vol. **70**, no. 4, pp. 539-551.

Lodge, D. J. & Grace, A. A. 2006, "The laterodorsal tegmentum is essential for burst firing of ventral tegmental area dopamine neurons", *Proc. Natl. Acad. Sci. USA*, vol. **103**, no. 13, pp. 5167-5172.

Logan, J., Fowler, J. S., Dewey, S. L., Volkow, N. D., & Gatley, S. J. 2001, "A consideration of the dopamine D2 receptor monomer-dimer equilibrium and the anomalous binding properties of the dopamine D2 receptor ligand, N-methyl spiperone", *J. Neural Transm.*, vol. **108**, no. 3, pp. 279-286.

Logan, J., Fowler, J. S., Volkow, N. D., Wolf, A. P., Dewey, S. L., Schlyer, D. J., MacGregor, R. R., Hitzemann, R., Bendriem, B., Gatley, S. J., *et al.* 1990, "Graphical analysis of reversible radioligand binding from time-activity measurements applied to [N-11C-methyl]-(-)-cocaine PET studies in human subjects", *J. Cereb. Blood Flow Metab.*, vol. **10**, no. 5, pp. 740-747.

Logan, J., Volkow, N. D., Fowler, J. S., Wang, G. J., Fischman, M. W., Foltin, R. W., Abumrad, N. N., Vitkun, S., Gatley, S. J., Pappas, N., Hitzemann, R., & Shea, C. E. 1997, "Concentration and occupancy of dopamine transporters in cocaine abusers with [11C]cocaine and PET", *Synapse*, vol. **27**, no. 4, pp. 347-356.

Lokkegaard, A., Werdelin, L. M., Regeur, L., Karlsborg, M., Jensen, S. R., Brodsgaard, E., Madsen, F. F., Lonsdale, M. N., & Friberg, L. 2007, "Dopamine transporter imaging and the effects of deep brain stimulation in patients with Parkinson's disease", *Eur. J. Nucl. Med. Mol. Imaging*, vol. **34**, no. 4, pp. 508-516.

Lopez-Martin, E., Rozas, G., Rodriguez, J., Guerra, M. J., & Labandeira-Garcia, J. L. 1998, "The corticostriatal system mediates the 'paradoxical' contraversive rotation but not the striatal hyperexpression of Fos induced by amphetamine early after 6-hydroxydopamine lesion of the nigrostriatal pathway", *Exp. Brain Res.*, vol. **120**, no. 2, pp. 153-163.

Lorberboym, M., Djaldetti, R., Melamed, E., Sadeh, M., & Lampl, Y. 2004, "123I-FP-CIT SPECT imaging of dopamine transporters in patients with cerebrovascular disease and clinical diagnosis of vascular parkinsonism", *J. Nucl. Med.*, vol. **45**, no. 10, pp. 1688-1693.

Lorberboym, M., Treves, T. A., Melamed, E., Lampl, Y., Hellmann, M., & Djaldetti, R. 2006, "[123I]-FP/CIT SPECT imaging for distinguishing drug-induced parkinsonism from Parkinson's disease", *Mov. Disord.*, vol. **21**, no. 4, pp. 510-514.

Lotta, T., Vidgren, J., Tilgmann, C., Ulmanen, I., Melen, K., Julkunen, I., & Taskinen, J. 1995, "Kinetics of human soluble and membrane-bound catechol O-methyltransferase: a revised mechanism and description of the thermolabile variant of the enzyme", *Biochemistry*, vol. **34**, no. 13, pp. 4202-4210.

Lovenberg, W., Barchas, J., Weissbach, H., & Udenfriend, S. 1963, "Characteristics of the inhibition of aromatic L-amino acid decarboxylase by alpha-methylamino acids", *Arch. Biochem. Biophys.*, vol. **103**, pp. 9–14.

Lovenberg, W., Weissbach, H., & Udenfriend, S. 1962, "Aromatic L-amino acid decarboxylase", *J. Biol. Chem.*, vol. **237**, pp. 89–93.

Ludecke, B., Knappskog, P. M., Clayton, P. T., Surtees, R. A., Clelland, J. D., Heales, S. J., Brand, M. P., Bartholome, K., & Flatmark, T. 1996, "Recessively inherited L-DOPA-responsive parkinsonism in infancy caused by a point mutation (L205P) in the tyrosine hydroxylase gene", *Hum. Mol. Genet.*, vol. **5**, no. 7, pp. 1023–1028.

Ludolph, A. G., Kassubek, J., Schmeck, K., Glaser, C., Wunderlich, A., Buck, A. K., Reske, S. N., Fegert, J. M., & Mottaghy, F. M. 2008, "Dopaminergic dysfunction in attention deficit hyperactivity disorder (ADHD), differences between pharmacologically treated and never treated young adults: a 3,4-dihdroxy-6-[18F] fluorophenyl-l-alanine PET study", *Neuroimage.*, vol. **41**, no. 3, pp. 718–727.

Lundkvist, C., Halldin, C., Ginovart, N., Swahn, C. G., & Farde, L. 1997, "[18F] beta-CIT-FP is superior to [11C] beta-CIT-FP for quantitation of the dopamine transporter", *Nucl. Med. Biol.*, vol. **24**, no. 7, pp. 621–627.

Lundquist, P., Blomquist, G., Hartvig, P., Hagberg, G. E., Torstenson, R., Hammarlund-Udenaes, M., & Langstrom, B. 2006, "Validation studies on the 5-hydroxy-L-[beta-11C]-tryptophan/PET method for probing the decarboxylase step in serotonin synthesis", *Synapse*, vol. **59**, no. 8, pp. 521–531.

Lyon, R. A., Titeler, M., Frost, J. J., Whitehouse, P. J., Wong, D. F., Wagner, H. N., Jr., Dannals, R. F., Links, J. M., & Kuhar, M. J. 1986, "3H-3-N-methylspiperone labels D2 dopamine receptors in basal ganglia and S2 serotonin receptors in cerebral cortex", *J. Neurosci.*, vol. **6**, no. 10, pp. 2941–2949.

Ma, S. Y., Roytt, M., Collan, Y., & Rinne, J. O. 1999, "Unbiased morphometrical measurements show loss of pigmented nigral neurones with ageing", *Neuropathol. Appl. Neurobiol.*, vol. **25**, no. 5, pp. 394–399.

Mach, R. H., Ehrenkaufer, R. L., Greenberg, J. H., Shao, L., Morton, T. E., Evora, P. H., Nowak, P. A., Luedtke, R. R., Cohen, D., & Reivich, M. 1995, "PET imaging studies of dopamine D2 receptors: comparison of [18F]N-methylspiperone and the benzamide analogues [18F]MABN and [18F]MBP in baboon brain", *Synapse*, vol. **19**, no. 3, pp. 177–187.

Mackay, A. V., Davies, P., Dewar, A. J., & Yates, C. M. 1978, "Regional distribution of enzymes associated with neurotransmission by monoamines, acetylcholine and GABA in the human brain", *J. Neurochem.*, vol. **30**, no. 4, pp. 827–839.

MacKenzie, R. G. & Zigmond, M. J. 1984, "High- and low-affinity states of striatal D2 receptors are not affected by 6-hydroxydopamine or chronic haloperidol treatment", *J. Neurochem.*, vol. **43**, no. 5, pp. 1310–1318.

MacRae, P. G., Spirduso, W. W., Walters, T. J., Farrar, R. P., & Wilcox, R. E. 1987, "Endurance training effects on striatal D2 dopamine receptor binding and striatal dopamine metabolites in presenescent older rats", *Psychopharmacology (Berl)*, vol. **92**, no. 2, pp. 236–240.

MacRae, P. G., Spirduso, W. W., & Wilcox, R. E. 1988, "Reaction time and nigrostriatal dopamine function: the effects of age and practice", *Brain Res.*, vol. **451**, no. 1–2, pp. 139–146.

Madras, B. K., Fahey, M. A., Bergman, J., Canfield, D. R., & Spealman, R. D. 1989, "Effects of cocaine and related drugs in nonhuman primates. I. [3H]cocaine binding sites in caudate-putamen", *J. Pharmacol. Exp. Ther.*, vol. **251**, no. 1, pp. 131–141.

Madras, B. K., Fahey, M. A., Goulet, M., Lin, Z., Bendor, J., Goodrich, C., Meltzer, P. C., Elmaleh, D. R., Livni, E., Bonab, A. A., & Fischman, A. J. 2006, "Dopamine transporter (DAT) inhibitors alleviate specific parkinsonian deficits in monkeys: association with DAT occupancy in vivo", *J. Pharmacol. Exp. Ther.*, vol. **319**, no. 2, pp. 570–585.

Madras, B. K., Gracz, L. M., Fahey, M. A., Elmaleh, D., Meltzer, P. C., Liang, A. Y., Stopa, E. G., Babich, J., & Fischman, A. J. 1998, "Altropane, a SPECT or PET imaging probe for dopamine neurons: III. Human dopamine transporter in postmortem normal and Parkinson's diseased brain", *Synapse*, vol. **29**, no. 2, pp. 116–127.

Maggos, C. E., Tsukada, H., Kakiuchi, T., Nishiyama, S., Myers, J. E., Kreuter, J., Schlussman, S. D., Unterwald, E. M., Ho, A., & Kreek, M. J. 1998, "Sustained withdrawal allows normalization of in vivo [11C]N-methylspiperone dopamine D2 receptor binding after chronic binge cocaine: a positron emission tomography study in rats", *Neuropsychopharmacology*, vol. **19**, no. 2, pp. 146–153.

Major, L. J., Murphy, D. L., Lipper, S., & Gordon, E. 1979, "Effects of clorgyline and pargyline on deaminated metabolites of norepinephrine, dopamine and serotonin in human cerebrospinal fluid", *J. Neurochem.*, vol. **32**, no. 1, pp. 229–231.

Malison, R. T., Best, S. E., van Dyck, C. H., McCance, E. F., Wallace, E. A., Laruelle, M., Baldwin, R. M., Seibyl, J. P., Price, L. H., Kosten, T. R., & Innis, R. B. 1998a, "Elevated striatal dopamine transporters during acute cocaine abstinence as measured by [123I] beta-CIT SPECT", *Am. J. Psychiatry*, vol. **155**, no. 6, pp. 832–834.

Malison, R. T., Best, S. E., Wallace, E. A., McCance, E., Laruelle, M., Zoghbi, S. S., Baldwin, R. M., Seibyl, J. S., Hoffer, P. B., Price, L. H., *et al.* 1995a, "Euphorigenic doses of cocaine reduce [123I]beta-CIT SPECT measures of dopamine transporter availability in human cocaine addicts", *Psychopharmacology (Berl)*, vol. **122**, no. 4, pp. 358–362.

Malison, R. T., McCance, E., Carpenter, L. L., Baldwin, R. M., Seibyl, J. P., Price, L. H., Kosten, T. R., & Innis, R. B. 1998b, "[123I]beta-CIT SPECT imaging of dopamine transporter availability after mazindol administration in human cocaine addicts", *Psychopharmacology (Berl)*, vol. **137**, no. 4, pp. 321–325.

Malison, R. T., McDougle, C. J., van Dyck, C. H., Scahill, L., Baldwin, R. M., Seibyl, J. P., Price, L. H., Leckman, J. F., & Innis, R. B. 1995b, "[123I]beta-CIT SPECT imaging of striatal dopamine transporter binding in Tourette's disorder", *Am. J. Psychiatry*, vol. **152**, no. 9, pp. 1359–1361.

Mallajosyula, J. K., Kaur, D., Chinta, S. J., Rajagopalan, S., Rane, A., Nicholls, D. G., Di Monte, D. A., Macarthur, H., & Andersen, J. K. 2008, "MAO-B elevation in mouse brain astrocytes results in Parkinson's pathology", *PLoS ONE*, vol. **3**, no. 2, pp. e1616.

Mamelak, M., Chiu, S., & Mishra, R. K. 1993, "High- and low-affinity states of dopamine D1 receptors in schizophrenia", *Eur. J. Pharmacol.*, vol. **233**, no. 1, pp. 175–176.

Mamo, D., Kapur, S., Shammi, C. M., Papatheodorou, G., Mann, S., Therrien, F., & Remington, G. 2004a, "A PET study of dopamine D2 and serotonin 5-HT2 receptor occupancy in patients with schizophrenia treated with therapeutic doses of ziprasidone", *Am. J. Psychiatry*, vol. **161**, no. 5, pp. 818–825.

Mamo, D., Remington, G., Nobrega, J., Hussey, D., Chirakal, R., Wilson, A. A., Baker, G., Houle, S., & Kapur, S. 2004b, "Effect of acute antipsychotic administration on dopamine synthesis in rodents and human subjects using 6-[18F]-L-m-tyrosine", *Synapse*, vol. **52**, no. 2, pp. 153–162.

Mann, S. P. & Hill, M. W. 1983, "Activation and inactivation of striatal tyrosine hydroxylase: the effects of pH, ATP and cyclic AMP, S-adenosylmethionine and S-adenosylhomocysteine", *Biochem. Pharmacol.*, vol. **32**, no. 22, pp. 3369–3374.

Marek, K., Jennings, D., & Seibyl, J. 2002, "Do dopamine agonists or levodopa modify Parkinson's disease progression?", *Eur. J. Neurol.*, vol. **9** (Suppl. 3), pp. 15–22.

Marshall, J. F., O'Dell, S. J., Navarrete, R., & Rosenstein, A. J. 1990, "Dopamine high-affinity transport site topography in rat brain: major differences between dorsal and ventral striatum", *Neuroscience*, vol. **37**, no. 1, pp. 11–21.

Marshall, V. L., Patterson, J., Hadley, D. M., Grosset, K. A., & Grosset, D. G. 2006, "Two-year follow-up in 150 consecutive cases with normal dopamine transporter imaging", *Nucl. Med. Commun.*, vol. **27**, no. 12, pp. 933–937.

Martikainen, I. K., Hagelberg, N., Mansikka, H., Hietala, J., Nagren, K., Scheinin, H., & Pertovaara, A. 2005, "Association of striatal dopamine D2/D3 receptor binding potential with pain but not tactile sensitivity or placebo analgesia", *Neurosci. Lett.*, vol. **376**, no. 3, pp. 149–153.

Martin, W. R., Palmer, M. R., Patlak, C. S., & Calne, D. B. 1989, "Nigrostriatal function in humans studied with positron emission tomography", *Ann. Neurol.*, vol. **26**, no. 4, pp. 535–542.

Martin, W. R., Wieler, M., Stoessl, A. J., & Schulzer, M. 2008, "Dihydrotetrabenazine positron emission tomography imaging in early, untreated Parkinson's disease", *Ann. Neurol.*, vol. **63**, no. 3, pp. 388–394.

Martinez, D., Broft, A., Foltin, R. W., Slifstein, M., Hwang, D. R., Huang, Y., Perez, A., Frankle, W. G., Cooper, T., Kleber, H. D., Fischman, M. W., & Laruelle, M. 2004, "Cocaine dependence and d2 receptor availability in the functional subdivisions of the striatum: relationship with cocaine-seeking behavior", *Neuropsychopharmacology*, vol. **29**, no. 6, pp. 1190–1202.

Martinez, D., Gelernter, J., Abi-Dargham, A., van Dyck, C. H., Kegeles, L., Innis, R. B., & Laruelle, M. 2001, "The variable number of tandem repeats polymorphism of the dopamine transporter gene is not associated with significant change in dopamine transporter phenotype in humans", *Neuropsychopharmacology*, vol. **24**, no. 5, pp. 553–560.

Martinez, D., Gil, R., Slifstein, M., Hwang, D. R., Huang, Y., Perez, A., Kegeles, L., Talbot, P., Evans, S., Krystal, J., Laruelle, M., & Abi-Dargham, A. 2005, "Alcohol dependence is associated with blunted dopamine transmission in the ventral striatum", *Biol. Psychiatry*, vol. **58**, no. 10, pp. 779–786.

Martinez, D., Narendran, R., Foltin, R. W., Slifstein, M., Hwang, D. R., Broft, A., Huang, Y., Cooper, T. B., Fischman, M. W., Kleber, H. D., & Laruelle, M. 2007, "Amphetamine-induced dopamine release: markedly blunted in cocaine dependence and predictive of the choice to self-administer cocaine", *Am. J. Psychiatry*, vol. **164**, no. 4, pp. 622–629.

Martinez, D., Slifstein, M., Broft, A., Mawlawi, O., Hwang, D. R., Huang, Y., Cooper, T., Kegeles, L., Zarahn, E., Abi-Dargham, A., Haber, S. N., & Laruelle, M. 2003, "Imaging human mesolimbic dopamine transmission with positron emission tomography. Part II: amphetamine-induced dopamine release in the functional subdivisions of the striatum", *J. Cereb. Blood Flow Metab.*, vol. **23**, no. 3, pp. 285–300.

Mata, I., Arranz, M. J., Staddon, S., Lopez-Ilundain, J. M., Tabares-Seisdedos, R., & Murray, R. M. 2006, "The high-activity Val allele of the catechol-O-methyltransferase gene predicts greater cognitive deterioration in patients with psychosis", *Psychiatr. Genet.*, vol. **16**, no. 5, pp. 213–216.

Mateo, Y., Budygin, E. A., John, C. E., & Jones, S. R. 2004, "Role of serotonin in cocaine effects in mice with reduced dopamine transporter function", *Proc. Natl. Acad. Sci. USA*, vol. **101**, no. 1, pp. 372–377.

Matsumoto, M., Weickert, C. S., Beltaifa, S., Kolachana, B., Chen, J., Hyde, T. M., Herman, M. M., Weinberger, D. R., & Kleinman, J. E. 2003, "Catechol O-methyltransferase (COMT) mRNA expression in the dorsolateral prefrontal cortex of patients with schizophrenia", *Neuropsychopharmacology*, vol. **28**, no. 8, pp. 1521–1530.

May, T., Rommelspacher, H., & Pawlik, M. 1991, "[3H]Harman binding experiments. I: A reversible and selective radioligand for monoamine oxidase subtype A in the CNS of the rat", *J. Neurochem.*, vol. **56**, no. 2, pp. 490–499.

Maycock, A. L., Aster, S. D., & Patchett, A. A. 1980, "Inactivation of 3-(3,4-dihydroxyphenyl)alanine decarboxylase by 2-(fluoromethyl)-3-(3,4-dihydroxyphenyl)alanine", *Biochemistry*, vol. **19**, no. 4, pp. 709–718.

Mayfield, R. D., Jones, B. A., Miller, H. A., Simosky, J. K., Larson, G. A., & Zahniser, N. R. 1999, "Modulation of endogenous GABA release by an antagonistic adenosine A1/dopamineD1 receptor interaction in rat brain limbic regions but not basal ganglia", *Synapse*, vol. **33**, no. 4, pp. 274–281.

Mazei-Robison, M. S., Bowton, E., Holy, M., Schmudermaier, M., Freissmuth, M., Sitte, H. H., Galli, A., & Blakely, R. D. 2008, "Anomalous dopamine release associated with a human dopamine transporter coding variant", *J. Neurosci.*, vol. **28**, no. 28, pp. 7040–7046.

McCann, U. D., Wong, D. F., Yokoi, F., Villemagne, V., Dannals, R. F., & Ricaurte, G. A. 1998, "Reduced striatal dopamine transporter density in abstinent methamphetamine and methcathinone users: evidence from positron emission tomography studies with [11C]WIN-35428", *J. Neurosci.*, vol. **18**, no. 20, pp. 8417–8422.

McCormick, P. N., Kapur, S., Seeman, P., Wilson, A. A. 2008, "Dopamine D2 receptor radiotracers [(11)C](+)-PHNO and [(3)H]raclopride are indistinguishably inhibited by D2 agonists and antagonists ex vivo", *Nucl. Med. Biol.*, vol. **35**, no. 1, pp. 11–17.

McGowan, S., Lawrence, A. D., Sales, T., Quested, D., & Grasby, P. 2004, "Presynaptic dopaminergic dysfunction in schizophrenia: a positron emission tomographic [18F]fluorodopa study", *Arch. Gen. Psychiatry*, vol. **61**, no. 2, pp. 134–142.

McKenna, D. J., Towers, G. H., & Abbott, F. 1984, "Monoamine oxidase inhibitors in South American hallucinogenic plants: tryptamine and beta-carboline constituents of ayahuasca", *J. Ethnopharmacol.*, vol. **10**, no. 2, pp. 195–223.

McMillen, B. A. & Shore, P. A. 1980, "Role of dopamine storage function in the control of rat striatal tyrosine hydroxylase activity", *Naunyn Schmiedebergs Arch. Pharmacol.*, vol. **313**, no. 1, pp. 39–44.

Meek, J. K. & Neff, N. H. 1973, "Biogenic amines and their metabolites as substrates for phenol sulphotransferase (EC 2.8.2.1) of brain and liver", *J. Neurochem.*, vol. **21**, no. 1, pp. 1–9.

Melamed, E., Hefti, F., & Wurtman, R. J. 1980, "Tyrosine administration increases striatal dopamine release in rats with partial nigrostriatal lesions", *Proc. Natl. Acad. Sci. USA*, vol. **77**, no. 7, pp. 4305–4309.

Melega, W. P., Lacan, G., Desalles, A. A., & Phelps, M. E. 2000, "Long-term methamphetamine-induced decreases of [(11)C]WIN 35,428 binding in striatum are reduced by GDNF: PET studies in the vervet monkey", *Synapse*, vol. **35**, no. 4, pp. 243–249.

Melega, W. P., Raleigh, M. J., Stout, D. B., DeSalles, A. A., Cherry, S. R., Blurton-Jones, M., Morton, G. G., Huang, S. C., & Phelps, M. E. 1996, "Longitudinal behavioral and 6-[18F]fluoro-L-DOPA-PET assessment in MPTP-hemiparkinsonian monkeys", *Exp. Neurol.*, vol. **141**, no. 2, pp. 318–329.

Melis, M. R. & Gale, K. 1984, "Intranigral application of substance P antagonists prevents the haloperidol-induced activation of striatal tyrosine hydroxylase", *Naunyn Schmiedebergs Arch. Pharmacol.*, vol. **326**, no. 1, pp. 83–86.

Mellick, G. D., Buchanan, D. D., McCann, S. J., James, K. M., Johnson, A. G., Davis, D. R., Liyou, N., Chan, D., & Le Couteur, D. G. 1999, "Variations in the monoamine oxidase B (MAOB) gene are associated with Parkinson's disease", *Mov. Disord.*, vol. **14**, no. 2, pp. 219–224.

Menza, M. A., Mark, M. H., Burn, D. J., & Brooks, D. J. 1995, "Personality correlates of [18F]dopa striatal uptake: results of positron-emission tomography in Parkinson's disease", *J. Neuropsychiatry Clin. Neurosci.*, vol. **7**, no. 2, pp. 176–179.

Merickel, A., Rosandich, P., Peter, D., & Edwards, R. H. 1995, "Identification of residues involved in substrate recognition by a vesicular monoamine transporter", *J. Biol. Chem.*, vol. **270**, no. 43, pp. 25798–25804.

Meshgin-Azarian, S., Chang, W., Cugier, D. L., Vincent, M. S., & Near, J. A. 1988, "Distribution of [3H]dihydrotetrabenazine binding in bovine striatal subsynaptic fractions: enrichment of higher affinity binding in a synaptic vesicle fraction", *J. Neurochem.*, vol. **50**, no. 3, pp. 824–830.

Meyer, J. H., Ginovart, N., Boovariwala, A., Sagrati, S., Hussey, D., Garcia, A., Young, T., Praschak-Rieder, N., Wilson, A. A., & Houle, S. 2006a, "Elevated monoamine oxidase a levels in the brain: an explanation for the monoamine imbalance of major depression", *Arch. Gen. Psychiatry*, vol. **63**, no. 11, pp. 1209–1216.

Meyer, J. H., Kruger, S., Wilson, A. A., Christensen, B. K., Goulding, V. S., Schaffer, A., Minifie, C., Houle, S., Hussey, D., & Kennedy, S. H. 2001, "Lower dopamine transporter binding potential in striatum during depression", *Neuroreport*, vol. **12**, no. 18, pp. 4121–4125.

Meyer, J. H., McNeely, H. E., Sagrati, S., Boovariwala, A., Martin, K., Verhoeff, N. P., Wilson, A. A., & Houle, S. 2006b, "Elevated putamen D(2) receptor binding potential in major depression with motor retardation: an [11C]raclopride positron emission tomography study", *Am. J. Psychiatry*, vol. **163**, no. 9, pp. 1594–1602.

Meyer, P., Bohnen, N. I., Minoshima, S., Koeppe, R. A., Wernette, K., Kilbourn, M. R., Kuhl, D. E., Frey, K. A., & Albin, R. L. 1999, "Striatal presynaptic monoaminergic vesicles are not increased in Tourette's syndrome", *Neurology*, vol. **53**, no. 2, pp. 371–374.

Meyer-Lindenberg, A., Miletich, R. S., Kohn, P. D., Esposito, G., Carson, R. E., Quarantelli, M., Weinberger, D. R., & Berman, K. F. 2002, "Reduced prefrontal activity predicts exaggerated striatal dopaminergic function in schizophrenia", *Nat. Neurosci.*, vol. **5**, no. 3, pp. 267–271.

Mignot, E. & Laude, D. 1985, "Study of dopamine turnover by monitoring the decline of dopamine metabolites in rat CSF after alpha-methyl-p-tyrosine", *J. Neurochem.*, vol. **45**, no. 5, pp. 1527–1533.

Mignot, E., Laude, D., & Elghozi, J. L. 1984, "Kinetics of drug-induced changes in dopamine and serotonin metabolite concentrations in the CSF of the rat", *J. Neurochem.*, vol. **42**, no. 3, pp. 819–825.

Milner, J. D., Irie, K., & Wurtman, R. J. 1986, "Effects of phenylalanine on the release of endogenous dopamine from rat striatal slices", *J. Neurochem.*, vol. **47**, no. 5, pp. 1444–1448.

Minuzzi, L., Nomikos, G. G., Wade, M. R., Jensen, S. B., Olsen, A. K., & Cumming, P. 2005, "Interaction between LSD and dopamine D2/3 binding sites in pig brain", *Synapse*, vol. **56**, no. 4, pp. 198–204.

Minuzzi, L., Olsen, A. K., Bender, D., Arnfred, S., Grant, R., Danielsen, E. H., & Cumming, P. 2006, "Quantitative autoradiography of ligands for dopamine receptors and transporters in brain of Gottingen minipig: comparison with results in vivo", *Synapse*, vol. **59**, no. 4, pp. 211–219.

Mireylees, S. E., Brammer, N. T., & Buckley, G. A. 1986, "A kinetic study of the in vitro uptake of [3H]dopamine over a wide range of concentrations by rat striatal preparations", *Biochem. Pharmacol.*, vol. **35**, no. 22, pp. 4065–4071.

Miwa, S., Gillberg, P. G., Bjurling, P., Yumoto, N., Odano, I., Watanabe, Y., & Langstrom, B. 1992, "Assessment of dopamine and its metabolites in the intracellular and extracellular compartments of the rat striatum after peripheral administration of L-[11C]dopa", *Brain Res.*, vol. **578**, no. 1-2, pp. 122–128.

Miwa, S., Watanabe, Y., & Hayaishi, O. 1985, "6R-L-erythro-5,6,7,8-tetrahydrobiopterin as a regulator of dopamine and serotonin biosynthesis in the rat brain", *Arch. Biochem. Biophys.*, vol. **239**, no. 1, pp. 234–241.

Miyamoto, J. K., Uezu, E., Jiang, P. J., & Miyamoto, A. T. 1993, "H(+)-ATPase and transport of DOPAC, HVA, and 5-HIAA in monoamine neurons", *Physiol. Behav.*, vol. **53**, no. 1, pp. 65–74.

Miyamoto, J. K., Uezu, E., & Terashima, S. 1991, "Active transport pumps of HVA and DOPAC in dopaminergic nerve terminals", *Physiol. Behav.*, vol. **49**, no. 1, pp. 141–147.

Miyamoto, J. K., Uezu, E., Yusa, T., & Terashima, S. 1990, "Efflux of 5-HIAA from 5-HT neurons: a membrane potential-dependent process", *Physiol. Behav.*, vol. **47**, no. 4, pp. 767–772.

Moghaddam, B. & Bunney, B. S. 1989, "Ionic composition of microdialysis perfusing solution alters the pharmacological responsiveness and basal outflow of striatal dopamine", *J. Neurochem.*, vol. **53**, no. 2, pp. 652–654.

Mogi, M., Harada, M., Kiuchi, K., Kojima, K., Kondo, T., Narabayashi, H., Rausch, D., Riederer, P., Jellinger, K., & Nagatsu, T. 1988, "Homospecific activity (activity per enzyme protein) of tyrosine hydroxylase increases in parkinsonian brain", *J. Neural Transm.*, vol. **72**, no. 1, pp. 77–82.

Mollard, P., Seward, E. P., & Nowycky, M. C. 1995, "Activation of nicotinic receptors triggers exocytosis from bovine chromaffin cells in the absence of membrane depolarization", *Proc. Natl. Acad. Sci. USA*, vol. **92**, no. 7, pp. 3065–3069.

Monchi, O., Ko, J. H., & Strafella, A. P. 2006, "Striatal dopamine release during performance of executive functions: A [(11)C]raclopride PET study", *Neuroimage*, vol. **33**, no. 3, pp. 907–912.

Montague, D. M., Lawler, C. P., Mailman, R. B., & Gilmore, J. H. 1999, "Developmental regulation of the dopamine D1 receptor in human caudate and putamen", *Neuropsychopharmacology*, vol. **21**, no. 5, pp. 641–649.

Montgomery, A. J., Asselin, M. C., Farde, L., & Grasby, P. M. 2007a, "Measurement of methylphenidate-induced change in extrastriatal dopamine concentration using [11C]FLB 457 PET", *J. Cereb. Blood Flow Metab.*, vol. **27**, no. 2, pp. 369–377.

Montgomery, A. J., Lingford-Hughes, A. R., Egerton, A., Nutt, D. J., & Grasby, P. M. 2007b, "The effect of nicotine on striatal dopamine release in man: a [11C]raclopride PET study", *Synapse*, vol. **61**, no. 8, pp. 637–645.

Montgomery, A. J., Mehta, M. A., & Grasby, P. M. 2006, "Is psychological stress in man associated with increased striatal dopamine levels? A [11C]raclopride PET study", *Synapse*, vol. **60**, no. 2, pp. 124–131.

Montgomery, A. J., Stokes, P., Kitamura, Y., & Grasby, P. M. 2007, "Extrastriatal D(2) and striatal D(2) receptors in depressive illness: Pilot PET studies using [(11)C]FLB 457 and [(11)C]raclopride", *J. Affect. Disord.*, vol. **101**, no. 1–3, pp. 113–122.

Morgan, M. E., Yamamoto, B. K., & Freed, C. R. 1984, "Unilateral activation of caudate tyrosine hydroxylase during voluntary circling behavior", *J. Neurochem.*, vol. **43**, no. 3, pp. 737–741.

Moriyama, Y., Amakatsu, K., & Futai, M. 1993, "Uptake of the neurotoxin, 4-methylphenylpyridinium, into chromaffin granules and synaptic vesicles: a proton gradient drives its uptake through monoamine transporter", *Arch. Biochem. Biophys.*, vol. **305**, no. 2, pp. 271–277.

Moron, J. A., Brockington, A., Wise, R. A., Rocha, B. A., & Hope, B. T. 2002, "Dopamine uptake through the norepinephrine transporter in brain regions with low levels of the dopamine transporter: evidence from knock-out mouse lines", *J. Neurosci.*, vol. **22**, no. 2, pp. 389–395.

Morris, E. D., Babich, J. W., Alpert, N. M., Bonab, A. A., Livni, E., Weise, S., Hsu, H., Christian, B. T., Madras, B. K., & Fischman, A. J. 1996, "Quantification of dopamine transporter density in monkeys by dynamic PET imaging of multiple injections of 11C-CFT", *Synapse*, vol. **24**, no. 3, pp. 262–272.

Morris, E. D., Chefer, S. I., Lane, M. A., Muzic, R. F., Jr., Wong, D. F., Dannals, R. F., Matochik, J. A., Bonab, A. A., Villemagne, V. L., Grant, S. J., Ingram, D. K., Roth, G. S., & London, E. D. 1999, "Loss of D2 receptor binding with age in rhesus monkeys: importance of correction for differences in striatal size", *J. Cereb. Blood Flow Metab.*, vol. **19**, no. 2, pp. 218–229.

Morris, E. D., & Yoder, K. K. 2007, "Positron emission tomography displacement sensitivity: predicting binding potential change for positron emission tomography tracers based on their kinetic characteristics", *J. Cereb. Blood Flow Metab.*, vol. **27**, no. 3, pp. 606–617.

Morrish, P. K., Sawle, G. V., & Brooks, D. J. 1995, "Clinical and [18F] dopa PET findings in early Parkinson's disease", *J. Neurol. Neurosurg. Psychiatry*, vol. **59**, no. 6, pp. 597–600.

Morrish, P. K., Sawle, G. V., & Brooks, D. J. 1996, "An [18F]dopa-PET and clinical study of the rate of progression in Parkinson's disease", *Brain*, vol. **119** (Pt 2), pp. 585–591.

Moser, T. & Neher, E. 1997, "Estimation of mean exocytic vesicle capacitance in mouse adrenal chromaffin cells", *Proc. Natl. Acad. Sci. USA*, vol. **94**, no. 13, pp. 6735–6740.

Mozley, P. D., Acton, P. D., Barraclough, E. D., Plossl, K., Gur, R. C., Alavi, A., Mathur, A., Saffer, J., & Kung, H. F. 1999, "Effects of age on dopamine transporters in healthy humans", *J. Nucl. Med.*, vol. **40**, no. 11, pp. 1812–1817.

Mueller, R. A., Thoenen, H., & Axelrod, J. 1969, "Adrenal tyrosine hydroxylase: compensatory increase in activity after chemical sympathectomy", *Science*, vol. **163**, no. 866, pp. 468–469.

Mukherjee, J., Yang, Z. Y., Lew, R., Brown, T., Kronmal, S., Cooper, M. D., & Seiden, L. S. 1997, "Evaluation of d-amphetamine effects on the binding of dopamine D-2 receptor radioligand, 18F-fallypride in nonhuman primates using positron emission tomography", *Synapse*, vol. **27**, no. 1, pp. 1–13.

Munro, C. A., McCaul, M. E., Wong, D. F., Oswald, L. M., Zhou, Y., Brasic, J., Kuwabara, H., Kumar, A., Alexander, M., Ye, W., & Wand, G. S. 2006, "Sex differences in striatal dopamine release in healthy adults", *Biol. Psychiatry*, vol. **59**, no. 10, pp. 966–974.

Nagai, Y., Obayashi, S., Ando, K., Inaji, M., Maeda, J., Okauchi, T., Ito, H., & Suhara, T. 2007, "Progressive changes of pre- and post-synaptic dopaminergic biomarkers in conscious MPTP-treated cynomolgus monkeys measured by positron emission tomography", *Synapse*, vol. **61**, no. 10, pp. 809–819.

Nagatsu, I., Sakai, M., Takeuchi, T., Arai, R., Karasawa, N., Yamada, K., & Nagatsu, T. 1997, "Tyrosine hydroxylase (TH)-only-immunoreactive non-catecholaminergic neurons in the brain of wild mice or the human TH transgenic mice do not contain GTP cyclohydrolase I", *Neurosci. Lett.*, vol. **228**, no. 1, pp. 55–57.

Nakahara, D., Hashiguti, H., Kaneda, N., Sasaoka, T., & Nagatsu, T. 1993, "Normalization of tyrosine hydroxylase activity in vivo in the striatum of transgenic mice carrying human tyrosine hydroxylase gene: a microdialysis study", *Neurosci. Lett.*, vol. **158**, no. 1, pp. 44–46.

Nakashima, A., Mori, K., Suzuki, T., Kurita, H., Otani, M., Nagatsu, T., & Ota, A. 1999, "Dopamine inhibition of human tyrosine hydroxylase type 1 is controlled by the specific portion in the N-terminus of the enzyme", *J. Neurochem.*, vol. **72**, no. 5, pp. 2145–2153.

Narendran, R., Hwang, D. R., Slifstein, M., Hwang, Y., Huang, Y., Ekelund, J., Guillin, O., Scher, E., Martinez, D., & Laruelle, M. 2005, "Measurement of the proportion of D2 receptors configured in state of high affinity for agonists in vivo: a positron emission tomography study using [11C]N-propyl-norapomorphine and [11C]raclopride in baboons", *J. Pharmacol. Exp. Ther.*, vol. **315**, no. 1, pp. 80–90.

Narendran, R., Hwang, D. R., Slifstein, M., Talbot, P. S., Erritzoe, D., Huang, Y., Cooper, T. B., Martinez, D., Kegeles, L. S., Abi-Dargham, A., & Laruelle, M. 2004, "In vivo vulnerability to competition by endogenous dopamine: comparison of the D2 receptor agonist radiotracer (-)-N-[11C]propyl-norapomorphine ([11C]NPA) with the D2 receptor antagonist radiotracer [11C]-raclopride", *Synapse*, vol. **52**, no. 3, pp. 188–208.

Narendran, R., Slifstein, M., Guillin, O., Hwang, Y., Hwang, D. R., Scher, E., Reeder, S., Rabiner, E., & Laruelle, M. 2006, "Dopamine (D2/3) receptor agonist positron emission tomography radiotracer [11C]-(+)-PHNO is a D3 receptor preferring agonist in vivo", *Synapse*, vol. **60**, no. 7, pp. 485–495.

Naudon, L., Dourmap, N., Leroux-Nicollet, I., & Costentin, J. 1992, "Kainic acid lesion of the striatum increases dopamine release but reduces 3-methoxytyramine level", *Brain Res.*, vol. **572**, no. 1–2, pp. 247–249.

Naumann, M., Pirker, W., Reiners, K., Lange, K. W., Becker, G., & Brucke, T. 1998, "Imaging the pre- and postsynaptic side of striatal dopaminergic synapses in idiopathic cervical dystonia: a SPECT study using [123I] epidepride and [123I] beta-CIT", *Mov. Disord.*, vol. **13**, no. 2, pp. 319–323.

Near, J. A. 1986, "[3H]Dihydrotetrabenazine binding to bovine striatal synaptic vesicles", *Mol. Pharmacol.*, vol. **30**, no. 3, pp. 252–257.

Near, J. A., & Mahler, H. R. 1983, "Reserpine labels the catecholamine transporter in synaptic vesicles from bovine caudate nucleus", *FEBS Lett.*, vol. **158**, no. 1, pp. 31–35.

Neff, N. H. & Tozer, T. N. 1968, "In vivo measurement of brain serotonin turnover", *Adv. Pharmacol.*, vol. **6** (Pt A), pp. 97–109.

Nelson, T. J. & Kaufman, S. 1987, "Activation of rat caudate tyrosine hydroxylase phosphatase by tetrahydropterins", *J. Biol. Chem.*, vol. **262**, no. 34, pp. 16470–16475.

Neve, K. A., Altar, C. A., Wong, C. A., & Marshall, J. F. 1984, "Quantitative analysis of [3H]spiroperidol binding to rat forebrain sections: plasticity of neostriatal dopamine receptors after nigrostriatal injury", *Brain Res.*, vol. **302**, no. 1, pp. 9–18.

Neve, K. A. & Neve, R. L. 1997, "Molecular biology of dopamine receptors," in *The Dopamine Receptors*, K. A. Neve & R. L. Neve, eds., Humana Press, Totawa, NJ.

Newberg, A., Amsterdam, J., & Shults, J. 2007, "Dopamine transporter density may be associated with the depressed affect in healthy subjects", *Nucl. Med. Commun.*, vol. **28**, no. 1, pp. 3–6.

Newberg, A., Lerman, C., Wintering, N., Ploessl, K., & Mozley, P. D. 2007, "Dopamine transporter binding in smokers and nonsmokers", *Clin. Nucl. Med.*, vol. **32**, no. 6, pp. 452–455.

Newton, A. P. & Justice, J. B., Jr. 1994, "Temporal response of microdialysis probes to local perfusion of dopamine and cocaine followed with one-minute sampling", *Anal. Chem.*, vol. **66**, no. 9, pp. 1468–1472.

Ng, G. Y., O'Dowd, B. F., Lee, S. P., Chung, H. T., Brann, M. R., Seeman, P., & George, S. R. 1996, "Dopamine D2 receptor dimers and receptor-blocking peptides", *Biochem. Biophys. Res. Commun.*, vol. **227**, no. 1, pp. 200–204.

Ng, G. Y., Trogadis, J., Stevens, J., Bouvier, M., O'Dowd, B. F., & George, S. R. 1995, "Agonist-induced desensitization of dopamine D1 receptor-stimulated adenylyl cyclase activity is temporally and biochemically separated from D1 receptor internalization", *Proc. Natl. Acad. Sci. USA*, vol. **92**, no. 22, pp. 10157–10161.

Niddam, R., Arbilla, S., Scatton, B., Dennis, T., & Langer, S. Z. 1985, "Amphetamine induced release of endogenous dopamine in vitro is not reduced following pretreatment with reserpine", *Naunyn Schmiedebergs Arch. Pharmacol.*, vol. **329**, no. 2, pp. 123–127.

Nimura, T., Yamaguchi, K., Ando, T., Shibuya, S., Oikawa, T., Nakagawa, A., Shirane, R., Itoh, M., & Tominaga, T. 2005, "Attenuation of fluctuating striatal synaptic dopamine levels in patients with Parkinson disease in response to subthalamic nucleus stimulation: a positron emission tomography study", *J. Neurosurg*, vol. **103**, no. 6, pp. 968–973.

Nishino, J., Suzuki, H., Sugiyama, D., Kitazawa, T., Ito, K., Hanano, M., & Sugiyama, Y. 1999, "Transepithelial transport of organic anions across the choroid plexus: possible involvement of organic anion transporter and multidrug resistance-associated protein", *J. Pharmacol. Exp. Ther.*, vol. **290**, no. 1, pp. 289–294.

Nissbrandt, H. & Carlsson, A. 1987, "Turnover of dopamine and dopamine metabolites in rat brain: comparison between striatum and substantia nigra", *J. Neurochem.*, vol. **49**, no. 3, pp. 959–967.

Nissbrandt, H., Engberg, G., Wikstrom, H., Magnusson, T., & Carlsson, A. 1988, "NSD 1034: an amino acid decarboxylase inhibitor with a stimulatory action on dopamine synthesis not mediated by classical dopamine receptors", *Naunyn Schmiedebergs Arch. Pharmacol.*, vol. **338**, no. 2, pp. 148–161.

Nissbrandt, H., Pileblad, E., & Carlsson, A. 1985, "Evidence for dopamine release and metabolism beyond the control of nerve impulses and dopamine receptors in rat substantia nigra", *J. Pharm. Pharmacol.*, vol. **37**, no. 12, pp. 884–889.

Nissbrandt, H., Sundstrom, E., Jonsson, G., Hjorth, S., & Carlsson, A. 1989, "Synthesis and release of dopamine in rat brain: comparison between substantia nigra pars compacts, pars reticulata, and striatum", *J. Neurochem.*, vol. **52**, no. 4, pp. 1170–1182.

Nobrega, J. N. & Seeman, P. 1994, "Dopamine D2 receptors mapped in rat brain with [3H](+)PHNO", *Synapse*, vol. **17**, no. 3, pp. 167–172.

Nordstrom, A. L., Farde, L., Eriksson, L., & Halldin, C. 1995, "No elevated D2 dopamine receptors in neuroleptic-naive schizophrenic patients revealed by positron emission tomography and [11C]N-methylspiperone", *Psychiatry Res.*, vol. **61**, no. 2, pp. 67–83.

Nurmi, E., Ruottinen, H. M., Bergman, J., Haaparanta, M., Solin, O., Sonninen, P., & Rinne, J. O. 2001, "Rate of progression in Parkinson's disease: a 6-[18F] fluoro-L-dopa PET study", *Mov. Disord.*, vol. **16**, no. 4, pp. 608–615.

Nurmi, E., Bergman, J., Eskola, O., Solin, O., Vahlberg, T., Sonninen, P., & Rinne, J. O. 2003, "Progression of dopaminergic hypofunction in striatal subregions in Parkinson's disease using [18F]CFT PET", *Synapse.*, vol. **48**, no. 3, pp. 109–115.

Nuutila, J., Kaakkola, S., & Mannisto, P. T. 1987, "Potentiation of central effects of L-dopa by an inhibitor of catechol-O-methyltransferase", *J. Neural Transm.*, vol. **70**, no. 3–4, pp. 233–240.

Nygaard, T. G. 1995, "Dopa-responsive dystonia", *Curr. Opin. Neurol.*, vol. **8**, no. 4, pp. 310–313.

Oberhauser, A. F., Robinson, I. M., & Fernandez, J. M. 1996, "Simultaneous capacitance and amperometric measurements of exocytosis: a comparison", *Biophys. J.*, vol. **71**, no. 2, pp. 1131–1139.

O'Brien, J. T., Colloby, S., Fenwick, J., Williams, E. D., Firbank, M., Burn, D., Aarsland, D., & McKeith, I. G. 2004, "Dopamine transporter loss visualized with FP-CIT SPECT in the differential diagnosis of dementia with Lewy bodies", *Arch. Neurol.*, vol. **61**, no. 6, pp. 919–925.

O'Donnell, P. & Grace, A. A. 1993, "Dopaminergic modulation of dye coupling between neurons in the core and shell regions of the nucleus accumbens", *J. Neurosci.*, vol. **13**, no. 8, pp. 3456–3471.

Oh, J. D., Chartisathian, K., Ahmed, S. M., & Chase, T. N. 2003, "Cyclic AMP responsive element binding protein phosphorylation and persistent expression of levodopa-induced response alterations in unilateral nigrostriatal 6-OHDA lesioned rats", *J. Neurosci. Res.*, vol. **72**, no. 6, pp. 768–780.

Ohnishi, T., Hayashi, T., Okabe, S., Nonaka, I., Matsuda, H., Iida, H., Imabayashi, E., Watabe, H., Miyake, Y., Ogawa, M., Teramoto, N., Ohta, Y., Ejima, N., Sawada, T., & Ugawa, Y. 2004, "Endogenous dopamine release induced by repetitive transcranial magnetic stimulation over the primary motor cortex: an

[11C]raclopride positron emission tomography study in anesthetized macaque monkeys", *Biol. Psychiatry*, vol. **55**, no. 5, pp. 484–489.

Ohtsuki, S. 2004, "New aspects of the blood-brain barrier transporters; its physiological roles in the central nervous system", *Biol. Pharm. Bull.*, vol. **27**, no. 10, pp. 1489–1496.

Oiwa, Y., Eberling, J. L., Nagy, D., Pivirotto, P., Emborg, M. E., & Bankiewicz, K. S. 2003, "Overlesioned hemiparkinsonian non human primate model: correlation between clinical, neurochemical and histochemical changes", *Front Biosci.*, vol. **8**, pp. a155–a166.

Oka, K., Ashiba, G., Sugimoto, T., Matsuura, S., & Nagatsu, T. 1982, "Kinetic properties of tyrosine hydroxylase purified from bovine adrenal medulla and bovine caudate nucleus", *Biochim. Biophys. Acta*, vol. **706**, no. 2, pp. 188–196.

Okauchi, T., Suhara, T., Maeda, J., Kawabe, K., Obayashi, S., & Suzuki, K. 2001, "Effect of endogenous dopamine on endogenous dopamine on extrastriated [(11)C]FLB 457 binding measured by PET", *Synapse*, vol. **41**, no. 2, pp. 87–95.

Okuno, S. & Fujisawa, H. 1985, "A new mechanism for regulation of tyrosine 3-monooxygenase by end product and cyclic AMP-dependent protein kinase", *J. Biol. Chem.*, vol. **260**, no. 5, pp. 2633–2635.

Olanow, C. W. 2006, "Rationale for considering that propargylamines might be neuroprotective in Parkinson's disease", *Neurology*, vol. **66**, no. 10 (Suppl. 4), pp. S69–S79.

Oldendorf, W. H. & Szabo, J. 1976, "Amino acid assignment to one of three blood-brain barrier amino acid carriers", *Am. J. Physiol*, vol. **230**, no. 1, pp. 94–98.

Olsson, H., Halldin, C., & Farde, L. 2004, "Differentiation of extrastriatal dopamine D2 receptor density and affinity in the human brain using PET", *Neuroimage*, vol. **22**, no. 2, pp. 794–803.

Olsson, H., Halldin, C., Swahn, C. G., & Farde, L. 1999, "Quantification of [11C]FLB 457 binding to extrastriatal dopamine receptors in the human brain", *J. Cereb. Blood Flow Metab.*, vol. **19**, no. 10, pp. 1164–1173.

Oswald, L. M., Wong, D. F., McCaul, M., Zhou, Y., Kuwabara, H., Choi, L., Brasic, J., & Wand, G. S. 2005, "Relationships among ventral striatal dopamine release, cortisol secretion, and subjective responses to amphetamine", *Neuropsychopharmacology*, vol. **30**, no. 4, pp. 821–832.

Oswald, L. M., Wong, D. F., Zhou, Y., Kumar, A., Brasic, J., Alexander, M., Ye, W., Kuwabara, H., Hilton, J., & Wand, G. S. 2007, "Impulsivity and chronic stress are associated with amphetamine-induced striatal dopamine release", *Neuroimage*, vol. **36**, no. 1, pp. 153–166.

Otsuka, M., Ichiya, Y., Kuwabara, Y., Hosokawa, S., Sasaki, M., Fukumura, T., Masuda, K., Goto, I., & Kato, M. 1993, "Cerebral glucose metabolism and striatal 18F-dopa uptake by PET in cases of chorea with or without dementia", *J. Neurol. Sci.*, vol. **115**, no. 2, pp. 153–157.

Ouchi, Y., Yoshikawa, E., Futatsubashi, M., Okada, H., Torizuka, T., & Sakamoto, M. 2002, "Effect of simple motor performance on regional dopamine release in the striatum in Parkinson disease patients and healthy subjects: a positron emission tomography study", *J. Cereb. Blood Flow Metab.*, vol. **22**, no. 6, pp. 746–752.

Ouchi, Y., Yoshikawa, E., Okada, H., Futatsubashi, M., Sekine, Y., Iyo, M., & Sakamoto, M. 1999, "Alterations in binding site density of dopamine transporter in the striatum, orbitofrontal cortex, and amygdala in early Parkinson's disease: compartment analysis for beta-CFT binding with positron emission tomography", *Ann. Neurol.*, vol. **45**, no. 5, pp. 601–610.

Pardridge, W. M. & Oldendorf, W. H. 1977, "Transport of metabolic substrates through the blood-brain barrier", *J. Neurochem.*, vol. **28**, no. 1, pp. 5–12.

Parkinson Study Group, 2002, "Dopamine transporter brain imaging to assess the effects of pramipexole vs levodopa on Parkinson disease progression", *JAMA*, vol. **287**, no. 13, pp. 1653–1661.

Parsey, R. V., Oquendo, M. A., Zea-Ponce, Y., Rodenhiser, J., Kegeles, L. S., Pratap, M., Cooper, T. B., Van, H. R., Mann, J. J., & Laruelle, M. 2001, "Dopamine D(2) receptor availability and amphetamine-induced dopamine release in unipolar depression", *Biol. Psychiatry*, vol. **50**, no. 5, pp. 313–322.

Parsons, L. H. & Justice, J. B., Jr. 1992, "Extracellular concentration and in vivo recovery of dopamine in the nucleus accumbens using microdialysis", *J. Neurochem.*, vol. **58**, no. 1, pp. 212–218.

Parsons, L. H., Smith, A. D., & Justice, J. B., Jr. 1991, "The in vivo microdialysis recovery of dopamine is altered independently of basal level by 6-hydroxydopamine lesions to the nucleus accumbens", *J. Neurosci. Methods*, vol. **40**, no. 2–3, pp. 139–147.

Parsons, T. D., Coorssen, J. R., Horstmann, H., & Almers, W. 1995, "Docked granules, the exocytic burst, and the need for ATP hydrolysis in endocrine cells", *Neuron*, vol. **15**, no. 5, pp. 1085–1096.

Parvizi, N. & Wuttke, W. 1983, "Catecholestrogens affect catecholamine turnover rates in the anterior part of the mediobasal hypothalamus and medial preoptic area in the male and female castrated rat", *Neuroendocrinology*, vol. **36**, no. 1, pp. 21–26.

Pasinetti, G. M., Morgan, D. G., Johnson, S. A., Millar, S. L., & Finch, C. E. 1990, "Tyrosine hydroxylase mRNA concentration in midbrain dopaminergic neurons is differentially regulated by reserpine", *J. Neurochem.*, vol. **55**, no. 5, pp. 1793–1799.

Pasqualini, C., Olivier, V., Guibert, B., Frain, O., & Leviel, V. 1995, "Acute stimulatory effect of estradiol on striatal dopamine synthesis", *J. Neurochem.*, vol. **65**, no. 4, pp. 1651–1657.

Pate, B. D., Kawamata, T., Yamada, T., McGeer, E. G., Hewitt, K. A., Snow, B. J., Ruth, T. J., & Calne, D. B. 1993, "Correlation of striatal fluorodopa uptake in the MPTP monkey with dopaminergic indices", *Ann. Neurol.*, vol. **34**, no. 3, pp. 331–338.

Patlak, C. S. & Blasberg, R. G. 1985, "Graphical evaluation of blood-to-brain transfer constants from multiple-time uptake data. Generalizations", *J. Cereb. Blood Flow Metab.*, vol. **5**, no. 4, pp. 584–590.

Patlak, C. S., Blasberg, R. G., & Fenstermacher, J. D. 1983, "Graphical evaluation of blood-to-brain transfer constants from multiple-time uptake data", *J. Cereb. Blood Flow Metab.*, vol. **3**, no. 1, pp. 1–7.

Paulson, P. E. & Robinson, T. E. 1994, "Relationship between circadian changes in spontaneous motor activity and dorsal versus ventral striatal dopamine neurotransmission assessed with on-line microdialysis", *Behav. Neurosci.*, vol. **108**, no. 3, pp. 624–635.

Pavese, N., Evans, A. H., Tai, Y. F., Hotton, G., Brooks, D. J., Lees, A. J., & Piccini, P. 2006, "Clinical correlates of levodopa-induced dopamine release in Parkinson disease: a PET study", *Neurology*, vol. **67**, no. 9, pp. 1612–1617.

Pedersen, K., Simonsen, M., Ostergaard, S. D., Lajord, M. O., Rosa-Neto, P., Olsen, A. K., Jensen, S. B., Moller, A., & Cumming, P. 2007, "Mapping the amphetamine-evoked changes in [11C]raclopride binding in living rat using small animal PET: modulation by MAO-inhibition", *Neuroimage*, vol. **35**, no. 1, pp. 38–46.

Pellevoisin, C., Chalon, S., Zouakia, A., Dognon, A. M., Frangin, Y., Baulieu, J. L., Besnard, J. C., & Guilloteau, D. 1993, "Comparison of two radioiodinated ligands of dopamine D2 receptors in animal models: iodobenzamide and iodoethylspiperone", *Life Sci.*, vol. **52**, no. 23, pp. 1851–1860.

Pepper, J. P., Baumann, M. H., Ayestas, M., & Rothman, R. B. 2001, "Inhibition of MAO-A fails to alter cocaine-induced increases in extracellular dopamine and norepinephrine in rat nucleus accumbens", *Brain Res. Mol. Brain Res.*, vol. **87**, no. 2, pp. 184–189.

Perlmutter, J. S., Stambuk, M. K., Markham, J., Black, K. J., McGee-Minnich, L., Jankovic, J., & Moerlein, S. M. 1998, "Decreased [18F]spiperone binding in putamen in dystonia", *Adv. Neurol.*, vol. **78**, pp. 161–168.

Perrone-Capano, C., Tino, A., Amadoro, G., Pernas-Alonso, R., & di Porzio, U. 1996, "Dopamine transporter gene expression in rat mesencephalic dopaminergic neurons is increased by direct interaction with target striatal cells in vitro", *Brain Res. Mol. Brain Res.*, vol. **39**, no. 1–2, pp. 160–166.

Pertovaara, A., Martikainen, I. K., Hagelberg, N., Mansikka, H., Nagren, K., Hietala, J., & Scheinin, H. 2004, "Striatal dopamine D2/D3 receptor availability correlates with individual response characteristics to pain", *Eur. J. Neurosci.*, vol. **20**, no. 6, pp. 1587–1592.

Peter, D., Jimenez, J., Liu, Y., Kim, J., & Edwards, R. H. 1994, "The chromaffin granule and synaptic vesicle amine transporters differ in substrate recognition and sensitivity to inhibitors", *J. Biol. Chem.*, vol. **269**, no. 10, pp. 7231–7237.

Pettersson, G., Johannessen, K., Hulthe, P., & Engel, J. A. 1990, "Effect of amperozide on the synthesis and turnover of monoamines in rat brain", *Pharmacol. Toxicol.*, vol. **66** (Suppl. 1), pp. 40–44.

Pfaus, J. G., Damsma, G., Nomikos, G. G., Wenkstern, D. G., Blaha, C. D., Phillips, A. G., & Fibiger, H. C. 1990, "Sexual behavior enhances central dopamine transmission in the male rat", *Brain Res.*, vol. **530**, no. 2, pp. 345–348.

Pfaus, J. G., Damsma, G., Wenkstern, D., & Fibiger, H. C. 1995, "Sexual activity increases dopamine transmission in the nucleus accumbens and striatum of female rats", *Brain Res.*, vol. **693**, no. 1–2, pp. 21–30.

Phelps, M. E., Huang, S. C., Hoffman, E. J., Selin, C., Sokoloff, L., & Kuhl, D. E. 1979, "Tomographic measurement of local cerebral glucose metabolic rate in humans with (F-18)2-fluoro-2-deoxy-D-glucose: validation of method", *Ann. Neurol.*, vol. **6**, no. 5, pp. 371–388.

Philippu, A. & Beyer, J. 1973, "Dopamine and noradrenaline transport into subcellular vesicles of the striatum", *Naunyn Schmiedebergs Arch. Pharmacol.*, vol. **278**, no. 4, pp. 387–402.

Pierce, R. C., Duffy, P., & Kalivas, P. W. 1995, "Sensitization to cocaine and dopamine autoreceptor subsensitivity in the nucleus accumbens", *Synapse*, vol. **20**, no. 1, pp. 33–36.

Pierce, R. C. & Kalivas, P. W. 1995, "Amphetamine produces sensitized increases in locomotion and extracellular dopamine preferentially in the nucleus accumbens shell of rats administered repeated cocaine", *J. Pharmacol. Exp. Ther.*, vol. **275**, no. 2, pp. 1019–1029.

Pifl, C., Giros, B., & Caron, M. G. 1993, "Dopamine transporter expression confers cytotoxicity to low doses of the parkinsonism-inducing neurotoxin 1-methyl-4-phenylpyridinium", *J. Neurosci.*, vol. **13**, no. 10, pp. 4246–4253.

Piggott, M. A., Marshall, E. F., Thomas, N., Lloyd, S., Court, J. A., Jaros, E., Burn, D., Johnson, M., Perry, R. H., McKeith, I. G., Ballard, C., & Perry, E. K. 1999a, "Striatal dopaminergic markers in dementia with Lewy bodies, Alzheimer's and Parkinson's diseases: rostrocaudal distribution", *Brain*, vol. **122** (Pt 8), pp. 1449–1468.

Piggott, M. A., Marshall, E. F., Thomas, N., Lloyd, S., Court, J. A., Jaros, E., Costa, D., Perry, R. H., & Perry, E. K. 1999b, "Dopaminergic activities in the human striatum: rostrocaudal gradients of uptake sites and of D1 and D2 but not of D3 receptor binding or dopamine", *Neuroscience*, vol. **90**, no. 2, pp. 433–445.

Pinborg, L. H., Videbaek, C., Ziebell, M., Mackeprang, T., Friberg, L., Rasmussen, H., Knudsen, G. M., & Glenthoj, B. Y. 2007, "[123I]epidepride binding to cerebellar dopamine D2/D3 receptors is displaceable: implications for the use of cerebellum as a reference region", *Neuroimage*, vol. **34**, no. 4, pp. 1450–1453.

Pinborg, L. H., Ziebell, M., Frokjaer, V. G., de Nijs, R., Svarer, C., Haugbol, S., Yndgaard, S., & Knudsen, G. M. 2005, "Quantification of 123I-PE2I binding to dopamine transporter with SPECT after bolus and bolus/infusion", *J. Nucl. Med.*, vol. **46**, no. 7, pp. 1119–1127.

Pinna, A., Morelli, M., Drukarch, B., & Stoof, J. C. 1997, "Priming of 6-hydroxydopamine-lesioned rats with L-DOPA or quinpirole results in an increase in dopamine D1 receptor-dependent cyclic AMP production in striatal tissue", *Eur. J. Pharmacol.*, vol. **331**, no. 1, pp. 23–26.

Pirker, W., Asenbaum, S., Hauk, M., Kandlhofer, S., Tauscher, J., Willeit, M., Neumeister, A., Praschak-Rieder, N., Angelberger, P., & Brucke, T. 2000, "Imaging serotonin and dopamine transporters with 123I-beta-CIT SPECT: binding kinetics and effects of normal aging", *J. Nucl. Med.*, vol. **41**, no. 1, pp. 36–44.

Pogarell, O., Koch, W., Popperl, G., Tatsch, K., Jakob, F., Zwanzger, P., Mulert, C., Rupprecht, R., Moller, H. J., Hegerl, U., & Padberg, F. 2006, "Striatal dopamine release after prefrontal repetitive transcranial magnetic stimulation in major depression: preliminary results of a dynamic [123I] IBZM SPECT study", *J. Psychiatr. Res.*, vol. **40**, no. 4, pp. 307–314.

Pohjalainen, T., Rinne, J. O., Nagren, K., Lehikoinen, P., Anttila, K., Syvalahti, E. K., & Hietala, J. 1998a, "The A1 allele of the human D2 dopamine receptor gene predicts low D2 receptor availability in healthy volunteers", *Mol. Psychiatry*, vol. **3**, no. 3, pp. 256–260.

Pohjalainen, T., Rinne, J. O., Nagren, K., Syvalahti, E., & Hietala, J. 1998b, "Sex differences in the striatal dopamine D2 receptor binding characteristics in vivo", *Am. J. Psychiatry*, vol. **155**, no. 6, pp. 768–773.

Poyot, T., Conde, F., Gregoire, M. C., Frouin, V., Coulon, C., Fuseau, C., Hinnen, F., Dolle, F., Hantraye, P., & Bottlaender, M. 2001, "Anatomic and biochemical correlates of the dopamine transporter ligand 11C-PE2I in normal and parkinsonian primates: comparison with 6-[18F]fluoro-L-dopa", *J. Cereb. Blood Flow Metab.*, vol. **21**, no. 7, pp. 782–792.

Pradhan, S., Alphs, L., & Lovenberg, W. 1981, "Characterization of haloperidol-mediated effects on rat striatal tyrosine hydroxylase", *Neuropharmacology*, vol. **20**, no. 2, pp. 149–154.

Pruessner, J. C., Champagne, F., Meaney, M. J., & Dagher, A. 2004, "Dopamine release in response to a psychological stress in humans and its relationship to early life maternal care: a positron emission tomography study using [11C]raclopride", *J. Neurosci.*, vol. **24**, no. 11, pp. 2825–2831.

Przedborski, S., Levivier, M., Jiang, H., Ferreira, M., Jackson-Lewis, V., Donaldson, D., & Togasaki, D. M. 1995, "Dose-dependent lesions of the dopaminergic nigrostriatal pathway induced by intrastriatal injection of 6-hydroxydopamine", *Neuroscience*, vol. **67**, no. 3, pp. 631–647.

Racette, B. A., Good, L., Antenor, J. A., Gee-Minnich, L., Moerlein, S. M., Videen, T. O., & Perlmutter, J. S. 2006, "[18F]FDOPA PET as an endophenotype for Parkinson's Disease linkage studies", *Am. J. Med. Genet. B Neuropsychiatr. Genet.*, vol. **141**, no. 3, pp. 245–249.

Rakshi, J. S., Uema, T., Ito, K., Bailey, D. L., Morrish, P. K., Ashburner, J., Dagher, A., Jenkins, I. H., Friston, K. J., & Brooks, D. J. 1999, "Frontal, midbrain and striatal dopaminergic function in early and advanced Parkinson's disease A 3D [(18)F] dopa-PET study", *Brain*, vol. **122** (Pt 9), pp. 1637–1650.

Ramsey, A. J., Hillas, P. J., & Fitzpatrick, P. F. 1996, "Characterization of the active site iron in tyrosine hydroxylase. Redox states of the iron", *J. Biol. Chem.*, vol. **271**, no. 40, pp. 24395–24400.

Rao, S. K., Vakil, S. D., Calne, D. B., & Hilson, A. 1972, "Augmenting the action of levodopa", *Postgrad. Med. J.*, vol. **48**, no. 565, pp. 653–656.

Rashid, A. J., So, C. H., Kong, M. M., Furtak, T., El-Ghundi, M., Cheng, R., O'Dowd, B. F., & George, S. R. 2007, "D1-D2 dopamine receptor heterooligomers with unique pharmacology are coupled to rapid activation of Gq/11 in the striatum", *Proc. Natl. Acad. Sci. USA*, vol. **104**, no. 2, pp. 654–659.

Reches, A., Wagner, H. R., Jackson-Lewis, V., & Fahn, S. 1985, "Presynaptic inhibition of dopamine synthesis in rat striatum: effects of chronic dopamine depletion and receptor blockade", *Brain Res.*, vol. **347**, no. 2, pp. 346–349.

Reenila, I., Tuomainen, P., Soinila, S., & Mannisto, P. T. 1997, "Increase of catechol-O-methyltransferase activity in rat brain microglia after intrastriatal infusion of fluorocitrate, a glial toxin", *Neurosci. Lett.*, vol. **230**, no. 3, pp. 155–158.

Reeves, S. J., Grasby, P. M., Howard, R. J., Bantick, R. A., Asselin, M. C., & Mehta, M. A. 2005, "A positron emission tomography (PET) investigation of the role of striatal dopamine (D2) receptor availability in spatial cognition", *Neuroimage*, vol. **28**, no. 1, pp. 216–226.

Reeves, S. J., Mehta, M. A., Montgomery, A. J., Amiras, D., Egerton, A., Howard, R. J., & Grasby, P. M. 2007, "Striatal dopamine (D2) receptor availability predicts socially desirable responding", *Neuroimage*, vol. **34**, no. 4, pp. 1782–1789.

Reinhard, J. F., Jr. & O'Callaghan, J. P. 1991, "Measurement of tyrosine hydroxylase apoenzyme protein by enzyme-linked immunosorbent assay (ELISA): effects of 1-methyl-4-phenyl-1,2,3,6-tetrahydropyridine (MPTP) on striatal tyrosine hydroxylase activity and content", *Anal. Biochem.*, vol. **196**, no. 2, pp. 296–301.

Reith, J., Benkelfat, C., Sherwin, A., Yasuhara, Y., Kuwabara, H., Andermann, F., Bachneff, S., Cumming, P., Diksic, M., Dyve, S. E., Etienne, P., Evans, A. C., Lal, S., Shevell, M., Savard, G., Wong, D. F., Chouinard, G., & Gjedde, A. 1994, "Elevated dopa decarboxylase activity in living brain of patients with psychosis", *Proc. Natl. Acad. Sci. USA*, vol. **91**, no. 24, pp. 11651–11654.

Reith, J., Cumming, P., & Gjedde, A. 1998, "Enhanced [3H]DOPA and [3H]dopamine turnover in striatum and frontal cortex in vivo linked to glutamate receptor antagonism", *J. Neurochem.*, vol. **70**, no. 5, pp. 1979–1985.

Renskers, K. J., Feor, K. D., & Roth, J. A. 1980, "Sulfation of dopamine and other biogenic amines by human brain phenol sulfotransferase", *J. Neurochem.*, vol. **34**, no. 6, pp. 1362–1368.

Riba, J., Valle, M., Urbano, G., Yritia, M., Morte, A., & Barbanoj, M. J. 2003, "Human pharmacology of ayahuasca: subjective and cardiovascular effects, monoamine metabolite excretion, and pharmacokinetics", *J. Pharmacol. Exp. Ther.*, vol. **306**, no. 1, pp. 73–83.

Riccardi, P., Baldwin, R., Salomon, R., Anderson, S., Ansari, M. S., Li, R., Dawant, B., Bauernfeind, A., Schmidt, D., & Kessler, R. 2007, "Estimation of Baseline Dopamine D(2) Receptor Occupancy in Striatum and Extrastriatal Regions in Humans With Positron Emission Tomography With [(18)F] Fallypride", *Biol. Psychiatry.*, vol. **15**, no. 2, pp. 241–244.

Riccardi, P., Zald, D., Li, R., Park, S., Ansari, M. S., Dawant, B., Anderson, S., Woodward, N., Schmidt, D., Baldwin, R., & Kessler, R. 2006, "Sex differences in amphetamine-induced displacement of [(18)F]fallypride in striatal and extrastriatal regions: a PET study", *Am. J. Psychiatry*, vol. **163**, no. 9, pp. 1639–1641.

Richardson, J. R., Caudle, W. M., Guillot, T. S., Watson, J. L., Nakamaru-Ogiso, E., Seo, B. B., Sherer, T. B., Greenamyre, J. T., Yagi, T., Matsuno-Yagi, A., & Miller, G. W. 2007, "Obligatory Role for Complex I Inhibition in the Dopaminergic Neurotoxicity of 1-methyl-4-phenyl-1,2,3,6-tetrahydropyridine (MPTP)", *Toxicol. Sci.*, vol. **95**, no. 1, pp. 196–204.

Richfield, E. K. 1991, "Quantitative autoradiography of the dopamine uptake complex in rat brain using [3H]GBR 12935: binding characteristics", *Brain Res.*, vol. **540**, no. 1–2, pp. 1–13.

Richfield, E. K., Penney, J. B., & Young, A. B. 1989, "Anatomical and affinity state comparisons between dopamine D1 and D2 receptors in the rat central nervous system", *Neuroscience*, vol. **30**, no. 3, pp. 767–777.

Richter, A., Ebert, U., Nobrega, J. N., Vallbacka, J. J., Fedrowitz, M., & Loscher, W. 1999, "Immunohistochemical and neurochemical studies on nigral and striatal functions in the circling (ci) rat, a genetic animal model with spontaneous rotational behavior", *Neuroscience*, vol. **89**, no. 2, pp. 461–471.

Ridd, M. J., Kitchen, I., & Fosbraey, P. 1998, "The effect of acute kainic acid treatment on dopamine D2 receptors in rat brain", *Neurosci. Res.*, vol. **30**, no. 3, pp. 201–211.

Rinne, J. O., Hietala, J., Ruotsalainen, U., Sako, E., Laihinen, A., Nagren, K., Lehikoinen, P., Oikonen, V., & Syvalahti, E. 1993, "Decrease in human striatal dopamine D2 receptor density with age: a PET study with [11C]raclopride", *J. Cereb. Blood Flow Metab.*, vol. **13**, no. 2, pp. 310–314.

Rinne, J. O., Laihinen, A., Lonnberg, P., Marjamaki, P., & Rinne, U. K. 1991, "A post-mortem study on striatal dopamine receptors in Parkinson's disease", *Brain Res.*, vol. **556**, no. 1, pp. 117–122.

Rinne, J. O., Laihinen, A., Ruottinen, H., Ruotsalainen, U., Nagren, K., Lehikoinen, P., Oikonen, V., & Rinne, U. K. 1995, "Increased density of dopamine D2 receptors in the putamen, but not in the caudate nucleus in early Parkinson's disease: a PET study with [11C]raclopride", *J. Neurol. Sci.*, vol. **132**, no. 2, pp. 156–161.

Rinne, J. O., Lonnberg, P., & Marjamaki, P. 1990, "Age-dependent decline in human brain dopamine D1 and D2 receptors", *Brain Res.*, vol. **508**, no. 2, pp. 349–352.

Rinne, J. O., Portin, R., Ruottinen, H., Nurmi, E., Bergman, J., Haaparanta, M., & Solin, O. 2000, "Cognitive impairment and the brain dopaminergic system in Parkinson disease: [18F]fluorodopa positron emission tomographic study", *Arch. Neurol.*, vol. **57**, no. 4, pp. 470–475.

Rinne, J. O., Ruottinen, H. M., Nagren, K., Aberg, L. E., & Santavuori, P. 2002, "Positron emission tomography shows reduced striatal dopamine D1 but not D2 receptors in juvenile neuronal ceroid lipofuscinosis", *Neuropediatrics*, vol. **33**, no. 3, pp. 138–141.

Rinne, U. K., Larsen, J. P., Siden, A., & Worm-Petersen, J. 1998, "Entacapone enhances the response to levodopa in parkinsonian patients with motor fluctuations. Nomecomt Study Group", *Neurology*, vol. **51**, no. 5, pp. 1309–1314.

Rios, M., Habecker, B., Sasaoka, T., Eisenhofer, G., Tian, H., Landis, S., Chikaraishi, D., & Roffler-Tarlov, S. 1999, "Catecholamine synthesis is mediated by tyrosinase in the absence of tyrosine hydroxylase", *J. Neurosci.*, vol. **19**, no. 9, pp. 3519–3526.

Ritchie, T. & Noble, E. P. 2003, "Association of seven polymorphisms of the D2 dopamine receptor gene with brain receptor-binding characteristics", *Neurochem. Res.*, vol. **28**, no. 1, pp. 73–82.

Rivera, A., Alberti, I., Martin, A. B., Narvaez, J. A., de la Calle, A., & Moratalla, R. 2002, "Molecular phenotype of rat striatal neurons expressing the dopamine D5 receptor subtype", *Eur. J. Neurosci.*, vol. **16**, no. 11, pp. 2049–2058.

Rivett, A. J., Eddy, B. J., & Roth, J. A. 1982, "Contribution of sulfate conjugation, deamination, and O-methylation to metabolism of dopamine and norepinephrine in human brain", *J. Neurochem.*, vol. **39**, no. 4, pp. 1009–1016.

Rivett, A. J., Francis, A., & Roth, J. A. 1983, "Distinct cellular localization of membrane-bound and soluble forms of catechol-O-methyltransferase in brain", *J. Neurochem.*, vol. **40**, no. 1, pp. 215–219.

Rivett, A. J., Francis, A., Whittemore, R., & Roth, J. A. 1984, "Sulfate conjugation of dopamine in rat brain: regional distribution of activity and evidence for neuronal localization", *J. Neurochem.*, vol. **42**, no. 5, pp. 1444–1449.

Rivett, A. J. & Roth, J. A. 1982, "Kinetic studies on the O-methylation of dopamine by human brain membrane-bound catechol O-methyltransferase", *Biochemistry*, vol. **21**, no. 8, pp. 1740–1742.

Roberts, D. C., Zis, A. P., & Fibiger, H. C. 1975, "Ascending catecholamine pathways and amphetamine-induced locomotor activity: importance of dopamine and apparent non-involvement of norepinephrine", *Brain Res.*, vol. **93**, no. 3, pp. 441–454.

Robinson, T. E., Noordhoorn, M., Chan, E. M., Mocsary, Z., Camp, D. M., & Whishaw, I. Q. 1994, "Relationship between asymmetries in striatal dopamine release and the direction of amphetamine-induced rotation during the first week following a unilateral 6-OHDA lesion of the substantia nigra", *Synapse*, vol. **17**, no. 1, pp. 16–25.

Rodriguez-Pascual, F., Ferrero, R., Miras-Portugal, M. T., & Torres, M. 1999, "Phosphorylation of tyrosine hydroxylase by cGMP-dependent protein kinase in intact bovine chromaffin cells", *Arch. Biochem. Biophys.*, vol. **366**, no. 2, pp. 207–214.

Rosa-Neto, P., Doudet, D. J., & Cumming, P. 2004, "Gradients of dopamine D1- and D2/3-binding sites in the basal ganglia of pig and monkey measured by PET", *Neuroimage*, vol. **22**, no. 3, pp. 1076–1083.

Rosa-Neto, P., Gjedde, A., Olsen, A. K., Jensen, S. B., Munk, O. L., Watanabe, H., & Cumming, P. 2004, "MDMA-evoked changes in [11C]raclopride and [11C]NMSP binding in living pig brain", *Synapse*, vol. **53**, no. 4, pp. 222–233.

Rosa-Neto, P., Lou, H. C., Cumming, P., Pryds, O., Karrebaek, H., Lunding, J., & Gjedde, A. 2005, "Methylphenidate-evoked changes in striatal dopamine correlate with inattention and impulsivity in adolescents with attention deficit hyperactivity disorder", *Neuroimage*, vol. **25**, no. 3, pp. 868–876.

Rosenberg, R. C. & Lovenberg, W. 1983, "Determination of some molecular parameters of tyrosine hydroxylase from rat adrenal, rat striatum, and human pheochromocytoma", *J. Neurochem.*, vol. **40**, no. 6, pp. 1529–1533.

Ross, S. B. 1991, "Synaptic concentration of dopamine in the mouse striatum in relationship to the kinetic properties of the dopamine receptors and uptake mechanism", *J. Neurochem.*, vol. **56**, no. 1, pp. 22–29.

Ross, S. B. & Jackson, D. M. 1989a, "Kinetic properties of the accumulation of 3H-raclopride in the mouse brain in vivo", *Naunyn Schmiedebergs Arch.Pharmacol.*, vol. **340**, no. 1, pp. 6–12.

Ross, S. B. & Jackson, D. M. 1989b, "Kinetic properties of the in vivo accumulation of 3H-(-)-N-n-propylnorapomorphine in mouse brain", *Naunyn Schmiedebergs Arch. Pharmacol.*, vol. **340**, no. 1, pp. 13–20.

Rossetti, Z., Krajnc, D., Neff, N. H., & Hadjiconstantinou, M. 1989, "Modulation of retinal aromatic L-amino acid decarboxylase via alpha 2 adrenoceptors", *J. Neurochem.*, vol. **52**, no. 2, pp. 647–652.

Rossetti, Z. L., Silvia, C. P., Krajnc, D., Neff, N. H., & Hadjiconstantinou, M. 1990, "Aromatic L-amino acid decarboxylase is modulated by D1 dopamine receptors in rat retina", *J. Neurochem.*, vol. **54**, no. 3, pp. 787–791.

Rousset, O. G., Deep, P., Kuwabara, H., Evans, A. C., Gjedde, A. H., & Cumming, P. 2000, "Effect of partial volume correction on estimates of the influx and cerebral metabolism of 6-[(18)F]fluoro-L-dopa studied with PET in normal control and Parkinson's disease subjects", *Synapse*, vol. **37**, no. 2, pp. 81–89.

Ruottinen, H. M., Partinen, M., Hublin, C., Bergman, J., Haaparanta, M., Solin, O., & Rinne, J. O. 2000, "An FDOPA PET study in patients with periodic limb movement disorder and restless legs syndrome", *Neurology.*, vol. **54**, no. 2, pp. 502–504.

Ruottinen, H. M., Rinne, J. O., Haaparanta, M., Solin, O., Bergman, J., Oikonen, V. J., Järvelä, I., & Santavuori, P. 1997, "[18F]fluorodopa PET shows striatal dopaminergic dysfunction in juvenile neuronal ceroid lipofuscinosis", *J. Neurol. Neurosirg. Psychiatry.*, vol. **62**, no. 6, pp. 622–625.

Ruprecht-Dorfler, P., Berg, D., Tucha, O., Benz, P., Meier-Meitinger, M., Alders, G. L., Lange, K. W., & Becker, G. 2003, "Echogenicity of the substantia nigra in relatives of patients with sporadic Parkinson's disease", *Neuroimage*, vol. **18**, no. 2, pp. 416–422.

Rushlow, W., Flumerfelt, B. A., & Naus, C. C. 1995, "Colocalization of somatostatin, neuropeptide Y, and NADPH-diaphorase in the caudate-putamen of the rat", *J. Comp Neurol.*, vol. **351**, no. 4, pp. 499–508.

Ryding, E., Lindstrom, M., Bradvik, B., Grabowski, M., Bosson, P., Traskman-Bendz, L., & Rosen, I. 2004, "A new model for separation between brain dopamine and serotonin transporters in 123I-beta-CIT SPECT measurements: normal values and sex and age dependence", *Eur. J. Nucl. Med. Mol. Imaging*, vol. **31**, no. 8, pp. 1114–1118.

Saigusa, T., Tuinstra, T., Koshikawa, N., & Cools, A. R. 1999, "High and low responders to novelty: effects of a catecholamine synthesis inhibitor on novelty-induced changes in behaviour and release of accumbal dopamine", *Neuroscience*, vol. **88**, no. 4, pp. 1153–1163.

Sakakibara, Y., Takami, Y., Nakayama, T., Suiko, M., & Liu, M. C. 1998, "Localization and functional analysis of the substrate specificity/catalytic domains of human M-form and P-form phenol sulfotransferases", *J. Biol. Chem.*, vol. **273**, no. 11, pp. 6242–6247.

Sakiyama, Y., Hatano, K., Kato, T., Tajima, T., Kawasumi, Y., & Ito, K. 2007, "Stimulation of adenosine A1 receptors decreases in vivo dopamine D1 receptor binding of [11C]SCH23390 in the cat striatum revealed by positron emission tomography", *Ann. Nucl. Med.*, vol. **21**, no. 8, pp. 447–453.

Salmon, E., Brooks, D. J., Leenders, K. L., Turton, D. R., Hume, S. P., Cremer, J. E., Jones, T., & Frackowiak, R. S. 1990, "A two-compartment description and kinetic procedure for measuring regional cerebral [11C]nomifensine uptake using positron emission tomography", *J. Cereb. Blood Flow Metab.*, vol. **10**, no. 3, pp. 307–316.

Salokangas, R. K., Vilkman, H., Ilonen, T., Taiminen, T., Bergman, J., Haaparanta, M., Solin, O., Alanen, A., Syvalahti, E., & Hietala, J. 2000, "High levels of dopamine activity in the basal ganglia of cigarette smokers", *Am. J. Psychiatry*, vol. **157**, no. 4, pp. 632–634.

Samii, A., Markopoulou, K., Wszolek, Z. K., Sossi, V., Dobko, T., Mak, E., Calne, D. B., & Stoessl, A. J. 1999, "PET studies of parkinsonism associated with mutation in the alpha-synuclein gene", *Neurology*, vol. **53**, no. 9, pp. 2097–2102.

Sandell, J. H., Graybiel, A. M., & Chesselet, M. F. 1986, "A new enzyme marker for striatal compartmentalization: NADPH diaphorase activity in the caudate nucleus and putamen of the cat", *J. Comp Neurol.*, vol. **243**, no. 3, pp. 326–334.

Sarchiapone, M., Carli, V., Camardese, G., Cuomo, C., Di, G. D., Calcagni, M. L., Focacci, C., & De, R. S. 2006, "Dopamine transporter binding in depressed patients with anhedonia", *Psychiatry Res.*, vol. **147**, no. 2–3, pp. 243–248.

Sardar, A., Juorio, A. V., & Boulton, A. A. 1987, "The concentration of p- and m-tyramine in the rat mesolimbic system: its regional distribution and effect of monoamine oxidase inhibition", *Brain Res.*, vol. **412**, no. 2, pp. 370–374.

Sarna, G. S., Hutson, P. H., & Curzon, G. 1984, "Effect of alpha-methyl fluorodopa on dopamine metabolites: importance of conjugation and egress", *Eur. J. Pharmacol.*, vol. **100**, no. 3–4, pp. 343–350.

Saunders, C., Ferrer, J. V., Shi, L., Chen, J., Merrill, G., Lamb, M. E., Leeb-Lundberg, L. M., Carvelli, L., Javitch, J. A., & Galli, A. 2000, "Amphetamine-induced loss of human dopamine transporter activity: an internalization-dependent and cocaine-sensitive mechanism", *Proc. Natl. Acad. Sci. USA*, vol. **97**, no. 12, pp. 6850–6855.

Savasta, M., Dubois, A., & Scatton, B. 1986, "Autoradiographic localization of D1 dopamine receptors in the rat brain with [3H]SCH 23390", *Brain Res.*, vol. **375**, no. 2, pp. 291–301.

Sawada, M., Hirata, Y., Arai, H., Iizuka, R., & Nagatsu, T. 1987, "Tyrosine hydroxylase, tryptophan hydroxylase, biopterin, and neopterin in the brains of normal controls and patients with senile dementia of Alzheimer type", *J. Neurochem.*, vol. **48**, no. 3, pp. 760–764.

Scanley, B. E., Baldwin, R. M., Laruelle, M., al-Tikriti, M. S., Zea-Ponce, Y., Zoghbi, S., Giddings, S. S., Charney, D. S., Hoffer, P. B., Wang, S., *et al.* 1994, "Active and inactive enantiomers of 2 beta-carbomethoxy-3 beta-(4-iodophenyl)tropane: comparison using homogenate binding and single photon emission computed tomographic imaging", *Mol. Pharmacol.*, vol. **45**, no. 1, pp. 136–141.

Scherfler, C., Boesch, S. M., Donnemiller, E., Seppi, K., Weirich-Schwaiger, H., Goebel, G., Virgolini, I., Wenning, G. K., & Poewe, W. 2006a, "Topography of cerebral monoamine transporter availability in families with SCA2 mutations: a voxel-wise [123I]beta-CIT SPECT analysis", *Eur. J. Nucl. Med. Mol. Imaging*, vol. **33**, no. 9, pp. 1084–1090.

Scherfler, C., Khan, N. L., Pavese, N., Lees, A. J., Quinn, N. P., Brooks, D. J., & Piccini, P. P. 2006b, "Upregulation of dopamine D2 receptors in dopaminergic drug-naive patients with Parkin gene mutations", *Mov. Disord.*, vol. **21**, no. 6, pp. 783–788.

Schiffer, W. K., Logan, J., & Dewey, S. L. 2003, "Positron emission tomography studies of potential mechanisms underlying phencyclidine-induced alterations in striatal dopamine", *Neuropsychopharmacology*, vol. **28**, no. 12, pp. 2192–2198.

Schmitt, G. J., Frodl, T., Dresel, S., la Fougère, C., Bottlender, R., Koutsouleris, N., Hahn, K., Moller, H. J., & Meisenzahl, E. M. 2006, "Striatal dopamine transporter availability is associated with the productive psychotic state in first episode, drug-naive schizophrenic patients", *Eur. Arch. Psychiatry Clin. Neurosci.*, vol. **256**, no. 2, pp. 115–121.

Schoepp, D. D. & Azzaro, A. J. 1981a, "Alteration of dopamine synthesis in rat striatum subsequent to selective type A monoamine oxidase inhibition", *J. Neurochem.*, vol. **37**, no. 2, pp. 527–530.

Schoepp, D. D. & Azzaro, A. J. 1981b, "Specificity of endogenous substrates for types A and B monoamine oxidase in rat striatum", *J. Neurochem.*, vol. **36**, no. 6, pp. 2025–2031.

Schoepp, D. D. & Azzaro, A. J. 1982, "Role of type A and type B monoamine oxidase in the metabolism of released [3H]dopamine from rat striatal slices", *Biochem. Pharmacol.*, vol. **31**, no. 18, pp. 2961–2968.

Schoepp, D. D. & Azzaro, A. J. 1983, "Effects of intrastriatal kainic acid injection on [3H]dopamine metabolism in rat striatal slices: evidence for postsynaptic glial cell metabolism by both the type A and B forms of monoamine oxidase", *J. Neurochem.*, vol. **40**, no. 5, pp. 1340–1348.

Schoots, O., Seeman, P., Guan, H. C., Paterson, A. D., & Van Tol, H. H. 1995, "Long-term haloperidol elevates dopamine D4 receptors by 2-fold in rats", *Eur. J. Pharmacol.*, vol. **289**, no. 1, pp. 67–72.

Schroder, J., Bubeck, B., Silvestri, S., Demisch, S., & Sauer, H. 1997, "Gender differences in D2 dopamine receptor binding in drug-naive patients with schizophrenia: an [123I]iodobenzamide single photon emission computed tomography study", *Psychiatry Res.*, vol. **75**, no. 2, pp. 115–123.

Schuldiner, S., Fishkes, H., & Kanner, B. I. 1978, "Role of a transmembrane pH gradient in epinephrine transport by chromaffin granule membrane vesicles", *Proc. Natl. Acad. Sci. USA*, vol. **75**, no. 8, pp. 3713–3716.

Schwarz, J., Antonini, A., Kraft, E., Tatsch, K., Vogl, T., Kirsch, C. M., Leenders, K. L., & Oertel, W. H. 1994, "Treatment with D-penicillamine improves dopamine D2-receptor binding and T2-signal intensity in de novo Wilson's disease", *Neurology*, vol. **44**, no. 6, pp. 1079–1082.

Schwarz, J., Oertel, W. H., & Tatsch, K. 1996, "Iodine-123-iodobenzamide binding in parkinsonism: reduction by dopamine agonists but not L-Dopa", *J. Nucl. Med.*, vol. **37**, no. 7, pp. 1112–1115.

Scott, D. J., Domino, E. F., Heitzeg, M. M., Koeppe, R. A., Ni, L., Guthrie, S., & Zubieta, J. K. 2007, "Smoking modulation of mu-opioid and dopamine D2 receptor-mediated neurotransmission in humans", *Neuropsychopharmacology*, vol. **32**, no. 2, pp. 450–457.

Scott, D. J., Heitzeg, M. M., Koeppe, R. A., Stohler, C. S., & Zubieta, J. K. 2006, "Variations in the human pain stress experience mediated by ventral and dorsal basal ganglia dopamine activity", *J. Neurosci.*, vol. **26**, no. 42, pp. 10789–10795.

Seeman, P. 1987, "The absolute density of neurotransmitter receptors in the brain. Example for dopamine receptors", *J. Pharmacol. Methods*, vol. **17**, no. 4, pp. 347–360.

Seeman, P., Bzowej, N. H., Guan, H. C., Bergeron, C., Becker, L. E., Reynolds, G. P., Bird, E. D., Riederer, P., Jellinger, K., Watanabe, S., *et al.* 1987, "Human brain dopamine receptors in children and aging adults", *Synapse*, vol. **1**, no. 5, pp. 399–404.

Seeman, P., Guan, H. C., & Niznik, H. B. 1989, "Endogenous dopamine lowers the dopamine D2 receptor density as measured by [3H]raclopride: implications for positron emission tomography of the human brain", *Synapse*, vol. **3**, no. 1, pp. 96–97.

Seeman, P., Guan, H. C., & van Tol, H. H. 1993, "Dopamine D4 receptors elevated in schizophrenia", *Nature*, vol. **365**, no. 6445, pp. 441–445.

Seeman, P., Ko, F., Willeit, M., McCormick, P., & Ginovart, N. 2005a, "Antiparkinson concentrations of pramipexole and PHNO occupy dopamine D2(high) and D3 (high) receptors", *Synapse*, vol. **58**, no. 2, pp. 122–128.

Seeman, P., McCormick, P. N., & Kapur, S. 2007, "Increased dopamine D2(High) receptors in amphetamine-sensitized rats, measured by the agonist [(3)H](+) PHNO", *Synapse*, vol. **61**, no. 5, pp. 263–267.

Seeman, P., Tallerico, T., & Ko, F. 2004, "Alcohol-withdrawn animals have a prolonged increase in dopamine D2 (High) receptors, reversed by general anesthesia: relation to relapse?", *Synapse*, vol. **52**, no. 2, pp. 77–83.

Seeman, P., Ulpian, C., Grigoriadis, D., Pri-Bar, I., & Buchman, O. 1985, "Conversion of dopamine D1 receptors from high to low affinity for dopamine", *Biochem. Pharmacol.*, vol. **34**, no. 1, pp. 151–154.

Seeman, P., Weinshenker, D., Quirion, R., Srivastava, L. K., Bhardwaj, S. K., Grandy, D. K., Premont, R. T., Sotnikova, T. D., Boksa, P., El-Ghundi, M., O'Dowd, B. F.,

George, S. R., Perreault, M. L., Mannisto, P. T., Robinson, S., Palmiter, R. D., & Tallerico, T. 2005b, "Dopamine supersensitivity correlates with D2High states, implying many paths to psychosis", *Proc. Natl. Acad. Sci. USA*, vol. 102, no. 9, pp. 3513–3518.

Segal, D. S., Kuczenski, R., & Okuda, C. 1992, "Clorgyline-induced increases in presynaptic DA: changes in the behavioral and neurochemical effects of amphetamine using in vivo microdialysis", *Pharmacol. Biochem. Behav.*, vol. **42**, no. 3, pp. 421–429.

Seibyl, J. P., Marek, K., Sheff, K., Zoghbi, S., Baldwin, R. M., Charney, D. S., van Dyck, C. H., & Innis, R. B. 1998, "Iodine-123-beta-CIT and iodine-123-FPCIT SPECT measurement of dopamine transporters in healthy subjects and Parkinson's patients", *J. Nucl. Med.*, vol. **39**, no. 9, pp. 1500–1508.

Sekine, Y., Minabe, Y., Ouchi, Y., Takei, N., Iyo, M., Nakamura, K., Suzuki, K., Tsukada, H., Okada, H., Yoshikawa, E., Futatsubashi, M., & Mori, N. 2003, "Association of dopamine transporter loss in the orbitofrontal and dorsolateral prefrontal cortices with methamphetamine-related psychiatric symptoms", *Am. J. Psychiatry*, vol. **160**, no. 9, pp. 1699–1701.

Semple, D. M., McIntosh, A. M., & Lawrie, S. M. 2005, "Cannabis as a risk factor for psychosis: systematic review", *J. Psychopharmacol.*, vol. **19**, no. 2, pp. 187–194.

Seneca, N., Finnema, S. J., Farde, L., Gulyas, B., Wikstrom, H. V., Halldin, C., & Innis, R. B. 2006, "Effect of amphetamine on dopamine D2 receptor binding in nonhuman primate brain: a comparison of the agonist radioligand [11C]MNPA and antagonist [11C]raclopride", *Synapse*, vol. **59**, no. 5, pp. 260–269.

Seneca, N., Zoghbi, S. S., Skinbjerg, M., Liow, J. S., Hong, J., Sibley, D. R., Pike, V. W., Halldin, C., & Innis, R. B. 2008, "Occupancy of dopamine D 2/3 receptors in rat brain by endogenous dopamine measured with the agonist positron emission tomography radioligand [11C]MNPA", *Synapse*, vol. **62**, no. 10, pp. 756–763.

Senogles, S. E. 1994, "The D2 dopamine receptor isoforms signal through distinct Gi alpha proteins to inhibit adenylyl cyclase. A study with site-directed mutant Gi alpha proteins", *J. Biol. Chem.*, vol. **269**, no. 37, pp. 23120–23127.

Senthilkumaran, B. & Joy, K. P. 1995, "A turnover study of hypothalamic monoamine oxidase (MAO) and effects of MAO inhibition on gonadotropin secretion in the female catfish, Heteropneustes fossilis", *Gen. Comp Endocrinol.*, vol. **97**, no. 1, pp. 1–12.

Seward, E. P. & Nowycky, M. C. 1996, "Kinetics of stimulus-coupled secretion in dialyzed bovine chromaffin cells in response to trains of depolarizing pulses", *J. Neurosci.*, vol. **16**, no. 2, pp. 553–562.

Shang, Y., Gibbs, M. A., Marek, G. J., Stiger, T., Burstein, A. H., Marek, K., Seibyl, J. P., & Rogers, J. F. 2007, "Displacement of serotonin and dopamine transporters by venlafaxine extended release capsule at steady state: a [123I]2beta-carbomethoxy-3beta-(4-iodophenyl)-tropane single photon emission computed tomography imaging study", *J. Clin. Psychopharmacol.*, vol. **27**, no. 1, pp. 71–75.

Shapiro, R. M., Glick, S. D., & Hough, L. B. 1986, "Striatal dopamine uptake asymmetries and rotational behavior in unlesioned rats: revising the model?", *Psychopharmacology (Berl)*, vol. **89**, no. 1, pp. 25–30.

Sharman, D. F. 1967, "A discussion of the modes of action of drugs which increase the concentration of 4-hydroxy-3-methoxyphenylacetic acid (homovanillic acid) in the striatum of the mouse", *Br. J. Pharmacol. Chemother.*, vol. **30**, no. 3, pp. 620–626.

Shih, J. C., Chen, K., & Ridd, M. J. 1999, "Monoamine oxidase: from genes to behavior", *Annu. Rev. Neurosci.*, vol. **22**, pp. 197–217.

Siessmeier, T., Kienast, T., Wrase, J., Larsen, J. L., Braus, D. F., Smolka, M. N., Buchholz, H. G., Schreckenberger, M., Rosch, F., Cumming, P., Mann, K., Bartenstein, P., & Heinz, A. 2006, "Net influx of plasma 6-[18F]fluoro-L-DOPA (FDOPA) to the ventral striatum correlates with prefrontal processing of affective stimuli", *Eur. J. Neurosci.*, vol. **24**, no. 1, pp. 305–313.

Siessmeier, T., Zhou, Y., Buchholz, H. G., Landvogt, C., Vernaleken, I., Piel, M., Schirrmacher, R., Rosch, F., Schreckenberger, M., Wong, D. F., Cumming, P., Grunder, G., & Bartenstein, P. 2005, "Parametric mapping of binding in human brain of D2 receptor ligands of different affinities", *J. Nucl. Med.*, vol. **46**, no. 6, pp. 964–972.

Sills, T. L., Onalaja, A. O., & Crawley, J. N. 1998, "Mesolimbic dopaminergic mechanisms underlying individual differences in sugar consumption and amphetamine hyperlocomotion in Wistar rats", *Eur. J. Neurosci.*, vol. **10**, no. 5, pp. 1895–1902.

Silvestri, S., Negrete, J. C., Seeman, M. V., Shammi, C. M., & Seeman, P. 2004, "Does nicotine affect D2 receptor upregulation? A case-control study", *Acta Psychiatr. Scand.*, vol. **109**, no. 4, pp. 313–317.

Singer, T. P. & Salach, J. I. 1981, "Interaction of suicide inhibitors with the active site of monoamine oxidase," in *Monoamine Oxidase Inhibitors: The State of the Art*, M. B. H. Youdim & E. S. Paykel, eds., John Wiley, New York, pp. 17–29.

Siow, Y. L. & Dakshinamurti, K. 1990, "Neuronal dopa decarboxylase", *Ann. N.Y. Acad. Sci.*, vol. **585**, pp. 173–188.

Slifstein, M., Hwang, D. R., Huang, Y., Guo, N., Sudo, Y., Narendran, R., Talbot, P., & Laruelle, M. 2004, "In vivo affinity of [18F]fallypride for striatal and extrastriatal dopamine D2 receptors in nonhuman primates", *Psychopharmacology*, vol. **175**, no. 3, pp. 274–286.

Slifstein, M., Kolachana, B., Simpson, E. H., Tabares, P., Cheng, B., Duvall, M., Frankle, W. G., Weinberger, D. R., Laruelle, M., & Abi-Dargham, A. 2008, "COMT genotype predicts cortical-limbic D1 receptor availability measured with [11C]NNC112 and PET", *Mol. Psychiatry.*, vol. **13**, no. 8, pp. 821–827.

Small, D. M., Jones-Gotman, M., & Dagher, A. 2003, "Feeding-induced dopamine release in dorsal striatum correlates with meal pleasantness ratings in healthy human volunteers", *Neuroimage*, vol. **19**, no. 4, pp. 1709–1715.

Smith, C. B., Sheldon, M. I., Bednarczyk, J. H., & Villarreal, J. E. 1972, "Morphine-induced increases in the incorporation of 14 C-tyrosine into 14 C-dopamine and

14 C-norepinephrine in the mouse brain: antagonism by naloxone and tolerance", *J. Pharmacol. Exp. Ther.*, vol. **180**, no. 3, pp. 547–557.

Smith, G. S., Dewey, S. L., Brodie, J. D., Logan, J., Vitkun, S. A., Simkowitz, P., Schloesser, R., Alexoff, D. A., Hurley, A., Cooper, T., & Volkow, N. D. 1997, "Serotonergic modulation of dopamine measured with [11C]raclopride and PET in normal human subjects", *Am. J. Psychiatry*, vol. **154**, no. 4, pp. 490–496.

Smith, Q. R., Momma, S., Aoyagi, M., & Rapoport, S. I. 1987, "Kinetics of neutral amino acid transport across the blood-brain barrier", *J. Neurochem.*, vol. **49**, no. 5, pp. 1651–1658.

Snow, B. J., Tooyama, I., McGeer, E. G., Yamada, T., Calne, D. B., Takahashi, H., & Kimura, H. 1993, "Human positron emission tomographic [18F]fluorodopa studies correlate with dopamine cell counts and levels", *Ann. Neurol.*, vol. **34**, no. 3, pp. 324–330.

So, C. H., Varghese, G., Curley, K. J., Kong, M. M., Alijaniaram, M., Ji, X., Nguyen, T., O'dowd, B. F., & George, S. R. 2005, "D1 and D2 dopamine receptors form heterooligomers and cointernalize after selective activation of either receptor", *Mol. Pharmacol.*, vol. **68**, no. 3, pp. 568–578.

Sokoloff, L., Reivich, M., Kennedy, C., Des Rosiers, M. H., Patlak, C. S., Pettigrew, K. D., Sakurada, O., & Shinohara, M. 1977, "The [14C]deoxyglucose method for the measurement of local cerebral glucose utilization: theory, procedure, and normal values in the conscious and anesthetized albino rat", *J. Neurochem.*, vol. **28**, no. 5, pp. 897–916.

Soliman, A., O'Driscoll, G. A., Pruessner, J., Holahan, A. L., Boileau, I., Gagnon, D., & Dagher, A. 2008, "Stress-induced dopamine release in humans at risk of psychosis: a [(11)C]raclopride PET study", *Neuropsychopharmacology*, vol. **33**, no. 8, pp. 2033–2041.

Sora, I., Wichems, C., Takahashi, N., Li, X. F., Zeng, Z., Revay, R., Lesch, K. P., Murphy, D. L., & Uhl, G. R. 1998, "Cocaine reward models: conditioned place preference can be established in dopamine- and in serotonin-transporter knockout mice", *Proc. Natl. Acad. Sci. USA*, vol. **95**, no. 13, pp. 7699–7704.

Sorg, B. A., & Kalivas, P. W. 1993, "Effects of cocaine and footshock stress on extracellular dopamine levels in the medial prefrontal cortex", *Neuroscience*, vol. **53**, no. 3, pp. 695–703.

Sossi, V., de la Fuente-Fernandez, R., Holden, J. E., Schulzer, M., Ruth, T. J., & Stoessl, J. 2004, "Changes of dopamine turnover in the progression of Parkinson's disease as measured by positron emission tomography: their relation to disease-compensatory mechanisms", *J. Cereb. Blood Flow Metab.*, vol. **24**, no. 8, pp. 869–876.

Sossi, V., Doudet, D. J., & Holden, J. E. 2001, "A reversible tracer analysis approach to the study of effective dopamine turnover", *J. Cereb. Blood Flow Metab.*, vol. **21**, no. 4, pp. 469–476.

Sossi, V., Holden, J. E., Topping, G. J., Camborde, M. L., Kornelsen, R. A., McCormick, S. E., Greene, J., Studenov, A. R., Ruth, T. J., & Doudet, D. J. 2007, "In vivo measurement of density and affinity of the monoamine vesicular transporter in a unilateral 6-hydroxydopamine rat model of PD", *J. Cereb. Blood Flow Metab.*, vol. **27**, no. 7, pp. 1407–1415.

Sotnikova, T. D., Beaulieu, J. M., Gainetdinov, R. R., & Caron, M. G. 2006, "Molecular biology, pharmacology and functional role of the plasma membrane dopamine transporter", *CNS Neurol. Disord. Drug Targets*, vol. **5**, no. 1, pp. 45–56.

Sovago, J., Farde, L., Halldin, C., Schukin, E., Schou, M., Laszlovszky, I., Kiss, B., & Gulyas, B. 2005, "Lack of effect of reserpine-induced dopamine depletion on the binding of the dopamine-D3 selective radioligand, [11C]RGH-1756", *Brain Res. Bull.*, vol. **67**, no. 3, pp. 219–224.

Sparks, D. L., Slevin, J. T., & Hunsaker, J. C., III 1986, "3-Methoxytyramine in the putamen as a gauge of the postmortem interval", *J. Forensic Sci.*, vol. **31**, no. 3, pp. 962–971.

Spector, R. & Shikuma, S. N. 1978, "The stability of vitamin B6 accumulation and pyridoxal kinase activity in rabbit brain and choroid plexus", *J. Neurochem.*, vol. **31**, no. 6, pp. 1403–1410.

Spector, S., Sjoerdsma, A., & Udenfriend, S. 1965, "Blockade of endogenous norepinephrine synthesis by alpha-methyl-tyrosine, an inhibitor of tyrosine hydroxylase", *J. Pharmacol. Exp. Ther.*, vol. **147**, pp. 86–95.

Spencer, T. J., Biederman, J., Ciccone, P. E., Madras, B. K., Dougherty, D. D., Bonab, A. A., Livni, E., Parasrampuria, D. A., & Fischman, A. J. 2006, "PET study examining pharmacokinetics, detection and likeability, and dopamine transporter receptor occupancy of short- and long-acting oral methylphenidate", *Am. J. Psychiatry*, vol. **163**, no. 3, pp. 387–395.

Spencer, T. J., Biederman, J., Madras, B. K., Dougherty, D. D., Bonab, A. A., Livni, E., Meltzer, P. C., Martin, J., Rauch, S., & Fischman, A. J. 2007, "Further evidence of dopamine transporter dysregulation in ADHD: a controlled PET imaging study using altropane", *Biol. Psychiatry*, vol. **62**, no. 9, pp. 1059–1061.

Staley, J. K., Basile, M., Flynn, D. D., & Mash, D. C. 1994, "Visualizing dopamine and serotonin transporters in the human brain with the potent cocaine analogue [125I]RTI-55: in vitro binding and autoradiographic characterization", *J. Neurochem.*, vol. **62**, no. 2, pp. 549–556.

Staley, J. K., Boja, J. W., Carroll, F. I., Seltzman, H. H., Wyrick, C. D., Lewin, A. H., Abraham, P., & Mash, D. C. 1995, "Mapping dopamine transporters in the human brain with novel selective cocaine analog [125I]RTI-121", *Synapse*, vol. **21**, no. 4, pp. 364–372.

Staley, J. K., Krishnan-Sarin, S., Zoghbi, S., Tamagnan, G., Fujita, M., Seibyl, J. P., Maciejewski, P. K., O'Malley, S., & Innis, R. B. 2001, "Sex differences in [123I]beta-CIT SPECT measures of dopamine and serotonin transporter availability in healthy smokers and nonsmokers", *Synapse*, vol. **41**, no. 4, pp. 275–284.

Stark, A. K. & Pakkenberg, B. 2004, "Histological changes of the dopaminergic nigrostriatal system in aging", *Cell Tissue Res.*, vol. **318**, no. 1, pp. 81–92.

Stein, W. D. 1986, *Transport and Diffusion Across Cell Membranes*, Academic Press, Orlando, FL.

Stepanov, V., Schou, M., Jarv, J., & Halldin, C. 2007, "Synthesis of 3H-labeled N-(3-iodoprop-2E-enyl)-2beta-carbomethoxy-3beta-(4-methylphenyl)nortropane (PE2I) and its interaction with mice striatal membrane fragments", *Appl. Radiat. Isot.*, vol. **65**, no. 3, pp. 293–300.

Stone, A. L. 1980, "Studies on a molecular basis for the heparin-induced regulation of enzymatic activity of mouse striatal tyrosine hydroxylase in vitro. Inhibition of heparin activation and of the enzyme by poly-L-lysyltyrosine and poly-L-lysylphenylalanine and their constituent peptides", *J. Neurochem.*, vol. **35**, no. 5, pp. 1137–1150.

Stone, J. M., Bressan, R. A., Erlandsson, K., Ell, P. J., & Pilowsky, L. S. 2005, "Non-uniform blockade of intrastriatal D2/D3 receptors by risperidone and amisulpride", *Psychopharmacology (Berl)*, vol. **180**, no. 4, pp. 664–669.

Stout, D. B., Huang, S. C., Melega, W. P., Raleigh, M. J., Phelps, M. E., & Barrio, J. R. 1998, "Effects of large neutral amino acid concentrations on 6-[F-18]fluoro-L-DOPA kinetics", *J. Cereb. Blood Flow Metab.*, vol. **18**, no. 1, pp. 43–51.

Strafella, A. P., Ko, J. H., Grant, J., Fraraccio, M., & Monchi, O. 2005, "Corticostriatal functional interactions in Parkinson's disease: a rTMS/[11C]raclopride PET study", *Eur. J. Neurosci.*, vol. **22**, no. 11, pp. 2946–2952.

Strafella, A. P., Ko, J. H., & Monchi, O. 2006, "Therapeutic application of transcranial magnetic stimulation in Parkinson's disease: the contribution of expectation", *Neuroimage*, vol. **31**, no. 4, pp. 1666–1672.

Strafella, A. P., Paus, T., Barrett, J., & Dagher, A. 2001, "Repetitive transcranial magnetic stimulation of the human prefrontal cortex induces dopamine release in the caudate nucleus", *J. Neurosci.*, vol. **21**, no. 15, p. RC157.

Strafella, A. P., Paus, T., Fraraccio, M., & Dagher, A. 2003, "Striatal dopamine release induced by repetitive transcranial magnetic stimulation of the human motor cortex", *Brain*, vol. **126** (Pt 12), pp. 2609–2615.

Strafella, A. P., Sadikot, A. F., & Dagher, A. 2003, "Subthalamic deep brain stimulation does not induce striatal dopamine release in Parkinson's disease", *Neuroreport*, vol. **14**, no. 9, pp. 1287–1289.

Suhara, T., Yasuno, F., Sudo, Y., Yamamoto, M., Inoue, M., Okubo, Y., & Suzuki, K. 2001, "Dopamine D2 receptors in the insular cortex and the personality trait of novelty seeking", *Neuroimage*, vol. **13**, no. 5, pp. 891–895.

Sun, W., Ginovart, N., Ko, F., Seeman, P., & Kapur, S. 2003, "In vivo evidence for dopamine-mediated internalization of D2-receptors after amphetamine: differential findings with [3H]raclopride versus [3H]spiperone", *Mol.Pharmacol.*, vol. **63**, no. 2, pp. 456–462.

Sunahara, R. K., Guan, H. C., O'Dowd, B. F., Seeman, P., Laurier, L. G., Ng, G., George, S. R., Torchia, J., Van Tol, H. H., & Niznik, H. B. 1991, "Cloning of the gene for a human dopamine D5 receptor with higher affinity for dopamine than D1", *Nature*, vol. **350**, no. 6319, pp. 614–619.

Suto, N., Austin, J. D., & Vezina, P. 2001, "Locomotor response to novelty predicts a rat's propensity to self-administer nicotine", *Psychopharmacology (Berl)*, vol. **158**, no. 2, pp. 175–180.

Suzuki, M., Hatano, K., Sakiyama, Y., Kawasumi, Y., Kato, T., & Ito, K. 2001, "Age-related changes of dopamine D1-like and D2-like receptor binding in the F344/N rat striatum revealed by positron emission tomography and in vitro receptor autoradiography", *Synapse*, vol. **41**, no. 4, pp. 285–293.

Suzuki, S., Watanabe, Y., Tsubokura, S., Kagamiyama, H., & Hayaishi, O. 1988, "Decrease in tetrahydrobiopterin content and neurotransmitter amine biosynthesis in rat brain by an inhibitor of guanosine triphosphate cyclohydrolase", *Brain Res.*, vol. **446**, no. 1, pp. 1–10.

Svenningsson, P., Fienberg, A. A., Allen, P. B., Moine, C. L., Lindskog, M., Fisone, G., Greengard, P., & Fredholm, B. B. 2000, "Dopamine D(1) receptor-induced gene transcription is modulated by DARPP-32", *J. Neurochem.*, vol. **75**, no. 1, pp. 248–257.

Svenningsson, P., Nishi, A., Fisone, G., Girault, J. A., Nairn, A. C., & Greengard, P. 2004, "DARPP-32: an integrator of neurotransmission", *Annu. Rev. Pharmacol. Toxicol.*, vol. **44**, pp. 269–296.

Svingos, A. L., Periasamy, S., & Pickel, V. M. 2000, "Presynaptic dopamine D(4) receptor localization in the rat nucleus accumbens shell", *Synapse*, vol. **36**, no. 3, pp. 222–232.

Szabo, D., Szabo, G., Jr., Ocsovszki, I., Aszalos, A., & Molnar, J. 1999, "Anti-psychotic drugs reverse multidrug resistance of tumor cell lines and human AML cells ex-vivo", *Cancer Lett.*, vol. **139**, no. 1, pp. 115–119.

Szostak, C., Jakubovic, A., Phillips, A. G., & Fibiger, H. C. 1986, "Bilateral augmentation of dopaminergic and serotonergic activity in the striatum and nucleus accumbens induced by conditioned circling", *J. Neurosci.*, vol. **6**, no. 7, pp. 2037–2044.

Tai, Y. F., Ahsan, R. L., de Yebenes, J. G., Pavese, N., Brooks, D. J., & Piccini, P. 2007, "Characterization of dopaminergic dysfunction in familial progressive supranuclear palsy: an 18F-dopa PET study", *J. Neural Transm.*, vol. **114**, no. 3, pp. 337–340.

Tajima, T., Hatano, K., Suzuki, M., Ogawa, M., Sakiyama, Y., Kato, T., Endo, H., Miura, H., Matsubara, M., & Ito, K. 2007, "Increased binding potential of [(11)C]raclopride during unilateral continuous microinjection of nicotine in rat striatum observed by positron emission tomography", *Synapse*, vol. **61**, no. 12, pp. 943–950.

Takahashi, H., Fujimura, Y., Hayashi, M., Takano, H., Kato, M., Okubo, Y., Kanno, I., Ito, H., & Suhara, T. 2008, "Enhanced dopamine release by nicotine in cigarette smokers: a double-blind, randomized, placebo-controlled pilot study", *Int. J. Neuropsychopharmacol.*, vol. **11**, no. 3, pp. 413–417.

Takahashi, H., Kato, M., Hayashi, M., Okubo, Y., Takano, A., Ito, H., & Suhara, T. 2007, "Memory and frontal lobe functions; possible relations with dopamine D2 receptors in the hippocampus", *Neuroimage*, vol. **34**, no. 4, pp. 1643–1649.

Takahashi, N., Miner, L. L., Sora, I., Ujike, H., Revay, R. S., Kostic, V., Jackson-Lewis, V., Przedborski, S., & Uhl, G. R. 1997, "VMAT2 knockout mice: heterozygotes display reduced amphetamine-conditioned reward, enhanced amphetamine locomotion, and enhanced MPTP toxicity", *Proc. Natl. Acad. Sci. USA*, vol. **94**, no. 18, pp. 9938–9943.

Talvik, M., Nordstrom, A. L., Okubo, Y., Olsson, H., Borg, J., Halldin, C., & Farde, L. 2006, "Dopamine D2 receptor binding in drug-naive patients with schizophrenia examined with raclopride-C11 and positron emission tomography", *Psychiatry Res.*, vol. **148**, no. 2–3, pp. 165–173.

Talvik, M., Nordstrom, A. L., Olsson, H., Halldin, C., & Farde, L. 2003, "Decreased thalamic D2/D3 receptor binding in drug-naive patients with schizophrenia: a PET study with [11C]FLB 457", *Int. J. Neuropsychopharmacol.*, vol. **6**, no. 4, pp. 361–370.

Tam, S. Y., Elsworth, J. D., Bradberry, C. W., & Roth, R. H. 1990, "Mesocortical dopamine neurons: high basal firing frequency predicts tyrosine dependence of dopamine synthesis", *J. Neural Transm. Gen. Sect.*, vol. **81**, no. 2, pp. 97–110.

Tanaka, Y., Meguro, K., Yamaguchi, S., Ishii, H., Watanuki, S., Funaki, Y., Yamaguchi, K., Yamadori, A., Iwata, R., & Itoh, M. 2003, "Decreased striatal D2 receptor density associated with severe behavioral abnormality in Alzheimer's disease", *Ann. Nucl. Med.*, vol. **17**, no. 7, pp. 567–573.

Tappaz, M. L. & Pujol, J. F. 1980, "Estimation of the rate of tryptophan hydroxylation in vivo: a sensitive microassay in discrete rat brain nuclei", *J. Neurochem.*, vol. **34**, no. 4, pp. 933–940.

Tarazi, F. I., Kula, N. S., & Baldessarini, R. J. 1997, "Regional distribution of dopamine D4 receptors in rat forebrain", *Neuroreport*, vol. **8**, no. 16, pp. 3423–3426.

Tauscher-Wisniewski, S., Kapur, S., Tauscher, J., Jones, C., Daskalakis, Z. J., Papatheodorou, G., Epstein, I., Christensen, B. K., & Zipursky, R. B. 2002, "Quetiapine: an effective antipsychotic in first-episode schizophrenia despite only transiently high dopamine-2 receptor blockade", *J. Clin. Psychiatry*, vol. **63**, no. 11, pp. 992–997.

Taylor, S. F., Koeppe, R. A., Tandon, R., Zubieta, J. K., & Frey, K. A. 2000, "In vivo measurement of the vesicular monoamine transporter in schizophrenia", *Neuropsychopharmacology*, vol. **23**, no. 6, pp. 667–675.

Tedroff, J., Pedersen, M., Aquilonius, S. M., Hartvig, P., Jacobsson, G., & Langstrom, B. 1996, "Levodopa-induced changes in synaptic dopamine in patients with Parkinson's disease as measured by [11C]raclopride displacement and PET", *Neurology*, vol. **46**, no. 5, pp. 1430–1436.

Telang, F. W., Volkow, N. D., Levy, A., Logan, J., Fowler, J. S., Felder, C., Wong, C., & Wang, G. J. 1999, "Distribution of tracer levels of cocaine in the human brain as assessed with averaged [11C]cocaine images", *Synapse*, vol. **31**, no. 4, pp. 290–296.

Teng, L., Crooks, P. A., & Dwoskin, L. P. 1998, "Lobeline displaces [3H] dihydrotetrabenazine binding and releases [3H]dopamine from rat striatal synaptic vesicles: comparison with d-amphetamine", *J. Neurochem.*, vol. **71**, no. 1, pp. 258–265.

Tenhunen, J., Salminen, M., Lundstrom, K., Kiviluoto, T., Savolainen, R., & Ulmanen, I. 1994, "Genomic organization of the human catechol O-methyltransferase gene and its expression from two distinct promoters", *Eur. J. Biochem.*, vol. **223**, no. 3, pp. 1049–1059.

Thanos, P. K., Michaelides, M., Benveniste, H., Wang, G. J., & Volkow, N. D. 2007a, "Effects of chronic oral methylphenidate on cocaine self-administration and striatal dopamine D2 receptors in rodents", *Pharmacol. Biochem. Behav.*, vol. **87**, no. 4, pp. 426–433.

Thanos, P. K., Michaelides, M., Piyis, Y. K., Wang, G. J., & Volkow, N. D. 2007b, "Food restriction markedly increases dopamine D2 receptor (D2R) in a rat model of obesity as assessed with in-vivo muPET imaging ([(11)C] raclopride) and in-vitro ([(3)H] spiperone) autoradiography", *Synapse*, vol. **62**, no. 1, pp. 50–61.

Thibaut, F., Faucheux, B. A., Marquez, J., Villares, J., Menard, J. F., Agid, Y., & Hirsch, E. C. 1995, "Regional distribution of monoamine vesicular uptake sites in the mesencephalon of control subjects and patients with Parkinson's disease: a postmortem study using tritiated tetrabenazine", *Brain Res.*, vol. **692**, no. 1–2, pp. 233–243.

Thierry, A. M., Tassin, J. P., Blanc, G., & Glowinski, J. 1976, "Selective activation of mesocortical DA system by stress", *Nature*, vol. **263**, no. 5574, pp. 242–244.

Thobois, S., Fraix, V., Savasta, M., Costes, N., Pollak, P., Mertens, P., Koudsie, A., Le Bass, D., Benabid, A. L., & Broussolle, E. 2003, "Chronic subthalamic nucleus stimulation and striatal D2 dopamine receptors in Parkinson's disease – A [(11)C]raclopride PET study", *J. Neurol.*, vol. **250**, no. 10, pp. 1219–1223.

Thobois, S., Hassoun, W., Ginovart, N., Garcia-Larrea, L., Le Cavorsin, M., Guillouet, S., Bonnefoi, F., Costes, N., Lavenne, F., Broussolle, E., & Leviel, V. 2004, "Effect of sensory stimulus on striatal dopamine release in humans and cats: a [(11)C]raclopride PET study", *Neurosci. Lett.*, vol. **368**, no. 1, pp. 46–51.

Tidey, J. W. & Miczek, K. A. 1996, "Social defeat stress selectively alters mesocorticolimbic dopamine release: an in vivo microdialysis study", *Brain Res.*, vol. **721**, no. 1–2, pp. 140–149.

Tiihonen, J., Kuikka, J., Bergstrom, K., Hakola, P., Karhu, J., Ryynanen, O. P., & Fohr, J. 1995, "Altered striatal dopamine re-uptake site densities in habitually violent and non-violent alcoholics", *Nat. Med.*, vol. **1**, no. 7, pp. 654–657.

Tiihonen, J., Kuikka, J., Bergstrom, K., Lepola, U., Koponen, H., & Leinonen, E. 1997, "Dopamine reuptake site densities in patients with social phobia", *Am. J. Psychiatry*, vol. **154**, no. 2, pp. 239–242.

Tiihonen, J., Kuoppamaki, M., Nagren, K., Bergman, J., Eronen, E., Syvalahti, E., & Hietala, J. 1996, "Serotonergic modulation of striatal D2 dopamine receptor binding in humans measured with positron emission tomography", *Psychopharmacology (Berl)*, vol. **126**, no. 4, pp. 277–280.

Tipton, K. F. & Mantle, T. J. 1981, "The inhibition of rat liver monoamine oxidase by clorgyline and deprenyl," in *Monoamine Oxidase Inhibitors: The State of the Art*, M. B. H. Youdim & E. S. Paykel, eds., John Wiley, New York, pp. 3–15.

Tomer, R., Goldstein, R. Z., Wang, G. J., Wong, C., & Volkow, N. D. 2008, "Incentive motivation is associated with striatal dopamine asymmetry", *Biol. Psychol.*, vol. **77**, no. 1, pp. 98–101.

Tong, J., Wilson, A. A., Boileau, I., Houle, S., & Kish, S. J. 2008, "Dopamine modulating drugs influence striatal (+)-[(11)C]DTBZ binding in rats: VMAT2 binding is sensitive to changes in vesicular dopamine concentration", *Synapse*, vol. **62**, no. 11, pp. 873–876.

Tonissaar, M., Herm, L., Rinken, A., & Harro, J. 2006, "Individual differences in sucrose intake and preference in the rat: circadian variation and association with dopamine D2 receptor function in striatum and nucleus accumbens", *Neurosci. Lett.*, vol. **403**, no. 1–2, pp. 119–124.

Torstenson, R., Tedroff, J., Hartvig, P., Fasth, K. J., & Langstrom, B. 1999, "A comparison of 11C-labeled L-DOPA and L-fluorodopa as positron emission tomography tracers for the presynaptic dopaminergic system", *J. Cereb. Blood Flow Metab.*, vol. **19**, no. 10, pp. 1142–1149.

Travis, E. R. & Wightman, R. M. 1998, "Spatio-temporal resolution of exocytosis from individual cells", *Annu. Rev. Biophys. Biomol. Struct.*, vol. **27**, pp. 77–103.

Tribl, G. G., Asenbaum, S., Happe, S., Bonelli, R. M., Zeitlhofer, J., & Auff, E. 2004, "Normal striatal D2 receptor binding in idiopathic restless legs syndrome with periodic leg movements in sleep", *Nucl. Med. Commun.*, vol. **25**, no. 1, pp. 55–60.

Trovero, F., Herve, D., Blanc, G., Glowinski, J., & Tassin, J. P. 1992, "In vivo partial inactivation of dopamine D1 receptors induces hypersensitivity of cortical dopamine-sensitive adenylate cyclase: permissive role of alpha 1-adrenergic receptors", *J. Neurochem.*, vol. **59**, no. 1, pp. 331–337.

Tsukada, H., Harada, N., Nishiyama, S., Ohba, H., & Kakiuchi, T. 2000a, "Cholinergic neuronal modulation alters dopamine D2 receptor availability in vivo by regulating receptor affinity induced by facilitated synaptic dopamine turnover: positron emission tomography studies with microdialysis in the conscious monkey brain", *J. Neurosci.*, vol. **20**, no. 18, pp. 7067–7073.

Tsukada, H., Harada, N., Nishiyama, S., Ohba, H., Sato, K., Fukumoto, D., & Kakiuchi, T. 2000b, "Ketamine decreased striatal [(11)C]raclopride binding with no alterations in static dopamine concentrations in the striatal extracellular fluid in the monkey brain: multiparametric PET studies combined with microdialysis analysis", *Synapse*, vol. **37**, no. 2, pp. 95–103.

Tsukada, H., Harada, N., Ohba, H., Nishiyama, S., & Kakiuchi, T. 2001, "Facilitation of dopaminergic neural transmission does not affect [(11)C]SCH23390 binding to the striatal D(1) dopamine receptors, but the facilitation enhances phosphodiesterase type-IV activity through D(1) receptors: PET studies in the conscious monkey brain", *Synapse*, vol. **42**, no. 4, pp. 258–265.

Tsukada, H., Kreuter, J., Maggos, C. E., Unterwald, E. M., Kakiuchi, T., Nishiyama, S., Futatsubashi, M., & Kreek, M. J. 1996, "Effects of binge pattern cocaine administration on dopamine D1 and D2 receptors in the rat brain: an in vivo study using positron emission tomography", *J. Neurosci.*, vol. **16**, no. 23, pp. 7670–7677.

Tsukada, H., Miyasato, K., Harada, N., Nishiyama, S., Fukumoto, D., & Kakiuchi, T. 2005, "Nicotine modulates dopamine synthesis rate as determined by L-[beta-11C]DOPA: PET studies compared with [11C]raclopride binding in the conscious monkey brain", *Synapse*, vol. **57**, no. 2, pp. 120–122.

Tsukada, H., Miyasato, K., Kakiuchi, T., Nishiyama, S., Harada, N., & Domino, E. F. 2002, "Comparative effects of methamphetamine and nicotine on the striatal [(11)C]raclopride binding in unanesthetized monkeys", *Synapse*, vol. **45**, no. 4, pp. 207–212.

Tsukada, H., Nishiyama, S., Kakiuchi, T., Ohba, H., Sato, K., & Harada, N. 1999, "Is synaptic dopamine concentration the exclusive factor which alters the in vivo binding of [11C]raclopride? PET studies combined with microdialysis in conscious monkeys", *Brain Res.*, vol. **841**, no. 1–2, pp. 160–169.

Tunbridge, E. M., Bannerman, D. M., Sharp, T., & Harrison, P. J. 2004, "Catechol-O-methyltransferase inhibition improves set-shifting performance and elevates stimulated dopamine release in the rat prefrontal cortex", *J. Neurosci.*, vol. **24**, no. 23, pp. 5331–5335.

Tune, L. E., Wong, D. F., Pearlson, G., Strauss, M., Young, T., Shaya, E. K., Dannals, R. F., Wilson, A. A., Ravert, H. T., Sapp, J., &. 1993, "Dopamine D2 receptor density estimates in schizophrenia: a positron emission tomography study with 11C-N-methylspiperone", *Psychiatry Res.*, vol. **49**, no. 3, pp. 219–237.

Tunnicliff, G., Brokaw, J. J., Hausz, J. A., Matheson, G. K., & White, G. W. 1992, "Influence of repeated treatment with buspirone on central 5-hydroxytryptamine and dopamine synthesis", *Neuropharmacology*, vol. **31**, no. 10, pp. 991–995.

Tuomainen, P., Tornwall, M., & Mannisto, P. T. 1996, "Minor effect of tolcapone, a catechol-O-methyltransferase inhibitor, on extracellular dopamine levels modified by amphetamine or pargyline: a microdialysis study in anaesthetized rats", *Pharmacol.Toxicol.*, vol. **78**, no. 6, pp. 392–396.

Tupala, E., Häkkinen, M., Storvik, M., Tiihonen, J. 2008, "Striatal dopaminergic terminals in type 1 and type 2 alcoholics measured with [3H]dihydrotetrabenazine and human whole hemisphere autoradiography", *Psychiatry Res.*, vol. **163**, no. 1, pp. 70–75.

Tupala, E., Kuikka, J. T., Hall, H., Bergström, K., Särkioja, T., Räsänen, P., Mantere, T., Hiltunen, J., Vepsäläinen, J., & Tiihonen, J. 2001, "Measurement of the striatal dopamine transporter density and heterogeneity in type 1 alcoholics using human whole hemisphere autoradiography", *Neuroimage*, vol. **14** (1 Pt 1), pp. 87–94.

Tuppurainen, H., Kuikka, J., Viinamaki, H., Husso-Saastamoinen, M., Bergstrom, K., & Tiihonen, J. 2003, "Extrastriatal dopamine D2/3 receptor density and distribution in drug-naive schizophrenic patients", *Mol. Psychiatry*, vol. **8**, no. 4, pp. 453–455.

Tuppurainen, H., Kuikka, J. T., Laakso, M. P., Viinamaki, H., Husso, M., & Tiihonen, J. 2006, "Midbrain dopamine D2/3 receptor binding in schizophrenia", *Eur. Arch. Psychiatry Clin. Neurosci.*, vol. **256**, no. 6, pp. 382–387.

Turjanski, N., Lees, A. J., & Brooks, D. J. 1997, "In vivo studies on striatal dopamine D1 and D2 site binding in L-dopa-treated Parkinson's disease patients with and without dyskinesias", *Neurology*, vol. **49**, no. 3, pp. 717–723.

Tyce, G. M., Messick, J. M., Yaksh, T. L., Byer, D. E., Danielson, D. R., & Rorie, D. K. 1986, "Amine sulfate formation in the central nervous system", *Fed.Proc.*, vol. **45**, no. 8, pp. 2247–2253.

Udenfriend, S., Zaltzman-Nirenberg, P., & Nagatsu, T. 1965, "Inhibitors of purified beef adrenal tyrosine hydroxylase", *Biochem. Pharmacol.*, vol. **14**, no. 5, pp. 837–845.

Udo de Haes, J. I., Kortekaas, R., van Waarde, A., Maguire, R. P., Pruim, J., & den Boer, J. A. 2005, "Assessment of methylphenidate-induced changes in binding of continuously infused [(11)C]raclopride in healthy human subjects: correlation with subjective effects", *Psychopharmacology (Berl)*, vol. **183**, no. 3, pp. 322–330.

Ujike, H., Akiyama, K., & Kuroda, S. 1996, "[3H]YM-09151-2 (nemonapride), a potent radioligand for both sigma 1 and sigma 2 receptor subtypes", *Neuroreport*, vol. **7**, no. 5, pp. 1057–1061.

Ulmanen, I., Peranen, J., Tenhunen, J., Tilgmann, C., Karhunen, T., Panula, P., Bernasconi, L., Aubry, J. P., & Lundstrom, K. 1997, "Expression and intracellular localization of catechol O-methyltransferase in transfected mammalian cells", *Eur. J. Biochem.*, vol. **243**, no. 1–2, pp. 452–459.

Ungerstedt, U. & Arbuthnott, G. W. 1970, "Quantitative recording of rotational behavior in rats after 6-hydroxy-dopamine lesions of the nigrostriatal dopamine system", *Brain Res.*, vol. **24**, no. 3, pp. 485–493.

Urwyler, S. & Coward, D. 1987, "Binding of 3H-spiperone and 3H-(-)-sulpiride to dopamine D2 receptors in rat striatal membranes: methodological considerations and demonstration of the identical nature of the binding sites for the two ligands", *Naunyn Schmiedebergs Arch. Pharmacol.*, vol. **335**, no. 2, pp. 115–122.

Valette, H., Bottlaender, M., Dolle, F., Coulon, C., Ottaviani, M., & Syrota, A. 2005, "Acute inhibition of cardiac monoamine oxidase A after tobacco smoke inhalation: validation study of [11C]befloxatone in rats followed by a positron emission tomography application in baboons", *J. Pharmacol. Exp. Ther.*, vol. **314**, no. 1, pp. 431–436.

van den Munckhof P., Luk, K. C., Ste-Marie, L., Montgomery, J., Blanchet, P. J., Sadikot, A. F., & Drouin, J. 2003, "Pitx3 is required for motor activity and for survival of a subset of midbrain dopaminergic neurons", *Development*, vol. **130**, no. 11, pp. 2535–2542.

van der Werf, J. F., Sebens, J. B., & Korf, J. 1984, "In vivo binding of N-n-propylnorapomorphine in the rat striatum: quantification after lesions produced by kainate, 6-hydroxydopamine and decortication", *Eur. J. Pharmacol.*, vol. **102**, no. 2, pp. 251–259.

van der Werf, J. F., Sebens, J. B., & Korf, J. 1986, "Tracer and maximal specific binding of tritiated spiperone or N-n-propylnorapomorphine to quantify dopamine receptors in rat brain regions in vivo", *Life Sci.*, vol. **39**, no. 2, pp. 155–160.

van der Werf, J. F., Sebens, J. B., Vaalburg, W., & Korf, J. 1983, "In vivo binding of N-n-propylnorapomorphine in the rat brain: regional localization, quantification in striatum and lack of correlation with dopamine metabolism", *Eur. J. Pharmacol.*, vol. **87**, no. 2–3, pp. 259–270.

van Dyck, C. H., Avery, R. A., Macavoy, M. G., Marek, K. L., Quinlan, D. M., Baldwin, R. M., Seibyl, J. P., Innis, R. B., & Arnsten, A. F. 2008, "Striatal dopamine transporters correlate with simple reaction time in elderly subjects", *Neurobiol. Aging.*, vol. **29**, no. 8, pp. 1237–1246.

van Dyck, C. H., Malison, R. T., Jacobsen, L. K., Seibyl, J. P., Staley, J. K., Laruelle, M., Baldwin, R. M., Innis, R. B., & Gelernter, J. 2005, "Increased dopamine transporter availability associated with the 9-repeat allele of the SLC6A3 gene", *J.Nucl.Med.*, vol. **46**, no. 5, pp. 745–751.

van Dyck, C. H., Seibyl, J. P., Malison, R. T., Laruelle, M., Wallace, E., Zoghbi, S. S., Zea-Ponce, Y., Baldwin, R. M., Charney, D. S., & Hoffer, P. B. 1995, "Age-related decline in striatal dopamine transporter binding with iodine-123-beta-CIT-SPECT", *J. Nucl. Med.*, vol. **36**, no. 7, pp. 1175–1181.

van Laere, K., de Ceuninck, L., Dom, R., van den Eyden, J., Vanbilloen, H., Cleynhens, J., Dupont, P., Bormans, G., Verbruggen, A., & Mortelmans, L. 2004, "Dopamine transporter SPECT using fast kinetic ligands: 123I-FP-beta-CIT versus 99mTc-TRODAT-1", *Eur. J. Nucl. Med. Mol. Imaging*, vol. **31**, no. 8, pp. 1119–1127.

van Oostrom, J. C., Maguire, R. P., Verschuuren-Bemelmans, C. C., van der Veenma, D. L., Pruim, J., Roos, R. A., & Leenders, K. L. 2005, "Striatal dopamine D2 receptors, metabolism, and volume in preclinical Huntington disease", *Neurology*, vol. **65**, no. 6, pp. 941–943.

van Valkenburg C., van der Krogt, J., Moleman, P., van Beerkum, H., Tjaden, U., & de Jong, J. 1984, "A procedure to measure the specific activities of dopamine and its metabolites in rat striatum, based on HPLC, electrochemical detection and liquid scintillation counting", *J. Neurosci. Methods*, vol. **11**, no. 1, pp. 29–38.

van Zwieten-Boot, B. J. & Noach, E. L. 1975, "The effect of blocking dopamine release on synthesis rate of dopamine in the striatum of the rat", *Eur. J. Pharmacol.*, vol. **33**, no. 2, pp. 247–254.

Vander Borght, T., Kilbourn, M., Desmond, T., Kuhl, D., & Frey, K. 1995, "The vesicular monoamine transporter is not regulated by dopaminergic drug treatments", *Eur. J. Pharmacol.*, vol. **294**, no. 2–3, pp. 577–583.

Vander Borght, T. M., Kilbourn, M. R., Koeppe, R. A., DaSilva, J. N., Carey, J. E., Kuhl, D. E., & Frey, K. A. 1995a, "In vivo imaging of the brain vesicular monoamine transporter", *J. Nucl. Med.*, vol. **36**, no. 12, pp. 2252–2260.

Vander Borght, T. M., Sima, A. A., Kilbourn, M. R., Desmond, T. J., Kuhl, D. E., & Frey, K. A. 1995b, "[3H]methoxytetrabenazine: a high specific activity ligand for estimating monoaminergic neuronal integrity", *Neuroscience*, vol. **68**, no. 3, pp. 955–962.

Vasdev, N., Natesan, S., Galineau, L., Garcia, A., Stableford, W. T., McCormick, P., Seeman, P., Houle, S., & Wilson, A. A. 2006, "Radiosynthesis, ex vivo and in vivo evaluation of [11C]preclamol as a partial dopamine D2 agonist radioligand for positron emission tomography", *Synapse*, vol. **60**, no. 4, pp. 314–318.

Vasdev, N., Seeman, P., Garcia, A., Stableford, W. T., Nobrega, J. N., Houle, S., & Wilson, A. A. 2007, "Syntheses and in vitro evaluation of fluorinated naphthoxazines as dopamine D2/D3 receptor agonists: radiosynthesis, ex vivo biodistribution and autoradiography of [(18)F]F-PHNO", *Nucl. Med. Biol.*, vol. **34**, no. 2, pp. 195–203.

Vassout, A., Bruinink, A., Krauss, J., Waldmeier, P., & Bischoff, S. 1993, "Regulation of dopamine receptors by bupropion: comparison with antidepressants and CNS stimulants", *J. Recept. Res.*, vol. **13**, no. 1–4, pp. 341–354.

Vaughn, D. M., Coleman, E., Simpson, S. T., Whitmer, B., & Satjawatcharaphong, C. 1988, "A rostrocaudal gradient for neurotransmitter metabolites and a caudorostral gradient for protein in canine cerebrospinal fluid", *Am. J. Vet. Res.*, vol. **49**, no. 12, pp. 2134–2137.

Venero, J. L., Machado, A., & Cano, J. 1991, "Turnover of dopamine and serotonin and their metabolites in the striatum of aged rats", *J. Neurochem.*, vol. **56**, no. 6, pp. 1940–1948.

Verhoeff, N. P., Hussey, D., Lee, M., Tauscher, J., Papatheodorou, G., Wilson, A. A., Houle, S., & Kapur, S. 2002, "Dopamine depletion results in increased neostriatal D(2), but not D(1), receptor binding in humans", *Mol. Psychiatry*, vol. **7**, no. 3, pp. 233, 322–328.

Verma, V., Mann, A., Costain, W., Pontoriero, G., Castellano, J. M., Skoblenick, K., Gupta, S. K., Pristupa, Z., Niznik, H. B., Johnson, R. L., Nair, V. D., & Mishra, R. K. 2005, "Modulation of agonist binding to human dopamine receptor subtypes by L-prolyl-L-leucyl-glycinamide and a peptidomimetic analog", *J. Pharmacol. Exp. Ther.*, vol. **315**, no. 3, pp. 1228–1236.

Vermeulen, R. J., Drukarch, B., Verhoeff, N. P., Goosen, C., Sahadat, M. C., Wolters, E. C., van Royen, E. A., & Stoof, J. C. 1994, "No direct correlation between behaviorally active doses of the dopamine D2 agonist LY 171555 and displacement of [123I]IBZM as measured with SPECT in MPTP monkeys," *Synapse*, vol. **17**, no. 2, pp. 115–124.

Vernaleken, I., Buchholz, H. G., Kumakura, Y., Siessmeier, T., Stoeter, P., Bartenstein, P., Cumming, P., & Grunder, G. 2007a, " 'Prefrontal' cognitive performance of healthy subjects positively correlates with cerebral FDOPA influx: An exploratory [(18)F]-fluoro-L-DOPA-PET investigation", *Hum. Brain Mapp.*, vol. **28**, no. 10, pp. 931–939.

Vernaleken, I., Kumakura, Y., Cumming, P., Buchholz, H. G., Siessmeier, T., Stoeter, P., Muller, M. J., Bartenstein, P., & Grunder, G. 2006, "Modulation of [18F] fluorodopa (FDOPA) kinetics in the brain of healthy volunteers after acute haloperidol challenge", *Neuroimage*, vol. **30**, no. 4, pp. 1332–1339.

Vernaleken, I., Weibrich, C., Siessmeier, T., Buchholz, H. G., Rosch, F., Heinz, A., Cumming, P., Stoeter, P., Bartenstein, P., & Grunder, G. 2007b, "Asymmetry in dopamine D(2/3) receptors of caudate nucleus is lost with age", *Neuroimage*, vol. **34**, no. 3, pp. 870–878.

Veronese, M. E., Burgess, W., Zhu, X., & McManus, M. E. 1994, "Functional characterization of two human sulphotransferase cDNAs that encode monoamine- and phenol-sulphating forms of phenol sulphotransferase: substrate kinetics, thermal-stability and inhibitor-sensitivity studies", *Biochem.J.*, vol. **302** (Pt 2), pp. 497–502.

Villemagne, V. L., Wong, D. F., Yokoi, F., Stephane, M., Rice, K. C., Matecka, D., Clough, D. J., Dannals, R. F., & Rothman, R. B. 1999, "GBR12909 attenuates amphetamine-induced striatal dopamine release as measured by [(11)C]raclopride continuous infusion PET scans", *Synapse*, vol. **33**, no. 4, pp. 268–273.

Villemagne, V., Yuan, J., Wong, D. F., Dannals, R. F., Hatzidimitriou, G., Mathews, W. B., Ravert, H. T., Musachio, J., McCann, U. D., & Ricaurte, G. A. 1998, "Brain dopamine neurotoxicity in baboons treated with doses of methamphetamine comparable to those recreationally abused by humans: evidence from [11C]WIN-35,428 positron emission tomography studies and direct in vitro determinations", *J. Neurosci.*, vol. **18**, no. 1, pp. 419–427.

Vincent, S. R. 1989, "Histochemical localization of 1-methyl-4-phenyl-1,2,3,6-tetrahydropyridine oxidation in the mouse brain", *Neuroscience*, vol. **28**, no. 1, pp. 189–199.

Vitale, M. L., Seward, E. P., & Trifaro, J. M. 1995, "Chromaffin cell cortical actin network dynamics control the size of the release-ready vesicle pool and the initial rate of exocytosis", *Neuron*, vol. **14**, no. 2, pp. 353–363.

Volkow, N. D., Chang, L., Wang, G. J., Fowler, J. S., Ding, Y. S., Sedler, M., Logan, J., Franceschi, D., Gatley, J., Hitzemann, R., Gifford, A., Wong, C., & Pappas, N. 2001a, "Low level of brain dopamine D2 receptors in methamphetamine abusers: association with metabolism in the orbitofrontal cortex", *Am. J. Psychiatry*, vol. **158**, no. 12, pp. 2015–2021.

Volkow, N. D., Chang, L., Wang, G. J., Fowler, J. S., Franceschi, D., Sedler, M., Gatley, S. J., Miller, E., Hitzemann, R., Ding, Y. S., & Logan, J. 2001b, "Loss of dopamine transporters in methamphetamine abusers recovers with protracted abstinence", *J. Neurosci.*, vol. **21**, no. 23, pp. 9414–9418.

Volkow, N. D., Chang, L., Wang, G. J., Fowler, J. S., Leonido-Yee, M., Franceschi, D., Sedler, M. J., Gatley, S. J., Hitzemann, R., Ding, Y. S., Logan, J., Wong, C., & Miller, E. N. 2001c, "Association of dopamine transporter reduction with psychomotor impairment in methamphetamine abusers", *Am. J. Psychiatry*, vol. **158**, no. 3, pp. 377–382.

Volkow, N. D., Ding, Y. S., Fowler, J. S., Wang, G. J., Logan, J., Gatley, J. S., Dewey, S., Ashby, C., Liebermann, J., Hitzemann, R., *et al.* 1995a, "Is methylphenidate like cocaine? Studies on their pharmacokinetics and distribution in the human brain", *Arch. Gen. Psychiatry*, vol. **52**, no. 6, pp. 456–463.

Volkow, N. D., Ding, Y. S., Fowler, J. S., Wang, G. J., Logan, J., Gatley, S. J., Hitzemann, R., Smith, G., Fields, S. D., & Gur, R. 1996a, "Dopamine transporters decrease with age", *J. Nucl. Med.*, vol. **37**, no. 4, pp. 554–559.

Volkow, N. D., Fowler, J. S., Gatley, S. J., Dewey, S. L., Wang, G. J., Logan, J., Ding, Y. S., Franceschi, D., Gifford, A., Morgan, A., Pappas, N., & King, P. 1999a, "Comparable changes in synaptic dopamine induced by methylphenidate and by cocaine in the baboon brain", *Synapse*, vol. **31**, no. 1, pp. 59–66.

Volkow, N. D., Fowler, J. S., Logan, J., Gatley, S. J., Dewey, S. L., MacGregor, R. R., Schlyer, D. J., Pappas, N., King, P., Wang, G. J., &. 1995b, "Carbon-11-cocaine binding compared at subpharmacological and pharmacological doses: a PET study", *J. Nucl. Med.*, vol. **36**, no. 7, pp. 1289–1297.

Volkow, N. D., Fowler, J. S., Wolf, A. P., Schlyer, D., Shiue, C. Y., Alpert, R., Dewey, S. L., Logan, J., Bendriem, B., Christman, D., *et al.* 1990, "Effects of chronic cocaine abuse on postsynaptic dopamine receptors", *Am. J. Psychiatry*, vol. **147**, no. 6, pp. 719–724.

Volkow, N. D., Gatley, S. J., Fowler, J. S., Chen, R., Logan, J., Dewey, S. L., Ding, Y. S., Pappas, N., King, P., MacGregor, R. R., &. 1995c, "Long-lasting inhibition of in vivo cocaine binding to dopamine transporters by 3 beta-(4-iodophenyl)tropane-2-carboxylic acid methyl ester: RTI-55 or beta CIT", *Synapse*, vol. **19**, no. 3, pp. 206–211.

Volkow, N. D., Gur, R. C., Wang, G. J., Fowler, J. S., Moberg, P. J., Ding, Y. S., Hitzemann, R., Smith, G., & Logan, J. 1998a, "Association between decline in brain dopamine activity with age and cognitive and motor impairment in healthy individuals", *Am. J. Psychiatry*, vol. **155**, no. 3, pp. 344–349.

Volkow, N. D., Wang, G. J., Begleiter, H., Porjesz, B., Fowler, J. S., Telang, F., Wong, C., Ma, Y., Logan, J., Goldstein, R., Alexoff, D., & Thanos, P. K. 2006, "High levels of dopamine D2 receptors in unaffected members of alcoholic families: possible protective factors", *Arch. Gen. Psychiatry*, vol. **63**, no. 9, pp. 999–1008.

Volkow, N. D., Wang, G. J., Fischman, M. W., Foltin, R. W., Fowler, J. S., Abumrad, N. N., Vitkun, S., Logan, J., Gatley, S. J., Pappas, N., Hitzemann, R., & Shea, C. E. 1997a, "Relationship between subjective effects of cocaine and dopamine transporter occupancy", *Nature*, vol. **386**, no. 6627, pp. 827–830.

Volkow, N. D., Wang, G. J., Fowler, J. S., Gatley, S. J., Logan, J., Ding, Y. S., Dewey, S. L., Hitzemann, R., Gifford, A. N., & Pappas, N. R. 1999b, "Blockade of striatal dopamine transporters by intravenous methylphenidate is not sufficient to induce self-reports of 'high' ", *J. Pharmacol. Exp. Ther.*, vol. **288**, no. 1, pp. 14–20.

Volkow, N. D., Wang, G. J., Fowler, J. S., Gatley, S. J., Logan, J., Ding, Y. S., Hitzemann, R., & Pappas, N. 1998b, "Dopamine transporter occupancies in the human brain induced by therapeutic doses of oral methylphenidate", *Am. J. Psychiatry, vol.* **155**, no. 10, pp. 1325–1331.

Volkow, N. D., Wang, G. J., Fowler, J. S., Logan, J., Franceschi, D., Maynard, L., Ding, Y. S., Gatley, S. J., Gifford, A., Zhu, W., & Swanson, J. M. 2002a, "Relationship between blockade of dopamine transporters by oral methylphenidate and the increases in extracellular dopamine: therapeutic implications", *Synapse*, vol. **43**, no. 3, pp. 181–187.

Volkow, N. D., Wang, G. J., Fowler, J. S., Logan, J., Gatley, S. J., Gifford, A., Hitzemann, R., Ding, Y. S., & Pappas, N. 1999c, "Prediction of reinforcing responses to psychostimulants in humans by brain dopamine D2 receptor levels", *Am. J. Psychiatry*, vol. **156**, no. 9, pp. 1440–1443.

Volkow, N. D., Wang, G. J., Fowler, J. S., Logan, J., Gatley, S. J., Hitzemann, R., Chen, A. D., Dewey, S. L., & Pappas, N. 1997b, "Decreased striatal dopaminergic responsiveness in detoxified cocaine-dependent subjects", *Nature*, vol. **386**, no. 6627, pp. 830–833.

Volkow, N. D., Wang, G. J., Fowler, J. S., Logan, J., Gatley, S. J., MacGregor, R. R., Schlyer, D. J., Hitzemann, R., & Wolf, A. P. 1996b, "Measuring age-related changes in dopamine D2 receptors with 11C-raclopride and 18F-N-methylspiroperidol", *Psychiatry Res.*, vol. **67**, no. 1, pp. 11–16.

Volkow, N. D., Wang, G. J., Fowler, J. S., Logan, J., Hitzemann, R., Ding, Y. S., Pappas, N., Shea, C., & Piscani, K. 1996c, "Decreases in dopamine receptors but not in dopamine transporters in alcoholics", *Alcohol Clin. Exp. Res.*, vol. **20**, no. 9, pp. 1594–1598.

Volkow, N. D., Wang, G. J., Fowler, J. S., Logan, J., Hitzemannn, R., Gatley, S. J., MacGregor, R. R., & Wolf, A. P. 1996d, "Cocaine uptake is decreased in the brain of detoxified cocaine abusers", *Neuropsychopharmacology*, vol. **14**, no. 3, pp. 159–168.

Volkow, N. D., Wang, G. J., Fowler, J. S., Logan, J., Jayne, M., Franceschi, D., Wong, C., Gatley, S. J., Gifford, A. N., Ding, Y. S., & Pappas, N. 2002b, " 'Nonhedonic' food motivation in humans involves dopamine in the dorsal striatum and methylphenidate amplifies this effect", *Synapse*, vol. **44**, no. 3, pp. 175–180.

Volkow, N. D., Wang, G. J., Fowler, J. S., Telang, F., Maynard, L., Logan, J., Gatley, S. J., Pappas, N., Wong, C., Vaska, P., Zhu, W., & Swanson, J. M. 2004, "Evidence that methylphenidate enhances the saliency of a mathematical task by increasing dopamine in the human brain", *Am. J. Psychiatry*, vol. **161**, no. 7, pp. 1173–1180.

Volkow, N. D., Wang, G. J., Maynard, L., Fowler, J. S., Jayne, B., Telang, F., Logan, J., Ding, Y. S., Gatley, S. J., Hitzemann, R., Wong, C., & Pappas, N. 2002c, "Effects of alcohol detoxification on dopamine D2 receptors in alcoholics: a preliminary study", *Psychiatry Res.*, vol. **116**, no. 3, pp. 163–172.

Volkow, N. D., Wang, G. J., Newcorn, J., Fowler, J. S., Telang, F., Solanto, M. V., Logan, J., Wong, C., Ma, Y., Swanson, J. M., Schulz, K., & Pradhan, K. 2007a, "Brain dopamine transporter levels in treatment and drug naive adults with ADHD", *Neuroimage*, vol. **34**, no. 3, pp. 1182–1190.

Volkow, N. D., Wang, G. J., Newcorn, J., Telang, F., Solanto, M. V., Fowler, J. S., Logan, J., Ma, Y., Schulz, K., Pradhan, K., Wong, C., & Swanson, J. M. 2007b, "Depressed dopamine activity in caudate and preliminary evidence of limbic involvement in adults with attention-deficit/hyperactivity disorder", *Arch. Gen. Psychiatry*, vol. **64**, no. 8, pp. 932–940.

Volkow, N. D., Wang, G. J., Telang, F., Fowler, J. S., Logan, J., Jayne, M., Ma, Y., Pradhan, K., & Wong, C. 2007c, "Profound decreases in dopamine release in striatum in detoxified alcoholics: possible orbitofrontal involvement", *J. Neurosci.*, vol. **27**, no. 46, pp. 12700–12706.

Vollenweider, F. X., Vontobel, P., Hell, D., & Leenders, K. L. 1999, "5-HT modulation of dopamine release in basal ganglia in psilocybin-induced psychosis in man – a PET study with [11C]raclopride", *Neuropsychopharmacology*, vol. **20**, no. 5, pp. 424–433.

Vollenweider, F. X., Vontobel, P., Oye, I., Hell, D., & Leenders, K. L. 2000, "Effects of (S)-ketamine on striatal dopamine: a [11C]raclopride PET study of a model psychosis in humans", *J. Psychiatr. Res.*, vol. **34**, no. 1, pp. 35–43.

Voltattorni, C. B., Minelli, A., & Dominici, P. 1983, "Interaction of aromatic amino acids in D and L forms with 3,4-dihydroxyphenylalanine decarboxylase from pig kidney", *Biochemistry*, vol. **22**, no. 9, pp. 2249–2254.

von Economo, C. 1931, *Encephalitis Lethargica. Its sequelae and Treatment*, Oxford University Press, London.

von Euler, G., van der Ploeg, I., Fredholm, B. B., & Fuxe, K. 1991, "Neurotensin decreases the affinity of dopamine D2 agonist binding by a G protein-independent mechanism", *J. Neurochem.*, vol. **56**, no. 1, pp. 178–183.

von Euler, G., van der Ploeg, I., Fredholm, B. B., & Fuxe, K. 1991, "Neurotensin decreases the affinity of dopamine D2 agonist binding by a G protein-independent mechanism", *J. Neurochem.*, vol. **56**, no. 1, pp. 178–183.

Vortherms, T. A., Nguyen, C. H., Bastepe, M., Juppner, H., & Watts, V. J. 2006, "D2 dopamine receptor-induced sensitization of adenylyl cyclase type 1 is G alpha(s) independent", *Neuropharmacology*, vol. **50**, no. 5, pp. 576–584.

Voruganti, L., Slomka, P., Zabel, P., Costa, G., So, A., Mattar, A., & Awad, A. G. 2001a, "Subjective effects of AMPT-induced dopamine depletion in schizophrenia: correlation between dysphoric responses and striatal D(2) binding ratios on SPECT imaging", *Neuropsychopharmacology*, vol. **25**, no. 5, pp. 642–650.

Voruganti, L. N., Slomka, P., Zabel, P., Mattar, A., & Awad, A. G. 2001b, "Cannabis induced dopamine release: an in-vivo SPECT study", *Psychiatry Res.*, vol. **107**, no. 3, pp. 173–177.

Vrana, K. E. & Roskoski, R., Jr. 1983, "Tyrosine hydroxylase inactivation following cAMP-dependent phosphorylation activation", *J. Neurochem.*, vol. **40**, no. 6, pp. 1692–1700.

Vrecko, K., Storga, D., Birkmayer, J. G., Moller, R., Tafeit, E., Horejsi, R., & Reibnegger, G. 1997, "NADH stimulates endogenous dopamine biosynthesis by enhancing the recycling of tetrahydrobiopterin in rat phaeochromocytoma cells", *Biochim. Biophys. Acta*, vol. **1361**, no. 1, pp. 59–65.

Wachtel, S. R. & Abercrombie, E. D. 1994, "L-3,4-dihydroxyphenylalanine-induced dopamine release in the striatum of intact and 6-hydroxydopamine-treated rats: differential effects of monoamine oxidase A and B inhibitors", *J. Neurochem.*, vol. **63**, no. 1, pp. 108–117.

Wagner, H. N., Jr., Burns, H. D., Dannals, R. F., Wong, D. F., Langstrom, B., Duelfer, T., Frost, J. J., Ravert, H. T., Links, J. M., Rosenbloom, S. B., Lukas, S. E., Kramer, A. V., & Kuhar, M. J. 1983, "Imaging dopamine receptors in the human brain by positron tomography", *Science*, vol. **221**, no. 4617, pp. 1264–1266.

Walker, Z., Costa, D. C., Walker, R. W., Lee, L., Livingston, G., Jaros, E., Perry, R., McKeith, I., & Katona, C. L. 2004, "Striatal dopamine transporter in dementia with Lewy bodies and Parkinson disease: a comparison", *Neurology*, vol. **62**, no. 9, pp. 1568–1572.

Wallace, D. R., Owens, J., & Booze, R. M. 1998, "[3H](+)-7-OH-DPAT and [3H] pramipexole binding in the striatum and nucleus accumbens of Sprague-Dawley and Fischer-344 rats", *Life Sci.*, vol. **63**, no. 19, pp. L275-L280.

Walters, J. R. & Roth, R. H. 1974, "Dopaminergic neurons: drug-induced antagonism of the increase in tyrosine hydroxylase activity produced by cessation of impulse flow", *J. Pharmacol. Exp. Ther.*, vol. **191**, no. 1, pp. 82–91.

Wand, G. S., Oswald, L. M., McCaul, M. E., Wong, D. F., Johnson, E., Zhou, Y., Kuwabara, H., & Kumar, A. 2007, "Association of amphetamine-induced striatal dopamine release and cortisol responses to psychological stress", *Neuropsychopharmacology*, vol. **32**, no. 11, pp. 2310–2320.

Wang, G. J., Chang, L., Volkow, N. D., Telang, F., Logan, J., Ernst, T., & Fowler, J. S. 2004, "Decreased brain dopaminergic transporters in HIV-associated dementia patients", *Brain*, vol. **127** (Pt 11), pp. 2452–2458.

Wang, G. J., Volkow, N. D., Fowler, J. S., Franceschi, D., Logan, J., Pappas, N. R., Wong, C. T., & Netusil, N. 2000, "PET studies of the effects of aerobic exercise on human striatal dopamine release", *J. Nucl. Med.*, vol. **41**, no. 8, pp. 1352–1356.

Wang, G. J., Volkow, N. D., Fowler, J. S., Logan, J., Abumrad, N. N., Hitzemann, R. J., Pappas, N. S., & Pascani, K. 1997, "Dopamine D2 receptor availability in opiate-dependent subjects before and after naloxone-precipitated withdrawal", *Neuropsychopharmacology*, vol. **16**, no. 2, pp. 174–182.

Wang, G. J., Volkow, N. D., Logan, J., Pappas, N. R., Wong, C. T., Zhu, W., Netusil, N., & Fowler, J. S. 2001, "Brain dopamine and obesity", *Lancet*, vol. **357**, no. 9253, pp. 354–357.

Watanabe, H. 1985, "Simple method for evaluation of stimulatory effect of drugs on presynaptic dopamine receptors in mice", *J. Pharmacol. Methods*, vol. **14**, no. 1, pp. 41–47.

Wee, S., Carroll, F. I., & Woolverton, W. L. 2006, "A reduced rate of in vivo dopamine transporter binding is associated with lower relative reinforcing efficacy of stimulants", *Neuropsychopharmacology*, vol. **31**, no. 2, pp. 351–362.

Wenkstern, D., Pfaus, J. G., & Fibiger, H. C. 1993, "Dopamine transmission increases in the nucleus accumbens of male rats during their first exposure to sexually receptive female rats", *Brain Res.*, vol. **618**, no. 1, pp. 41–46.

Wessel, T. C. & Joh, T. H. 1992, "Parallel upregulation of catecholamine-synthesizing enzymes in rat brain and adrenal gland: effects of reserpine and correlation with immediate early gene expression", *Brain Res. Mol. Brain Res.*, vol. **15**, no. 3-4, pp. 349–360.

Wester, P., Bergstrom, U., Eriksson, A., Gezelius, C., Hardy, J., & Winblad, B. 1990, "Ventricular cerebrospinal fluid monoamine transmitter and metabolite concentrations reflect human brain neurochemistry in autopsy cases", *J. Neurochem.*, vol. **54**, no. 4, pp. 1148–1156.

Westerink, B. H., Bosker, F. J., & Wirix, E. 1984, "Formation and metabolism of dopamine in nine areas of the rat brain: modifications by haloperidol", *J. Neurochem.*, vol. **42**, no. 5, pp. 1321–1327.

Westerink, B. H. & de Vries, J. B. 1991, "Effect of precursor loading on the synthesis rate and release of dopamine and serotonin in the striatum: a microdialysis study in conscious rats", *J. Neurochem.*, vol. **56**, no. 1, pp. 228–233.

Westerink, B. H., de Vries, J. B., & Duran, R. 1990, "Use of microdialysis for monitoring tyrosine hydroxylase activity in the brain of conscious rats", *J. Neurochem.*, vol. **54**, no. 2, pp. 381–387.

Westerink, B. H. & Kikkert, R. J. 1986, "Effect of various centrally acting drugs on the efflux of dopamine metabolites from the rat brain", *J. Neurochem.*, vol. **46**, no. 4, pp. 1145–1152.

Westerink, B. H. & Korf, J. 1976, "Turnover of acid dopamine metabolites in striatal and mesolimbic tissue of the rat brain", *Eur. J. Pharmacol.*, vol. **37**, no. 2, pp. 249–255.

Westerink, B. H. & Spaan, S. J. 1982a, "Simultaneous determination of the formation rate of dopamine and its metabolite 3,4-dihydroxyphenylacetic acid (DOPAC) in various rat brain areas", *Brain Res.*, vol. **252**, no. 2, pp. 239–245.

Westerink, B. H. & Spaan, S. J. 1982b, "Estimation of the turnover of 3-methoxytyramine in the rat striatum by HPLC with electrochemical detection: implications for the sequence in the cerebral metabolism of dopamine", *J. Neurochem.*, vol. **38**, no. 2, pp. 342–347.

Westerink, B. H. & Wirix, E. 1983, "On the significance of tyrosine for the synthesis and catabolism of dopamine in rat brain: evaluation by HPLC with electrochemical detection", *J. Neurochem.*, vol. **40**, no. 3, pp. 758–764.

Whittemore, R. M., Pearce, L. B., & Roth, J. A. 1985, "Purification and kinetic characterization of a dopamine-sulfating form of phenol sulfotransferase from human brain", *Biochemistry*, vol. **24**, no. 10, pp. 2477–2482.

Whittemore, R. M. & Roth, J. A. 1985, "Effect of phosphatase inhibition of in vitro dopamine sulfation and 3'-phosphoadenosine-5'-phosphosulfate catabolism in human brain", *Biochem. Pharmacol.*, vol. **34**, no. 21, pp. 3853–3856.

Whone, A. L., Bailey, D. L., Remy, P., Pavese, N., & Brooks, D. J. 2004, "A technique for standardized central analysis of 6-(18)F-fluoro-L-DOPA PET data from a multicenter study", *J. Nucl. Med.*, vol. **45**, no. 7, pp. 1135–1145.

Whone, A. L., Watts, R. L., Stoessl, A. J., Davis, M., Reske, S., Nahmias, C., Lang, A. E., Rascol, O., Ribeiro, M. J., Remy, P., Poewe, W. H., Hauser, R. A., & Brooks, D. J. 2003, "Slower progression of Parkinson's disease with ropinirole versus levodopa: The REAL-PET study", *Ann. Neurol.*, vol. **54**, no. 1, pp. 93–101.

Wiedemann, D. J., Garris, P. A., Near, J. A., & Wightman, R. M. 1992, "Effect of chronic haloperidol treatment on stimulated synaptic overflow of dopamine in the rat striatum", *J. Pharmacol. Exp. Ther.*, vol. **261**, no. 2, pp. 574–579.

Wightman, R. M., Jankowski, J. A., Kennedy, R. T., Kawagoe, K. T., Schroeder, T. J., Leszczyszyn, D. J., Near, J. A., Diliberto, E. J., Jr., & Viveros, O. H. 1991, "Temporally resolved catecholamine spikes correspond to single vesicle release from individual chromaffin cells", *Proc. Natl. Acad. Sci. USA*, vol. **88**, no. 23, pp. 10754–10758.

Wilcox, K. M., Lindsey, K. P., Votaw, J. R., Goodman, M. M., Martarello, L., Carroll, F. I., & Howell, L. L. 2002, "Self-administration of cocaine and the cocaine analog

RTI-113: relationship to dopamine transporter occupancy determined by PET neuroimaging in rhesus monkeys", *Synapse*, vol. **43**, no. 1, pp. 78–85.

Wilcox, R. E., Mudie, E., Mayfield, D., Young, R. K., & Spirduso, W. W. 1988, "Movement initiation characteristics in young adult rats in relation to the high- and low-affinity agonist states of the striatal D2 dopamine receptor", *Brain Res.*, vol. **443**, no. 1–2, pp. 190–198.

Willeit, M., Ginovart, N., Graff, A., Rusjan, P., Vitcu, I., Houle, S., Seeman, P., Wilson, A. A., & Kapur, S. 2008, "First human evidence of d-amphetamine induced displacement of a D(2/3) agonist radioligand: a [(11)C]-(+)-PHNO positron emission tomography Study", *Neuropsychopharmacology*, vol. **33**, no. 2, pp. 279–289.

Willeit, M., Ginovart, N., Kapur, S., Houle, S., Hussey, D., Seeman, P., & Wilson, A. A. 2006, "High-affinity states of human brain dopamine D2/3 receptors imaged by the agonist [11C]-(+)-PHNO", *Biol. Psychiatry*, vol. **59**, no. 5, pp. 389–394.

Wilson, J. M., Sanyal, S., & Van Tol, H. H. 1998, "Dopamine D2 and D4 receptor ligands: relation to antipsychotic action", *Eur. J. Pharmacol.*, vol. **351**, no. 3, pp. 273–286.

Winkler, H. & Westhead, E. 1980, "The molecular organization of adrenal chromaffin granules", *Neuroscience*, vol. **5**, no. 11, pp. 1803–1823.

Winogrodzka, A., Bergmans, P., Booij, J., van Royen, E. A., Stoof, J. C., & Wolters, E. C. 2003, "[(123)I]beta-CIT SPECT is a useful method for monitoring dopaminergic degeneration in early stage Parkinson's disease", *J. Neurol. Neurosurg. Psychiatry*, vol. **74**, no. 3, pp. 294–298.

Wirtshafter, D. 2000, "A comparison of the patterns of striatal Fos-like immunoreactivity induced by various dopamine agonists in rats", *Neurosci. Lett.*, vol. **289**, no. 2, pp. 99–102.

Wong, D. F., Gjedde, A., & Wagner, H. N., Jr. 1986, "Quantification of neuroreceptors in the living human brain. I. Irreversible binding of ligands", *J. Cereb. Blood Flow Metab.*, vol. **6**, no. 2, pp. 137–146.

Wong, D. F., Harris, J. C., Naidu, S., Yokoi, F., Marenco, S., Dannals, R. F., Ravert, H. T., Yaster, M., Evans, A., Rousset, O., Bryan, R. N., Gjedde, A., Kuhar, M. J., & Breese, G. R. 1996, "Dopamine transporters are markedly reduced in Lesch-Nyhan disease in vivo", *Proc. Natl. Acad. Sci. USA*, vol. **93**, no. 11, pp. 5539–5543.

Wong, D. F., Kuwabara, H., Schretlen, D. J., Bonson, K. R., Zhou, Y., Nandi, A., Brasic, J. R., Kimes, A. S., Maris, M. A., Kumar, A., Contoreggi, C., Links, J., Ernst, M., Rousset, O., Zukin, S., Grace, A. A., Lee, J. S., Rohde, C., Jasinski, D. R., Gjedde, A., & London, E. D. 2006, "Increased occupancy of dopamine receptors in human striatum during cue-elicited cocaine craving", *Neuropsychopharmacology*, vol. **31**, no. 12, pp. 2716–2727.

Wong, D. F., Pearlson, G. D., Tune, L. E., Young, L. T., Meltzer, C. C., Dannals, R. F., Ravert, H. T., Reith, J., Kuhar, M. J., & Gjedde, A. 1997a, "Quantification of neuroreceptors in the living human brain: IV. Effect of aging and elevations of D2-like receptors in schizophrenia and bipolar illness", *J. Cereb. Blood Flow Metab.*, vol. **17**, no. 3, pp. 331–342.

Wong, D. F., Singer, H. S., Brandt, J., Shaya, E., Chen, C., Brown, J., Kimball, A. W., Gjedde, A., Dannals, R. F., Ravert, H. T., Wilson, P. D., & Wagner, H. N., Jr. 1997b, "D2-like dopamine receptor density in Tourette syndrome measured by PET", *J. Nucl. Med.*, vol. **38**, no. 8, pp. 1243–1247.

Wong, D. F., Wagner, H. N., Jr., Tune, L. E., Dannals, R. F., Pearlson, G. D., Links, J. M., Tamminga, C. A., Broussolle, E. P., Ravert, H. T., Wilson, A. A., Toung, J. K., Malat, J., Williams, J. A., O'Tuama, L. A., Snyder, S. H., Kuhar, M. J., & Gjedde, A. 1986, "Positron emission tomography reveals elevated D2 dopamine receptors in drug-naive schizophrenics", *Science*, vol. **234**, no. 4783, pp. 1558–1563.

Wood, P. B., Schweinhardt, P., Jaeger, E., Dagher, A., Hakyemez, H., Rabiner, E. A., Bushnell, M. C., & Chizh, B. A. 2007, "Fibromyalgia patients show an abnormal dopamine response to pain", *Eur. J. Neurosci.*, vol. **25**, no. 12, pp. 3576–3582.

Woods, S. K. & Meyer, J. S. 1991, "Exogenous tyrosine potentiates the methylphenidate-induced increase in extracellular dopamine in the nucleus accumbens: a microdialysis study", *Brain Res.*, vol. **560**, no. 1–2, pp. 97–105.

Yamamoto, B. K. & Novotney, S. 1998, "Regulation of extracellular dopamine by the norepinephrine transporter", *J. Neurochem.*, vol. **71**, no. 1, pp. 274–280.

Yamamoto, K. K., Gonzalez, G. A., Biggs, W. H., III, & Montminy, M. R. 1988, "Phosphorylation-induced binding and transcriptional efficacy of nuclear factor CREB", *Nature*, vol. **334**, no. 6182, pp. 494–498.

Yang, H. Y. & Neff, N. H. 1973, "Beta-phenylethylamine: a specific substrate for type B monoamine oxidase of brain", *J. Pharmacol. Exp. Ther.*, vol. **187**, no. 2, pp. 365–371.

Yao, J., Erickson, J. D., & Hersh, L. B. 2004, "Protein kinase A affects trafficking of the vesicular monoamine transporters in PC12 cells", *Traffic.*, vol. **5**, no. 12, pp. 1006–1016.

Yassin, M. S., Cheng, H., Ekblom, J., & Oreland, L. 1998, "Inhibitors of catecholamine metabolizing enzymes cause changes in S-adenosylmethionine and S-adenosylhomocysteine in the rat brain", *Neurochem. Int.*, vol. **32**, no. 1, pp. 53–59.

Yatham, L. N., Liddle, P. F., Lam, R. W., Shiah, I. S., Lane, C., Stoessl, A. J., Sossi, V., & Ruth, T. J. 2002a, "PET study of the effects of valproate on dopamine D(2) receptors in neuroleptic- and mood-stabilizer-naive patients with nonpsychotic mania", *Am. J. Psychiatry*, vol. **159**, no. 10, pp. 1718–1723.

Yatham, L. N., Liddle, P. F., Shiah, I. S., Lam, R. W., Ngan, E., Scarrow, G., Imperial, M., Stoessl, J., Sossi, V., & Ruth, T. J. 2002b, "PET study of [(18)F]6-fluoro-L-dopa uptake in neuroleptic- and mood-stabilizer-naive first-episode nonpsychotic mania: effects of treatment with divalproex sodium", *Am. J. Psychiatry*, vol. **159**, no. 5, pp. 768–774.

Yavich, L., Forsberg, M. M., Karayiorgou, M., Gogos, J. A., & Mannisto, P. T. 2007, "Site-specific role of catechol-O-methyltransferase in dopamine overflow within prefrontal cortex and dorsal striatum", *J. Neurosci.*, vol. **27**, no. 38, pp. 10196–10209.

Yee, R. E., Huang, S. C., Stout, D. B., Irwin, I., Shoghi-Jadid, K., Togaski, D. M., DeLanney, L. E., Langston, J. W., Satyamurthy, N., Farahani, K. F., Phelps, M. E., &

Barrio, J.R. 2000, "Nigrostriatal reduction of aromatic L-amino acid decarboxylase activity in MPTP-treated squirrel monkeys: in vivo and in vitro investigations", *J. Neurochem.*, vol. **74**, no. 3, pp. 1147–1157.

Yee, R.E., Irwin, I., Milonas, C., Stout, D.B., Huang, S.C., Shoghi-Jadid, K., Satyamurthy, N., DeLanney, L.E., Togasaki, D.M., Farahani, K.F., Delfani, K., Janson, A.M., Phelps, M.E., Langston, J.W., & Barrio, J.R. 2001, "Novel observations with FDOPA-PET imaging after early nigrostriatal damage", *Mov. Disord.*, vol. **16**, no. 5, pp. 838–848.

Yen, T.C., Tzen, K.Y., Chen, M.C., Chou, Y.H., Chen, R.S., Chen, C.J., Wey, S.P., Ting, G., & Lu, C.S. 2002, "Dopamine transporter concentration is reduced in asymptomatic Machado-Joseph disease gene carriers", *J. Nucl. Med.*, vol. **43**, no. 2, pp. 153–159.

Yoder, K.K., Constantinescu, C.C., Kareken, D.A., Normandin, M.D., Cheng, T.E., O'Connor, S.J., & Morris, E.D. 2007, "Heterogeneous effects of alcohol on dopamine release in the striatum: a PET study", *Alcohol Clin. Exp. Res.*, vol. **31**, no. 6, pp. 965–973.

Yoder, K.K., Kareken, D.A., Seyoum, R.A., O'Connor, S.J., Wang, C., Zheng, Q.H., Mock, B., & Morris, E.D. 2005, "Dopamine D(2) receptor availability is associated with subjective responses to alcohol", *Alcohol Clin. Exp. Res.*, vol. **29**, no. 6, pp. 965–970.

Yokoi, F., Grunder, G., Biziere, K., Stephane, M., Dogan, A.S., Dannals, R.F., Ravert, H., Suri, A., Bramer, S., & Wong, D.F. 2002, "Dopamine D2 and D3 receptor occupancy in normal humans treated with the antipsychotic drug aripiprazole (OPC 14597): a study using positron emission tomography and [11C]raclopride", *Neuropsychopharmacology*, vol. **27**, no. 2, pp. 248–259.

Young, A.M., Joseph, M.H., & Gray, J.A. 1993, "Latent inhibition of conditioned dopamine release in rat nucleus accumbens", *Neuroscience*, vol. **54**, no. 1, pp. 5–9.

Young, E.A., Neff, N.H., & Hadjiconstantinou, M. 1993, "Evidence for cyclic AMP-mediated increase of aromatic L-amino acid decarboxylase activity in the striatum and midbrain", *J. Neurochem.*, vol. **60**, no. 6, pp. 2331–2333.

Young, L.T., Wong, D.F., Goldman, S., Minkin, E., Chen, C., Matsumura, K., Scheffel, U., & Wagner, H.N., Jr. 1991, "Effects of endogenous dopamine on kinetics of [3H] N-methylspiperone and [3H]raclopride binding in the rat brain", *Synapse*, vol. **9**, no. 3, pp. 188–194.

Yu, P.H., Rozdilsky, B., & Boulton, A.A. 1985, "Sulfate conjugation of monoamines in human brain: purification and some properties of an arylamine sulfotransferase from cerebral cortex", *J. Neurochem.*, vol. **45**, no. 3, pp. 836–843.

Zald, D.H., Boileau, I., El-Dearedy, W., Gunn, R., McGlone, F., Dichter, G.S., & Dagher, A. 2004, "Dopamine transmission in the human striatum during monetary reward tasks", *J. Neurosci.*, vol. **24**, no. 17, pp. 4105–4112.

Zallakian, M., Knoth, J., Metropoulos, G.E., & Njus, D. 1982, "Multiple effects of reserpine on chromaffin-granule in membranes", *Biochemistry*, vol. **21**, no. 5, pp. 1051–1055.

Zawarynski, P., Tallerico, T., Seeman, P., Lee, S. P., O'Dowd, B. F., & George, S. R. 1998, "Dopamine D2 receptor dimers in human and rat brain", *FEBS Lett.*, vol. **441**, no. 3, pp. 383–386.

Zerby, S. E. & Ewing, A. G. 1996, "Electrochemical monitoring of individual exocytotic events from the varicosities of differentiated PC12 cells", *Brain Res.*, vol. **712**, no. 1, pp. 1–10.

Zhang, M. R., Haradahira, T., Maeda, J., Okauchi, T., Kawabe, K., Noguchi, J., Kida, T., Suzuki, K., & Suhara, T. 2002, "Syntheses and pharmacological evaluation of two potent antagonists for dopamine D4 receptors: [11C]YM-50001 and N-[2-[4-(4-Chlorophenyl)-piperizin-1-yl]ethyl]-3-[11C]methoxybenzamide", *Nucl. Med. Biol.*, vol. **29**, no. 2, pp. 233–241.

Zhou, Q. Y., Quaife, C. J., & Palmiter, R. D. 1995, "Targeted disruption of the tyrosine hydroxylase gene reveals that catecholamines are required for mouse fetal development", *Nature*, vol. **374**, no. 6523, pp. 640–643.

Zhu, M. Y., Juorio, A. V., Paterson, I. A., & Boulton, A. A. 1993, "Regulation of striatal aromatic L-amino acid decarboxylase: effects of blockade or activation of dopamine receptors", *Eur. J. Pharmacol.*, vol. **238**, no. 2–3, pp. 157–164.

Zhu, S. J., Kavanaugh, M. P., Sonders, M. S., Amara, S. G., & Zahniser, N. R. 1997, "Activation of protein kinase C inhibits uptake, currents and binding associated with the human dopamine transporter expressed in Xenopus oocytes", *J. Pharmacol. Exp. Ther.*, vol. **282**, no. 3, pp. 1358–1365.

Zijlstra, S., van der Worp, H., Wiegman, T., Visser, G. M., Korf, J., & Vaalburg, W. 1993, "Synthesis and in vivo distribution in the rat of a dopamine agonist: N-([11C] methyl)norapomorphine", *Nucl. Med. Biol.*, vol. **20**, no. 1, pp. 7–12.

Zivkovic, B., Guidotti, A., & Costa, E. 1974, "Effects of neuroleptics on striatal tyrosine hydroxylase: Changes in affinity for the pteridine cofactor", *Mol. Pharmacol*, vol. **10**, pp. 727–735.

Index